Osteoporosis
SOURCEBOOK

SECOND EDITION

Osteoporosis
SOURCEBOOK

SECOND EDITION

Basic Consumer Information about Primary and Secondary Osteoporosis and Juvenile Osteoporosis and Related Conditions, Including Fibrous Dysplasia, Gaucher Disease, Hyperthyroidism, Hypophosphatasia, Myeloma, Osteopetrosis, Osteogenesis Imperfecta, and Paget Disease

Along with Information about Risk Factors, Treatments, Traditional and Nontraditional Pain Management, a Glossary of Related Terms, and a Directory of Resources

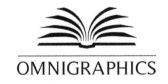

OMNIGRAPHICS

615 Griswold, Ste. 901, Detroit, MI 48226

Copyright © 2019 Omnigraphics

ISBN 978-0-7808-1685-5

E-ISBN 978-0-7808-1686-2

Library of Congress Cataloging-in-Publication Data

Names: Omnigraphics, Inc., issuing body.

Title: Osteoporosis sourcebook: basic consumer information about primary and secondary osteoporosis and juvenile osteoporosis and related conditions, including fibrous dysplasia, gaucher disease, hyperthyroidism, hypophosphatasia, myeloma, osteopetrosis, osteogenesis imperfecta, and paget disease, along with information about risk factors, treatments, along with traditional and nontraditional pain management.

Description: 2nd edition. | Detroit, MI: Omnigraphics, Inc., [2019]

Identifiers: LCCN 2018061585| ISBN 9780780816855 (hard cover: alk. paper) | ISBN 9780780816862 (ebook)

Subjects: LCSH: Osteoporosis--Popular works.

Classification: LCC RC931.O73 O777 2019 | DDC 616.7/16--dc23

LC record available at https://lccn.loc.gov/2018061585

Table of Contents

Part II: Osteoporosis in Women, Children, Men, and Older Adults

Part III: Osteoporosis and Related Conditions

Part IV: Risk Factors and Prevention of Osteoporosis

Part V: Diagnosis and Treatment of Osteoporosis

Part VI: Living with Osteoporosis

Preface

About This Book

Many people think of bones as simple, solid structures that make up the skeletal system. In truth, bones are complex, living tissues that go through a constant process of building up and tearing down. This process, called bone remodeling, rebuilds the bones as people grow and age. One of the main components of bone is calcium. In fact, the skeletal system contains 99 percent of the body's calcium. In osteoporosis, which literally means "porous bones," excessive bone loss results in a depletion of calcium. The gradual weakening of the bones over time makes them more susceptible to fractures and can lead to disfigurement and pain. Most people reach a peak bone mass between the ages of 25 and 35. By age 40, bone loss usually reaches 0.5 percent per year. Postmenopausal women can lose 2 to 3 percent per year and can have lost 50 percent of their bone mass by age 70 or 80. In osteoporosis, bone loss accelerates. Since the loss occurs over time, the effect may not be noticed until substantial bone loss has occurred, often signaled by an unexpected fracture. Osteoporosis cannot be detected by X-ray until the bone loss has reached 30 to 50 percent of bone mass, by which time the calcium depletion cannot be reversed. Because of this, prevention and early diagnosis are critical.

Osteoporosis Sourcebook, Second Edition provides information so that the layperson can identify the important risk factors of osteoporosis and the life-style changes needed to offset them. It provides answers to questions about calcium intake and supplements and other dietary needs, the drugs used to treat osteoporosis, and surgical options. It also suggests coping strategies for those suffering from the disease. The book concludes with a glossary of related terms and a directory of resources.

How to Use This Book

This book is divided into parts and chapters. Parts focus on broad areas of interest. Chapters are devoted to single topics within a part.

Part I: Osteoporosis: An Overview begins with an introduction to osteoporosis and gives a brief insight into the risk factors and preventive measures of the disease. It talks about the basic structure and functions of the bone and highlights the factors that influence/affect the bone health. It also distinguishes osteoporosis from arthritis and emphasizes the importance of proper diagnosis.

Part II: Osteoporosis in Women, Children, Men, and Older Adults outlines the impact of osteoporosis and its costs, both monetary and in terms of health effects, for various segments of population such as women, children, men, and older adults.

Part III: Osteoporosis and Related Conditions provides information about diseases and conditions that lead to or aggravate osteoporosis or that have symptoms similar to those produced by osteoporosis. The conditions include dripping candle wax bone disease, fibrous dysplasia, Gaucher disease, otosclerosis, hypercalcemia, hypocalcemia, hyperparathyroidism, hypophosphatasia, inflammatory bowel disease, multiple myeloma, oral health, osteopetrosis, osteogenesis imperfecta, and Paget Disease.

Part IV: Risk Factors and Prevention of Osteoporosis discusses in detail about the factors that lead to osteoporosis and suggests healthy lifestyle choices to minimize those factors.

Part V: Diagnosis and Treatment of Osteoporosis traces the process of diagnosing osteoporosis as early as possible and treating the condition effectively. It reviews the various options in drug and surgical therapies and points out their drawbacks and limitations. It also highlights some of the complementary and alternative medicines available for osteoporosis.

Part VI: Living with Osteoporosis deals with the impact to osteoporosis on an individual. It explains how lifestyle changes can help patients with osteoporosis lead a healthy life. The part also deals with the strategies to cope up with the chronic pain caused by the disease.

Part VII: Additional Help and Information provides a glossary of osteoporosis-related terminology and a list of resources for patients with osteoporosis or related conditions.

Bibliographic Note

This volume contains documents and excerpts from publications issued by the following U.S. government agencies: Agricultural Research Service (ARS); Centers for Disease Control and Prevention (CDC); Centers for Medicare & Medicaid Services (CMS); *Eunice Kennedy Shriver* National Institute of Child Health and Human Development (NICHD); Genetic and Rare Diseases Information Center (GARD); Genetics Home Reference (GHR); *Go4Life*; National Cancer Institute (NCI); National Center for Biotechnology Information (NCBI); National Institute of Arthritis and Musculoskeletal and Skin Diseases (NIAMS); National Institute of Diabetes and Digestive and Kidney Diseases (NIDDK); National Institute of Mental Health (NIMH); National Institute of Neurological Disorders and Stroke (NINDS); National Institute on Aging (NIA); National Institute on Alcohol Abuse and Alcoholism (NIAAA); National Institute on Deafness and Other Communication Disorders (NIDCD); National Institutes of Health (NIH); *NIH News in Health*; NIH Osteoporosis and Related Bone Diseases—National Resource Center (NIH ORBD—NRC); Office of Dietary Supplements (ODS); Office of Disease Prevention and Health Promotion (ODPHP); Office on Women's Health (OWH); U.S. Department of Energy (DOE); U.S. Department of Veterans Affairs (VA); and U.S. Food and Drug Administration (FDA).

It may also contain original material produced by Omnigraphics and reviewed by medical consultants

About the Health Reference Series

The *Health Reference Series* is designed to provide basic medical information for patients, families, caregivers, and the general public. Each volume takes a particular topic and provides comprehensive coverage. This is especially important for people who may be dealing with a newly diagnosed disease or a chronic disorder in themselves or in a family member. People looking for preventive guidance, information about disease warning signs, medical statistics, and risk factors for health problems will also find answers to their questions in the

Health Reference Series. The *Series*, however, is not intended to serve as a tool for diagnosing illness, in prescribing treatments, or as a substitute for the physician/patient relationship. All people concerned about medical symptoms or the possibility of disease are encouraged to seek professional care from an appropriate healthcare provider.

A Note about Spelling and Style

Health Reference Series editors use *Stedman's Medical Dictionary* as an authority for questions related to the spelling of medical terms and the *Chicago Manual of Style* for questions related to grammatical structures, punctuation, and other editorial concerns. Consistent adherence is not always possible, however, because the individual volumes within the *Series* include many documents from a wide variety of different producers, and the editor's primary goal is to present material from each source as accurately as is possible. This sometimes means that information in different chapters or sections may follow other guidelines and alternate spelling authorities. For example, occasionally a copyright holder may require that eponymous terms be shown in possessive forms (Crohn's disease vs. Crohn disease) or that British spelling norms be retained (leukaemia vs. leukemia).

Medical Review

Omnigraphics contracts with a team of qualified, senior medical professionals who serve as medical consultants for the *Health Reference Series*. As necessary, medical consultants review reprinted and originally written material for currency and accuracy. Citations including the phrase "Reviewed (month, year)" indicate material reviewed by this team. Medical consultation services are provided to the *Health Reference Series* editors by:

Dr. Vijayalakshmi, MBBS, DGO, MD
Dr. Senthil Selvan, MBBS, DCH, MD
Dr. K. Sivanandham, MBBS, DCH, MS (Research), PhD

Our Advisory Board

We would like to thank the following board members for providing initial guidance on the development of this series:

- Dr. Lynda Baker, Associate Professor of Library and Information Science, Wayne State University, Detroit, MI

- Nancy Bulgarelli, William Beaumont Hospital Library, Royal Oak, MI

- Karen Imarisio, Bloomfield Township Public Library, Bloomfield Township, MI

- Karen Morgan, Mardigian Library, University of Michigan-Dearborn, Dearborn, MI

- Rosemary Orlando, St. Clair Shores Public Library, St. Clair Shores, MI

Health Reference Series *Update Policy*

The inaugural book in the *Health Reference Series* was the first edition of *Cancer Sourcebook* published in 1989. Since then, the *Series* has been enthusiastically received by librarians and in the medical community. In order to maintain the standard of providing high-quality health information for the layperson the editorial staff at Omnigraphics felt it was necessary to implement a policy of updating volumes when warranted.

Medical researchers have been making tremendous strides, and it is the purpose of the *Health Reference Series* to stay current with the most recent advances. Each decision to update a volume is made on an individual basis. Some of the considerations include how much new information is available and the feedback we receive from people who use the books. If there is a topic you would like to see added to the update list, or an area of medical concern you feel has not been adequately addressed, please write to:

Managing Editor
Health Reference Series
Omnigraphics
615 Griswold, Ste. 901
Detroit, MI 48226

Part One

Osteoporosis: An Overview

Chapter 1

Introduction to Osteoporosis

Chapter Contents

3

Section 1.1

The Skeletal System and Bones

This section includes text excerpted from "Introduction to the Skeletal System," National Cancer Institute (NCI), July 1, 2002. Reviewed January 2019.

Humans are vertebrates, animals having a vertebral column or backbone. We rely on a sturdy internal frame that is centered on a prominent spine. The human skeletal system consists of bones, cartilage, ligaments, and tendons and accounts for about 20 percent of our body weight.

The living bones in our bodies use oxygen and give off waste products in metabolism. They contain active tissues that consume nutrients, require a blood supply and change shape or remodel in response to variations in mechanical stress.

Bones provide a rigid framework, known as the skeleton, that support and protect the soft organs of the body.

The skeleton supports the body against the pull of gravity. The large bones of the lower limbs support the trunk when standing.

The skeleton also protects the soft body parts. The fused bones of the cranium surround the brain to make it less vulnerable to injury. Vertebrae surround and protect the spinal cord and bones of the rib cage help protect the heart and lungs of the thorax.

Bones work together with muscles as simple mechanical lever systems to produce body movement.

Bones contain more calcium than any other organ. The intercellular matrix of bone contains large amounts of calcium salts, the most important being calcium phosphate.

When blood calcium levels decrease below normal, calcium is released from the bones so that there will be an adequate supply for metabolic needs. When blood calcium levels are increased, the excess calcium is stored in the bone matrix. The dynamic process of releasing and storing calcium goes on almost continuously.

Hematopoiesis, the formation of blood cells, mostly takes place in the red marrow of the bones.

In infants, red marrow is found in the bone cavities. With age, it is largely replaced by yellow marrow for fat storage. In adults, red marrow is limited to the spongy bone in the skull, ribs, sternum, clavicles, vertebrae, and pelvis. Red marrow functions in the formation of red blood cells, white blood cells, and blood platelets.

Structure of Bone Tissue

There are two types of bone tissue: compact and spongy. The names imply that the two types differ in density, or how tightly the tissue is packed together. There are three types of cells that contribute to bone homeostasis. Osteoblasts are bone-forming cell, osteoclasts resorb or break down bone, and osteocytes are mature bone cells. An equilibrium between osteoblasts and osteoclasts maintains bone tissue.

Compact Bone

Compact bone consists of closely packed osteons or haversian systems. The osteon consists of a central canal called the "osteonic" (haversian) canal, which is surrounded by concentric rings (lamellae) of matrix. Between the rings of matrix, the bone cells (osteocytes) are located in spaces called lacunae. Small channels (canaliculi) radiate from the lacunae to the osteonic (haversian) canal to provide passageways through the hard matrix. In compact bone, the haversian systems are packed tightly together to form what appears to be a solid mass. The osteonic canals contain blood vessels that are parallel to the long axis of the bone. These blood vessels interconnect, by way of perforating canals, with vessels on the surface of the bone.

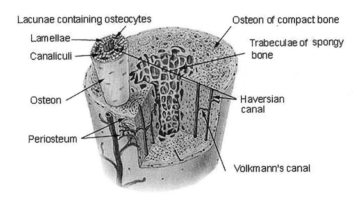

Figure 1.1. *Compact Bone and Spongy (Cancellous Bone)*

Spongy (Cancellous) Bone

Spongy (cancellous) bone is lighter and less dense than compact bone. Spongy bone consists of plates (trabeculae) and bars of bone adjacent to small, irregular cavities that contain red bone marrow.

The canaliculi connect to the adjacent cavities, instead of a central haversian canal, to receive their blood supply. It may appear that the trabeculae are arranged in a haphazard manner, but they are organized to provide maximum strength similar to braces that are used to support a building. The trabeculae of spongy bone follow the lines of stress and can realign if the direction of stress changes.

Bone Development and Growth

The terms "osteogenesis" and "ossification" are often used synonymously to indicate the process of bone formation. Parts of the skeleton form during the first few weeks after conception. By the end of the eighth week after conception, the skeletal pattern is formed in cartilage and connective tissue membranes and ossification begins.

Bone development continues throughout adulthood. Even after adult stature is attained, bone development continues for repair of fractures and for remodeling to meet changing lifestyles. Osteoblasts, osteocytes, and osteoclasts are the three cell types involved in the development, growth and remodeling of bones. Osteoblasts are bone-forming cells, osteocytes are mature bone cells and osteoclasts break down and reabsorb bone.

There are two types of ossification: intramembranous and endochondral.

Intramembranous

Intramembranous ossification involves the replacement of sheet-like connective tissue membranes with bony tissue. Bones formed in this manner are called "intramembranous" bones. They include certain flat bones of the skull and some of the irregular bones. The future bones are first formed as connective tissue membranes. Osteoblasts migrate to the membranes and deposit bony matrix around themselves. When the osteoblasts are surrounded by matrix they are called "osteocytes."

Endochondral Ossification

Endochondral ossification involves the replacement of hyaline cartilage with bony tissue. Most of the bones of the skeleton are formed in this manner. These bones are called "endochondral" bones. In this process, the future bones are first formed as hyaline cartilage models. During the third month after conception, the perichondrium that surrounds the hyaline cartilage "models" becomes infiltrated with blood vessels and osteoblasts and changes into a periosteum. The osteoblasts form a collar of compact bone around the diaphysis. At the same time, the cartilage in the center of the diaphysis begins to disintegrate. Osteoblasts penetrate the disintegrating cartilage and replace it with spongy bone. This forms a primary ossification center. Ossification continues from this center toward the ends of the bones. After spongy bone is formed in the diaphysis, osteoclasts break down the newly formed bone to open up the medullary cavity.

The cartilage in the epiphyses continues to grow so the developing bone increases in length. Later, usually after birth, secondary ossification centers form in the epiphyses. Ossification in the epiphyses is similar to that in the diaphysis except that the spongy bone is retained instead of being broken down to form a medullary cavity. When secondary ossification is complete, the hyaline cartilage is totally replaced by bone except in two areas. A region of hyaline cartilage remains over the surface of the epiphysis as the articular cartilage and another area of cartilage remains between the epiphysis and diaphysis. This is the epiphyseal plate or growth region.

Bone Growth

Bones grow in length at the epiphyseal plate by a process that is similar to endochondral ossification. The cartilage in the region of the epiphyseal plate next to the epiphysis continues to grow by mitosis. The chondrocytes, in the region next to the diaphysis, age and degenerate. Osteoblasts move in and ossify the matrix to form bone. This process continues throughout childhood and the adolescent years until the cartilage growth slows and finally stops. When cartilage growth ceases, usually in the early twenties, the epiphyseal plate completely ossifies so that only a thin epiphyseal line remains and the bones can no longer grow in length. Bone growth is under the influence of growth hormone from the anterior pituitary gland and sex hormones from the ovaries and testes.

- Even though bones stop growing in length in early adulthood, they can continue to increase in thickness or diameter throughout life in response to stress from increased muscle activity or to weight. The increase in diameter is called appositional growth. Osteoblasts in the periosteum form compact bone around the external bone surface. At the same time, osteoclasts in the endosteum break down bone on the internal bone surface, around the medullary cavity. These two processes together increase the diameter of the bone and, at the same time, keep the bone from becoming excessively heavy and bulky.

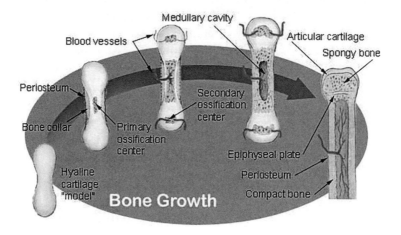

Figure 1.2. *Bone Growth*

Section 1.2

What Is Osteoporosis?

This section includes text excerpted from "Osteoporosis,"
National Institute of Arthritis and Musculoskeletal and
Skin Diseases (NIAMS), February 28, 2016.

Osteoporosis is a disease in which your bones become weak and are more likely to break. If you have osteoporosis you are more likely to break bones in your hip, spine, and wrist.

Our bones are alive. Every day, our body breaks down old bone and puts new bone in its place. As we get older, our bones break down more bone than they put back. It is normal to lose some bone as we age. But, if we do not take steps to keep our bones healthy, we can lose too much bone and get osteoporosis.

Who Gets Osteoporosis

In the United States, millions of people either already have osteoporosis or are at high risk due to low bone mass. Osteoporosis can occur in both men and women and at any age, but it is most common in older women. Because more women get osteoporosis than men, many men think they are not at risk for the disease. However, it is a real risk for older men and women from all backgrounds.

Also, people from certain ethnic backgrounds may be more likely to have other health problems that increase their risk for bone loss. In addition, some diseases and medications can increase the risk of osteoporosis.

What Are the Symptoms of Osteoporosis?

Osteoporosis is called the "silent disease" because bone loss does not have any symptoms until a bone breaks.

Section 1.3

Osteoporosis Risk Factors and Prevention

This section includes text excerpted from "Osteoporosis,"
National Institute on Aging (NIA), National
Institutes of Health (NIH), June 26, 2017.

Although osteoporosis can strike at any age, it is most common among older people, especially older women. Men also have this disease. White and Asian women are most likely to have osteoporosis. Other women at great risk include those who:

- Have a family history of broken bones or osteoporosis

- Have broken a bone after age 50

- Had surgery to remove their ovaries before their periods stopped

- Had early menopause

- Have not gotten enough calcium and/or vitamin D throughout their lives

- Had extended bed rest or were physically inactive
- Smoke (smokers may absorb less calcium from their diets)
- Take certain medications, including medicines for arthritis and asthma and some cancer drugs
- Used certain medicines for a long time
- Have a small body frame

The risk of osteoporosis grows as you get older. At the time of menopause, women may lose bone quickly for several years. After that, the loss slows down but continues. In men, the loss of bone mass is slower. But, by age 65 or 70, men and women are losing bone at the same rate.

What Is Osteopenia?

Whether your doctor calls it osteopenia or low bone mass, consider it a warning. Bone loss has started, but you can still take action to keep your bones strong and maybe prevent osteoporosis later in life. That way you will be less likely to break a wrist, hip, or vertebrae (bone in your spine) when you are older.

Can My Bones Be Tested?

For some people, the first sign of osteoporosis is to realize they are getting shorter or to break a bone easily. Don't wait until that happens to see if you have osteoporosis. You can have a bone density test to find out how strong your bones are.

The U.S. Preventive Service Task Force (USPSTF) recommends that women aged 65 and older be screened (tested) for osteoporosis, as well as women under age 65 who are at increased risk for an osteoporosis-related fracture.

A bone mineral density test compares your bone density to the bones of an average healthy young adult. The test result, known as a T-score, tells you how strong your bones are, whether you have osteoporosis or osteopenia, and your risk for having a fracture.

How Can I Keep My Bones Strong? Preventing Osteoporosis

There are things you should do at any age to prevent weakened bones. Eating foods that are rich in calcium and vitamin D is important.

So is regular weight-bearing exercise, such as weight training, walking, hiking, jogging, climbing stairs, tennis, and dancing.

If you have osteoporosis, avoid activities that involve twisting your spine or bending forward from the waist, such as conventional sit-ups, toe touches, or swinging a golf club. Learn how to exercise safety with *Go4Life* (go4life.nia.nih.gov), the exercise and physical activity campaign from the National Institute on Aging (NIA).

Those are the best ways to keep your bones strong and healthy.

What Can I Do for My Osteoporosis?

Treating osteoporosis means stopping the bone loss and rebuilding bone to prevent breaks. Healthy lifestyle choices such as proper diet, exercise, and medications can help prevent further bone loss and reduce the risk of fractures.

But, lifestyle changes may not be enough if you have lost a lot of bone density. There are also several medicines to think about. Some will slow your bone loss, and others can help rebuild bone. Talk with your doctor to see if medicines might work to treat your osteoporosis.

In addition, you'll want to learn how to fall-proof your home and change your lifestyle to avoid fracturing fragile bones.

Can I Avoid Falling?

When your bones are weak, a simple fall can cause a broken bone. This can mean a trip to the hospital and maybe surgery. It might also mean being laid up for a long time, especially in the case of a hip fracture. So, it is important to prevent falls.

Do Men Have Osteoporosis?

Osteoporosis is not just a woman's disease. Not as many men have it as women do, maybe because most men start with more bone density. As they age, men lose bone density more slowly than women. But, men need to be aware of osteoporosis.

Experts don't know as much about this disease in men as they do in women. However, many of the things that put men at risk are the same as those for women, including family history, not enough calcium or vitamin D, and too little exercise. Low levels of testosterone, too much alcohol, taking certain drugs, and smoking are other risk factors.

Older men who break a bone easily or are at risk for osteoporosis should talk with their doctors about testing and treatment.

Section 1.4

Types of Osteoporosis

This section includes text excerpted from "Bone Health and Osteoporosis: A Report of the Surgeon General," National Center for Biotechnology Information (NCBI), 2004. Reviewed January 2019.

Primary Osteoporosis

Primary osteoporosis is mainly a disease of the elderly, the result of the cumulative impact of bone loss and deterioration of bone structure that occurs as people age. This form of osteoporosis is sometimes referred to as age-related osteoporosis. Since postmenopausal women are at greater risk, the term "postmenopausal" osteoporosis is also used. Younger individuals (including children and young adults) rarely get primary osteoporosis, although it can occur on occasion. This rare form of the disease is sometimes referred to as "idiopathic" osteoporosis, since in many cases the exact causes of the disease are not known, or idiopathic. Since the exact mechanisms by which aging produces bone loss are not all understood (that is, it is not always clear why some postmenopausal women develop osteoporosis while others do not), age-related osteoporosis is also partially idiopathic.

Idiopathic Primary Osteoporosis

There are several different forms of idiopathic osteoporosis that can affect both children and adolescents, although these conditions are quite rare. Juvenile osteoporosis affects previously healthy children between the ages of 8 and 14. Over a period of several years, bone growth is impaired. The condition may be relatively mild, causing only one or two collapsed bones in the spine (vertebrae), or it may be severe, affecting virtually the entire spine. The disease almost always goes into remission (spontaneously) around the time of puberty with a resumption of normal bone growth at that time. Patients with mild or moderate forms of the disease may be left with a curvature of the spine (kyphosis) and short stature, but those with a more severe form of the disease may be incapacitated for life.

Primary osteoporosis is quite rare in young adults. In this age-group, the disease is usually caused by some other condition or factor, such as anorexia nervosa or glucocorticoid use. When idiopathic forms of primary osteoporosis do occur in young adults, they appear in men as often as they do in women (this is in contrast to age-related primary osteoporosis, which occurs more often in women). The characteristics of the disease can vary broadly and may involve more than one disorder. Some young adults with idiopathic primary osteoporosis may have a primary defect in the regulation of bone cell function, resulting in depressed bone formation, increased bone resorption, or both. Others with a mild form of the disease may simply have failed to achieve an adequate amount of skeletal mass during growth. In some patients, the disease runs a mild course, even without treatment, and the clinical manifestations are limited to asymptomatic spinal compression fractures. More typically, however, multiple spine fractures occur over a five-to-ten-year period leading to a height loss of up to six inches.

Age-Related Osteoporosis

Age-related osteoporosis is by far the most common form of the disease. There are many different causes of the ailment, but the bone loss that leads to the disease typically begins relatively early in life, at a time when corrective action (such as changes in diet and physical activity) could potentially slow down its course. While it occurs in both sexes, the disease is two to three times more common in women. This is partly due to the fact that women have two phases of age-related bone loss—a rapid phase that begins at menopause and lasts four to eight years, followed by a slower continuous phase that lasts throughout the rest of life. By contrast, men go through only the slow, continuous phase. As a result, women typically lose more bone than do men. The rapid phase of bone loss alone in women results in losses of 5 to 10 percent of cortical bone (which makes up the hard outer shell of the skeleton) and 20 to 30 percent of trabecular bone (which fills the ends of the limb bones and the vertebral bodies in the spine, the sites of most osteoporotic fractures). The slow phase of bone loss results in losses of 20 to 25 percent of cortical and trabecular bone in both men and women, but over a longer period of time.

Although other factors such as genetics and nutrition contribute, both the rapid phase of bone loss in postmenopausal women and the slow phase of bone loss in aging women and men appear to be largely the result of estrogen deficiency. (This is demonstrated by the fact that correction of estrogen deficiency can prevent these changes.) For women, the rapid phase of bone loss is initiated by a dramatic decline in estrogen production by the ovaries at menopause. The loss of estrogen action on estrogen receptors in bone results in large increases in bone resorption, combined with reduced bone formation. The end result is thinning of the cortical outer shell of bone and damage to the trabecular bone structure. There may be some countervailing forces on this process, as the outside diameter of the bone can increase with age, thus helping to maintain bone strength.

By contrast, the slower phase of bone loss is thought to be caused by a combination of factors including age-related impairment of bone formation, decreased calcium and vitamin D intake, decreased physical activity, and the loss of estrogen positive effects on calcium balance in the intestine and kidney as well as its effects on bone. This leads to further impairment of absorption of calcium by the intestine and reduced ability of the kidney to conserve calcium. If the amount of calcium absorbed from the diet is insufficient to make up for the obligatory calcium losses in the stool and urine, serum calcium begins to fall. Parathyroid hormone (PTH) levels will then increase, removing calcium from bone to make up for the loss. The net result of this process is an increase in bone resorption. It is important to realize that these mineral losses need not be great to result in osteoporosis. A negative balance of only 50 to 100 mg of calcium per day (far less than the 300 mg of calcium in a single glass of milk) over a long period of time is sufficient to produce the disease.

For aging men, sex steroid deficiency also appears to be a major factor in age-related osteoporosis. Although testosterone is the major sex steroid in men, some of it is converted by the aromatase enzyme into estrogen. In men, however, the deficiency is mainly due to an increase in sex hormone binding globulin, a substance that holds both testosterone and estrogen in a form that is not available for use by the body. Between 30 to 50 percent of elderly men are deficient in biologically active sex steroids. In fact, except for the lack of the early postmenopausal phase, the process of bone loss in older men is similar to that for older women. As with women, the loss of sex steroid activity in men has an effect on calcium absorption and conservation, leading to progressive secondary increases in parathyroid hormone levels. As in older women, the resulting imbalance between bone resorption and formation results in slow bone loss that continues over life. Since testosterone may stimulate bone formation more than estrogen does, however, decreased bone formation plays a relatively greater role in the bone loss experienced by elderly men.

Secondary Osteoporosis

Young adults and even older individuals who get osteoporosis often do so as a byproduct of another condition or medication use. In fact, there are a wide variety of diseases along with certain medications and toxic agents that can cause or contribute to the development of osteoporosis. Individuals who get the disease due to these "outside" causes are said to have "secondary" osteoporosis. They typically experience greater levels of bone loss than would be expected for a normal individual of the same age, gender, and race. Secondary causes of the disease are common in many premenopausal women and men with osteoporosis; in fact, by some estimates the majority of men with osteoporosis exhibit secondary causes of the disease. In addition, up to a third of postmenopausal women with osteoporosis also have other conditions that may contribute to their bone loss.

Chapter 2

Bone Basics

Chapter Contents

Section 2.1

What Is Bone?

This section includes text excerpted from "What Is Bone?" NIH
Osteoporosis and Related Bone Diseases—National Resource Center
(NIH ORBD—NRC), May 1, 2015. Reviewed January 2019.

To understand osteoporosis, it is important to learn about bone.
Made mostly of collagen, bone is living, growing tissue. Collagen is a
protein that provides a soft framework, and calcium phosphate is a
mineral that adds strength and hardens the framework. This combination of collagen and calcium makes bone strong and flexible enough
to withstand stress. More than 99 percent of the body's calcium is
contained in the bones and teeth. The remaining one percent is found
in the blood.

Two types of bone found in the body—cortical and trabecular. Cortical bone is dense and compact. It forms the outer layer of the bone. Trabecular bone makes up the inner layer of the bone and has a spongy,
honeycomb-like structure.

Bone Remodeling

Throughout life, bone is constantly renewed through a two-part
process called remodeling. This process consists of resorption and
formation. During resorption, special cells called osteoclasts break
down and remove old bone tissue. During bone formation, new bone
tissue is laid down to replace the old. Several hormones including
calcitonin, parathyroid hormone, vitamin D, estrogen (in women), and
testosterone (in men), among others, regulate osteoclast and osteoblast
function.

The Bone Bank Account

Think of bone as a bank account where you "deposit" and "withdraw" bone tissue. During childhood and the teenage years, new bone
is added to the skeleton faster than old bone is removed. As a result,
bones become larger, heavier, and denser. For most people, bone formation continues at a faster pace than removal until bone mass peaks
during the third decade of life.

After age 20, bone "withdrawals" can begin to exceed "deposits."
For many people, this bone loss can be prevented by continuing to
get calcium, vitamin D, and exercise and by avoiding tobacco and

excessive alcohol use. Osteoporosis develops when bone removal occurs too quickly, replacement occurs too slowly, or both. You are more likely to develop osteoporosis if you did not reach your maximum peak bone mass during your bone-building years.

Women, Men, and Osteoporosis

Women are more likely than men to develop osteoporosis. This is because women generally have smaller, thinner bones than men have and because women can lose bone tissue rapidly in the first four to eight years after menopause because of the sharp decline in production of the hormone estrogen. Produced by the ovaries, estrogen has been shown to have a protective effect on bone. Women usually go through menopause between age 45 and 55. After menopause, bone loss in women greatly exceeds that in men. However, by age 65, women and men tend to lose bone tissue at the same rate. Although men do not undergo the equivalent of menopause, production of the male hormone testosterone may decrease, and this can lead to increased bone loss and a greater risk of developing osteoporosis.

Section 2.2

Why Do We Have Bones?

This section includes text excerpted from "The Basics of Bone in Health and Disease," National Center for Biotechnology Information (NCBI), 2004. Reviewed January 2019.

The bony skeleton is a remarkable organ that serves both a structural function—providing mobility, support, and protection for the body—and a reservoir function, as the storehouse for essential minerals. It is not a static organ, but is constantly changing to better carry out its functions. The development of the bony skeleton likely began many eons ago, when animals left the calcium-rich ocean, first to live in freshwater where calcium was in short supply, and then on dry land where weight bearing put much greater stress on the skeleton. The architecture of the skeleton is remarkably adapted to provide adequate strength and mobility so that bones do not break when subjected to substantial impact, even the loads placed on bone during vigorous physical activity. The shape or structure of bone is at least as important as its mass in providing this strength.

The skeleton is also a storehouse for two minerals, calcium and phosphorus, that are essential for the functioning of other body systems, and this storehouse must be called upon in times of need. The maintenance of a constant level of calcium in the blood as well as an adequate supply of calcium and phosphorus in cells is critical for the function of all body organs, but particularly for the nerves and muscle.

Therefore, a complex system of regulatory hormones has developed that helps to maintain adequate supplies of these minerals in a variety of situations. These hormones act not only on bone but on other tissues, such as the intestine and the kidney, to regulate the supply of these elements. Thus one reason that bone health is difficult to maintain is that the skeleton is simultaneously serving two different functions that are in competition with each other.

First, bone must be responsive to changes in mechanical loading or weight bearing, both of which require strong bones that have ample supplies of calcium and phosphorus. When these elements are in short supply the regulating hormones take them out of the bone to serve vital functions in other systems of the body. Thus the skeleton can be likened to a bank where we can deposit calcium or phosphorus and then withdraw them later in times of need. However, too many withdrawals weaken the bone and can lead to the most common bone disorder, fractures.

Both the amount of bone and its architecture or shape are determined by the mechanical forces that act on the skeleton. Much of this is determined genetically so that each species, including humans, has a skeleton that is adapted to its functions. However, there can be great variation within a species, so that some individuals will have strong bones and others will have weak bones, largely because of differences in their genes. Moreover, bone mass and architecture are further modified throughout life as these functions and the mechanical forces required to fulfill them change. In other words, bones will weaken if they are not subjected to adequate amounts of loading and weight bearing for sufficient periods of time. If they are not (such as in the weightless condition of space travel), rapid bone loss can occur. In other words, as with muscle, it is "use it or lose it" with bone as well. Conversely, the amount and architecture of the bones can be improved by mechanical loading.

To respond to its dual roles of support and regulation of calcium and phosphorus, as well as to repair any damage to the skeleton, bone is constantly changing. Old bone breaks down and new bone is formed on a continuous basis. In fact, the tissue of the skeleton is replaced many times during life. This requires an exquisitely controlled regulatory system that involves specialized cells that communicate with each other. These cells must respond to many different signals, both internal and external, mechanical and hormonal, and systemic (affecting the whole skeleton) and local (affecting only a small region of the skeleton). It is not surprising that with so many different tasks to perform and so many different factors regulating how the skeleton grows, adapts, and responds to changing demands, there are many ways that these processes can go astray.

How Does Bones Work?

Bone is a composite material, consisting of crystals of mineral bound to protein. This provides both strength and resilience so that the skeleton can absorb impact without breaking. A structure made only of mineral would be more brittle and break more easily, while a structure made only of protein would be soft and bend too easily. The mineral phase of bone consists of small crystals containing calcium and phosphate, called hydroxyapatite. This mineral is bound in an orderly manner to a matrix that is made up largely of a single protein, collagen. Collagen is made by bone cells and assembled as long thin rods containing three intertwined protein chains, which are then assembled into larger fibers that are strengthened by chemical connections between them.

Other proteins in bone can help to strengthen the collagen matrix even further and to regulate its ability to bind mineral. Very small changes in the shape of the bone can act on the cells inside bone (the osteocytes), which produce chemical signals that allow the skeleton to respond to changes in mechanical loading. Abnormalities in the collagen scaffold can occur as a result of a genetic disorder called osteogenesis imperfecta, while the failure of mineral deposition can be the result of rickets and osteomalacia, conditions that result in marked weakening of the skeleton.

To provide the body with a frame that is both light and strong, bones are hollow. The outer dense shell is called cortical bone, which makes up roughly three-quarters of the total skeletal mass. Inside the cortical shell is a fine network of connecting plates and rods called trabecular bone that makes up the remaining 25 percent. Most bones are hollow structures in which the outer cortical bone shell defines the shape of the bone. This cortical shell is essential because it provides strength, sites for firm attachment of the tendons, and muscles and protection without excessive weight. The inner trabecular network has two important functions. It provides a large bone surface for mineral exchange.

In addition, trabecular bone helps to maintain skeletal strength and integrity, as it is particularly abundant in the spine and at the ends of the long bones, sites that are under continuous stress from motion and weight-bearing. Fractures are common at these sites when the bone is weakened. The rods and plates of trabecular bone are aligned in a pattern that provides maximal strength without too much bulk, much in the way that architects and engineers design buildings and bridges. The shape and size of both cortical and trabecular bone can respond to different kinds of stress produced by physical activity. For example, in most people, the cortex of their dominant arm is larger than that of their nondominant arm. The difference in cortex size is even larger for tennis players and other athletes who routinely use a dominant arm in their sporting activities.

Bones do not work in isolation, but rather are part of the musculoskeletal system, providing the "lever" that allows muscles to move (by pulling on the lever). Thus muscle activity is important for the normal function of the bone. When the mechanical force produced by muscle is lost—for example, in patients with muscular dystrophy or paralysis—bone mass and strength are also rapidly lost. Many bones in the skeleton also have connecting joints that provide greater flexibility of movement. These joints are sites of great mechanical stress and are subject to injury and to degeneration with aging. The most common type of joint degeneration is osteoarthritis, a painful, degenerative condition that affects the hip, knees, neck, lower back, and/or small joints of the hand. These joint diseases result from very different causes and require very different management than do bone diseases, and consequently, they are not covered in this section.

However, it is important to recognize that the bones, joints, and muscles are the key parts of an integrated "musculoskeletal system." Problems with any one component of this system can affect the other components. Thus, weakness of the muscles can lead to loss of bone and joint damage, while degeneration of the joints leads to changes in the underlying bone, such as the bony spurs or protuberances that occur in osteoarthritis.

Section 2.3

Bone Health for Life

This section contains text excerpted from the following sources: Text in this section begins with excerpts from "How Does Physical Activity Help Build Healthy Bones?" *Eunice Kennedy Shriver* National Institute of Child Health and Human Development (NICHD), December 1, 2016; Text beginning with the heading "What Can I Do to Make My Bones Healthier?" is excerpted from "Bone Health for Life: Health Information Basics for You and Your Family," NIH Osteoporosis and Related Bone Diseases—National Resource Center (NIH ORBD—NRC), July 2014. Reviewed January 2019.

Bones are living tissue. Weight-bearing physical activity causes new bone tissue to form, and this makes bones stronger. This kind of physical activity also makes muscles stronger. Bones and muscles both become stronger when muscles push and tug against bones during physical activity.

Weight-bearing physical activity keeps you on your feet so that your legs carry your body weight. Some examples of weight-bearing physical activities include:

- Walking, jogging, or running
- Playing tennis or racquetball
- Playing field hockey
- Climbing stairs
- Jumping rope and other types of jumping
- Playing basketball
- Dancing
- Hiking
- Playing soccer
- Lifting weights

Swimming and bicycling are not weight-bearing activities, so they do not directly help build bones. But swimming and bicycling do help build strong muscles, and having strong muscles helps build strong bones. These activities are also good for the heart and for overall health.

Bone-strengthening activities are especially important for children and teens because the greatest gains in bone mass occur just before and during puberty. They obtain their lifetime peak bone mass in their teens.

- Children and teens aged 6 to 17 years should get a total of 60 minutes of physical activity every day. Short bursts of activity throughout the day can add up to the recommended total.

- Children and teens should participate in bone-strengthening activities at least three days each week.

- Younger children, aged 2 to 5 years, should play actively several times every day.

What Can I Do to Make My Bones Healthier?

It is never too early or too late to take care of your bones. The following steps can help you improve your bone health:

- Eat a well-balanced diet rich in calcium and vitamin D. Good sources of calcium include low-fat dairy products, and, foods and drinks with added calcium. Good sources of vitamin D include egg yolks, saltwater fish, liver, and milk with vitamin D. Some people may need to take nutritional supplements in order to get enough calcium and vitamin D. The charts below show how much calcium and vitamin D you need each day. Fruits and vegetables also contribute other nutrients that are important for bone health.

- Get plenty of physical activity. Like muscles, bones become stronger with exercise. The best exercises for healthy bones are strength-building and weight-bearing, like walking, climbing stairs, lifting weights, and dancing. Try to get 30 minutes of exercise each day.

- Live a healthy lifestyle. Don't smoke, and, if you choose to drink alcohol, don't drink too much.

- Talk to your doctor about your bone health. Go over your risk factors with your doctor and ask if you should get a bone density test. If you need it, your doctor can order medicine to help prevent bone loss and reduce your chances of breaking a bone.

- Prevent falls. Falling down can cause a bone to break, especially in someone with osteoporosis. But most falls can be prevented.

Check your home for dangers like loose rugs and poor lighting. Have your vision checked? Increase your balance and strength by walking every day and taking classes like tai chi, yoga, or dancing.

Sources of Calcium

- Dairy products (e.g., milk, cheese, yogurt)
- Tofu (calcium fortified)
- Soy milk (calcium fortified)
- Green leafy vegetables (e.g., broccoli, brussels sprouts, mustard greens, kale)
- Chinese cabbage or bok choy
- Beans/legumes
- Tortillas
- Sardines/salmon with edible bones
- Shrimp
- Orange juice (calcium fortified)
- Pizza
- Bread
- Nuts/almonds

Will I Need to Take Medicine for My Bones?

There are medicines to help prevent and treat osteoporosis. Your doctor may want you to take medicine if your bone density test shows that your bones are weak and that you have a good chance of breaking a bone in the future. Your doctor is more likely to order medicine if you have other health concerns that increase your risk for breaking a bone, such as a tendency to fall or a low body weight.

Section 2.4

Boning Up

This section includes text excerpted from "Boning up on
Osteoporosis," Agricultural Research Service (ARS), U.S. Department
of Agriculture (USDA), March 2003. Reviewed January 2019.

When we eat beef, pork, lamb, chicken, or other foods from animals, our bodies take in proteins that may be rich in sulfur. That's unlike the proteins in plant foods—fruits, veggies, nuts, grains, or legumes like peas or dry beans. As we digest animal proteins, the sulfur in them forms acid. A slight, temporary acid overload—called acidosis—may result. To regain our natural balance of acidity to alkalinity, or pH, in the bloodstream, our bodies must buffer the influx of acid. One possible buffer is calcium phosphate, which the body can borrow from our bones—the body's main storage depot for this essential mineral.

Though calcium phosphate is an effective buffer and neutralizer, taking it from bones might increase our risk of osteoporosis. This unhealthy increase in the porosity of bones and resultant thinning leaves those afflicted with this disease especially vulnerable to fractures of the spine, hips, and wrists.

Estimates from the National Institutes of Health (NIH) indicate that ten million Americans, mainly women, already suffer from this disease. Another 28 million Americans are at risk. Other NIH analyses suggest that one in every two women and one in every eight men over age 50 in this country will have an osteoporosis-related fracture in their lifetime.

Does Animal Protein Play a Role?

The cause of osteoporosis is unknown. In exploring possible links between osteoporosis and what we eat, some researchers have developed a hypothesis and a model that point to sulfur-containing animal proteins as a culprit in the bone disease.

The theory has commanded the attention of nutrition researchers, including scientists at the ARS Western Human Nutrition Research Center (WHRC) in Davis, California. They have teamed up with university colleagues to crack some of the secrets of osteoporosis. In a novel study, they recruited women who eat both animal and plant foods—the omnivore regimen typical of most Americans—and women who only eat plant-derived foods. What better way to monitor the possible effect of sulfur-containing proteins than by comparing the bone health of vegan volunteers, who don't eat animal proteins, with that of omnivore volunteers, who do?

ARS physiologist Marta D. Van Loan of the Western Human Nutrition Research Center collaborated in the investigation with Anita M. Oberbauer of the University of California, Davis, (UCD) and with Lydia-Anne Stawasz, formerly at the Davis campus and now at the University of California, Irvine (UCI).

Forty-eight healthy, nonsmoking women, aged 18 to 40, volunteered for the 10-month study. At three intervals during the experiment, the women submitted records of the types and amounts of foods they had eaten during the previous three days. The records gave the researchers an indication of the amount of protein each volunteer had eaten.

The volunteers gave blood and urine specimens at each lab visit. The samples were analyzed for any of several standard indicators of bone health. These included bone formation, as indicated by the amount of a chemical called osteocalcin; and bone resorption, or the amount of calcium removed from bone and reabsorbed into the bloodstream, as measured by another biochemical, N-telopeptide. Other measures included renal net acid excretion and urinary calcium—both indicators of how much calcium was excreted from the body.

The model that other scientists developed predicts that to maintain the correct balance of calcium in the blood, or homeostasis, renal net acid excretion and urinary calcium increase as intake of sulfur-containing animal proteins increase.

But preliminary results suggest that osteoporosis may, in fact, be more complicated than the model predicts. The Davis scientists applied a statistical procedure—multivariate regression analysis—to determine the relative impact of each of the variables, or factors, they examined. As expected, they found that the vegan volunteers ate less protein than the omnivore volunteers. Also, as predicted by the model, renal net acid excretion and urinary calcium were higher in the volunteers who ate more protein (the omnivore women) than in those who ate less (the vegan participants).

Less Bone Formed

But two findings were unexpected. First, bone resorption—in which calcium is taken away from bones via the bloodstream—was the same for omnivore women as for vegan women.

"The current model predicts increased bone resorption for people who consume large amounts of animal protein, so it was somewhat surprising that bone resorption was the same for both groups of our volunteers," Van Loan notes.

Second, bone formation was significantly less in omnivore women than in vegan women. This happened even though the omnivore women had a higher calcium intake than did the vegan volunteers. (The volunteers did not differ in their intake of other nutrients that affect bone health, such as magnesium.)

Using the model as a basis, "one would not have predicted a significantly greater amount of bone formation for vegan volunteers than for omnivore volunteers," Van Loan adds.

The implication for people who eat high amounts of animal protein may be important: Specifically, over time, the net effect of a lower amount of bone formation would likely be a decrease in bone density. Explains Van Loan, "If you have less bone formation, the result is the same as if you had an increase in bone resorption. So, even though bone resorption was the same in both groups of volunteers, the lower amount of bone formation in the omnivore women could lead to a decrease in their bone density."

The findings, if borne out in larger studies, may lead to a modified model. What's more, the investigation may lead to other useful lines of inquiry for other studies.

Chapter 3

Osteoporosis in Your Family

If one of your parents has had a broken bone, especially a broken hip, you may need to be screened earlier for osteoporosis. This is a medical condition where bones become weak and are more likely to break. Share your family health history with your doctor. Your doctor can help you take steps to strengthen weak bones and prevent broken bones.

How Can Osteoporosis Affect My Health?

People with osteoporosis are more likely to break bones, most often in the hip, forearm, wrist, and spine. While most broken bones are caused by falls, osteoporosis can weaken bones to the point that a break can occur more easily, for example by coughing or bumping into something. As you get older, you are more likely to have osteoporosis and recovering from a broken bone becomes harder. Broken bones can have lasting effects including pain that does not go away. Osteoporosis can cause the bones in the spine to break and begin to collapse, so that some people with it get shorter and are not able to stand up straight.

This chapter contains text excerpted from the following sources: Text in this chapter begins with excerpts from "Does Osteoporosis Run in Your Family?" Centers for Disease Control and Prevention (CDC), May 3, 2018; Text under the heading "Bone Risks Linked to Genetic Variants" is excerpted from "Genetics of Bone Density," National Institutes of Health (NIH), April 23, 2012. Reviewed January 2019.

Broken hips are especially serious—afterward, many people are not able to live on their own and are more likely to die sooner.

How Can I Find Out If I Have Osteoporosis?

Osteoporosis is more common in women. It affects about 25 percent (1 in 4) of women aged 65 and over and about five percent (1 in 20) of men aged 65 and over. Many people with osteoporosis do not know they have it until they break a bone. Screening is important to find these people before this happens, so they can take steps to decrease the effects of osteoporosis.

Screening for osteoporosis is recommended for women who are 65 years old or older and for women who are 50 to 64 and have certain risk factors, which include having a parent who has broken a hip. You can use the Fracture Risk Assessment tool (FRAX) (www.sheffield.ac.uk/ FRAX) to learn if you should be screened. It uses several factors to determine how likely you are to have osteoporosis. Talk to your doctor if you have concerns about osteoporosis.

Screening for osteoporosis is commonly done using a type of low-level X-rays called dual-energy X-ray absorptiometry (DXA). Screening also can show if you have low bone mass, meaning your bones are weaker than normal, and are likely to develop osteoporosis.

How Can I Improve My Bone Health If I Have Osteoporosis?

There are steps you can take to improve your bone health and strengthen weak bones:

- Take medications to strengthen your bones and avoid medications that can make your bones weaker

- Eat a healthy diet that includes adequate amounts of calcium and vitamin D

- Perform weight-bearing exercises regularly

- Do not smoke

- Limit alcohol use

Don't wait until you have a broken bone to take steps to improve your bone health—you can start at any age! You can also take steps to prevent falls, including doing exercises to improve your leg strength and balance, having your eyes checked, and making your home safer.

Bone Risks Linked to Genetic Variants

Over 10 million people nationwide have osteoporosis, a disease in which bones become susceptible to fracture. Osteoporosis tends to run in families, and genetics is known to play an important role in bone mineral density, a major risk factor for fractures. Scientists have already identified many genetic factors associated with bone mineral density (BMD). But these factors likely represent just a small fraction of the underlying genetic variance.

Past efforts to link genetic variants with traits and diseases have largely uncovered common variants with relatively small effects. Studies have found less common noncoding variants with larger effects.

An international team of researchers led by Dr. Brent Richards at McGill University set out to examine the role of rare genetic variants in bone mineral density and fracture risk. The scientists used data from the UK10K Project—a massive, whole-genome sequence-based resource of the general European population; the National Institutes of Health (NIH)-funded 1000 Genomes Project, one of the world's earliest efforts to sequence the genomes of a large number of people; and data from several other studies.

The team first performed whole-genome sequencing of more than 2,800 people from the UK10K Project. They also sequenced the exomes (protein-coding regions) of more than 3,500 people. In a sophisticated analysis, the scientists compared these data with those from previous studies involving tens of thousands of other people. They then analyzed associations between the genetic variants and bone mineral density measurements taken in more than 53,000 people. Finally, they looked at data from more than 508,000 people to determine the relationship of the variants to actual bone fractures. Results appeared online on September 14, 2015, in *Nature.*

The team identified variants in a region near the *engrailed homeo-box-1 (EN1)* gene that were associated with bone mineral density in the lumbar area of the spine. One variant was also associated with bone mineral density in the thigh bone at the hip (the "neck" of the femur). Both are common sites of osteoporotic fractures. The effect of these variations, the researchers found, is greater than that of any previously reported genetic variants related to bone density.

Using a mouse model, the team genetically altered EN1 levels and confirmed that it plays an important role in bone physiology. Loss of EN1 results in low bone mass, probably due to high bone turnover.

"EN1 has never before been linked to osteoporosis in humans, so this opens up a brand new pathway to pursue in developing drugs to block the disease," Richards says.

The researchers also found several other variants associated with bone mineral density in specific areas, including three for forearm, 14 for femoral neck, and 19 for lumbar spine. These discoveries indicate that more comprehensive sequencing of diverse populations can lead to the discovery of rare variants influencing common diseases.

"Our findings enhance understanding of the genetics underlying the development of osteoporosis. A variant in a region of the genome that is not coding for a protein can have a relatively large effect on a gene regulating bone health," says Dr. Douglas Kiel, whose NIH-funded team at Hebrew SeniorLife and Harvard Medical School played a key role in the effort. "Ideally, genomic research will one day lead to more personalized interventions (precision medicine) that, in this case, will reduce bone loss and prevent fractures in older adults."

Chapter 4

Nutrition and Osteoporosis

Chapter Contents

Section 4.1

Role of Calcium in Bone Health

This section includes text excerpted from "Calcium Fact Sheet for Consumers," Office of Dietary Supplements (ODS), National Institutes of Health (NIH), November 17, 2016.

What Is Calcium and What Does It Do?

Calcium is a mineral found in many foods. The body needs calcium to maintain strong bones and to carry out many important functions. Almost all calcium is stored in bones and teeth, where it supports their structure and hardness.

The body also needs calcium for muscles to move and for nerves to carry messages between the brain and every body part. In addition, calcium is used to help blood vessels move blood throughout the body and to help release hormones and enzymes that affect almost every function in the human body.

How Much Calcium Do I Need?

The amount of calcium you need each day depends on your age. Average daily recommended amounts are listed below in milligrams (mg):

Table 4.1. Calcium Intake

Life Stage	Recommended Amount
Birth to 6 months	200 mg
Infants 7–12 months	260 mg
Children 1–3 years	700 mg
Children 4–8 years	1,000 mg
Children 9–13 years	1,300 mg
Teens 14–18 years	1,300 mg
Adults 19–50 years	1,000 mg
Adult men 51–70 years	1,000 mg
Adult women 51–70 years	1,200 mg
Adults 71 years and older	1,200 mg
Pregnant and breastfeeding teens	1,300 mg
Pregnant and breastfeeding adults	1,000 mg

What Foods Provide Calcium

Calcium is found in many foods. You can get recommended amounts of calcium by eating a variety of foods, including the following:

- Milk, yogurt, and cheese are the main food sources of calcium for the majority of people in the United States.

- Kale, broccoli, and Chinese cabbage are fine vegetable sources of calcium.

- Fish with soft bones that you eat, such as canned sardines and salmon, are fine animal sources of calcium.

- Most grains (such as breads, pastas, and unfortified cereals), while not rich in calcium, add significant amounts of calcium to the diet because people eat them often or in large amounts.

- Calcium is added to some breakfast cereals, fruit juices, soy and rice beverages, and tofu. To find out whether these foods have calcium, check the product labels.

What Kinds of Calcium Dietary Supplements Are Available?

Calcium is found in many multivitamin-mineral supplements, though the amount varies by product. Dietary supplements that contain only calcium or calcium with other nutrients such as vitamin D are also available. Check the Supplement Facts label to determine the amount of calcium provided.

The two main forms of calcium dietary supplements are carbonate and citrate. Calcium carbonate is inexpensive, but is absorbed best when taken with food. Some over-the-counter (OTC) antacid products, such as Tums® and Rolaids®, contain calcium carbonate. Each pill or chew provides 200 to 400 mg of calcium. Calcium citrate, a more expensive form of the supplement, is absorbed well on an empty or a full stomach. In addition, people with low levels of stomach acid (a condition more common in people older than 50) absorb calcium citrate more easily than calcium carbonate. Other forms of calcium in supplements and fortified foods include gluconate, lactate, and phosphate.

Calcium absorption is best when a person consumes no more than 500 mg at one time. So a person who takes 1,000 mg/day of calcium from supplements, for example, should split the dose rather than take it all at once.

Calcium supplements may cause gas, bloating, and constipation in some people. If any of these symptoms occur, try spreading out the calcium dose throughout the day, taking the supplement with meals, or changing the supplement brand or calcium form you take.

Am I Getting Enough Calcium?

Many people don't get recommended amounts of calcium from the foods they eat, including:

- Boys aged 9 to 13 years

- Girls aged 9 to 18 years

- Women older than 50 years

- Men older than 70 years

When total intakes from both food and supplements are considered, many people—particularly adolescent girls—still fall short of getting enough calcium, while some older women likely get more than the upper limit.

Certain groups of people are more likely than others to have trouble getting enough calcium:

- Postmenopausal women because they experience greater bone loss and do not absorb calcium as well. Sufficient calcium intake from food, and supplements if needed, can slow the rate of bone loss.

- Women of childbearing age whose menstrual periods stop (amenorrhea) because they exercise heavily, eat too little, or both. They need sufficient calcium to cope with the resulting decreased calcium absorption, increased calcium losses in the urine, and slowdown in the formation of new bone.

- People with lactose intolerance cannot digest this natural sugar found in milk and experience symptoms like bloating, gas, and diarrhea when they drink more than small amounts at a time. They usually can eat other calcium-rich dairy products that are low in lactose, such as yogurt and many cheeses, and drink lactose-reduced or lactose-free milk.

- Vegans (vegetarians who eat no animal products) and ovo-vegetarians (vegetarians who eat eggs but no dairy products), because they avoid the dairy products that are a major source of calcium in other people's diets.

Many factors can affect the amount of calcium absorbed from the digestive tract, including:

- **Age.** Efficiency of calcium absorption decreases as people age. Recommended calcium intakes are higher for people over age 70.

- **Vitamin D intake.** This vitamin, present in some foods and produced in the body when skin is exposed to sunlight, increases calcium absorption.

- **Other components in food.** Both oxalic acid (in some vegetables and beans) and phytic acid (in whole grains) can reduce calcium absorption. People who eat a variety of foods don't have to consider these factors. They are accounted for in the calcium recommended intakes, which take absorption into account.

Many factors can also affect how much calcium the body eliminates in urine, feces, and sweat. These include consumption of alcohol- and caffeine-containing beverages as well as intake of other nutrients (protein, sodium, potassium, and phosphorus). In most people, these factors have little effect on calcium status.

What Happens If I Don't Get Enough Calcium

Insufficient intakes of calcium do not produce obvious symptoms in the short term because the body maintains calcium levels in the blood by taking it from bone. Over the longterm, intakes of calcium below recommended levels have health consequences, such as causing low bone mass (osteopenia) and increasing the risks of osteoporosis and bone fractures.

Symptoms of serious calcium deficiency include numbness and tingling in the fingers, convulsions, and abnormal heart rhythms that can lead to death if not corrected. These symptoms occur almost always in people with serious health problems or who are undergoing certain medical treatments.

What Are Some Effects of Calcium on Health?

Scientists are studying calcium to understand how it affects health. Here are several examples of what this research has shown:

Bone Health and Osteoporosis

Bones need plenty of calcium and vitamin D throughout childhood and adolescence to reach their peak strength and calcium content by about age 30. After that, bones slowly lose calcium, but people can help reduce these losses by getting recommended amounts of calcium throughout adulthood and by having a healthy, active lifestyle that includes weight-bearing physical activity (such as walking and running).

Osteoporosis is a disease of the bones in older adults (especially women) in which the bones become porous, fragile, and more prone to fracture. Osteoporosis is a serious public health problem for more than 10 million adults over the age of 50 in the United States. Adequate calcium and vitamin D intakes as well as regular exercise are essential to keep bones healthy throughout life.

Taking calcium and vitamin D supplements reduce the risk of breaking a bone and the risk of falling in frail, elderly adults who live in nursing homes and similar facilities. But it's not clear if the supplements help prevent bone fractures and falls in older people who live at home.

Cancer

Studies have examined whether calcium supplements or diets high in calcium might lower the risks of developing cancer of the colon or rectum or increase the risk of prostate cancer. The research to date provides no clear answers. Given that cancer develops over many years, longer-term studies are needed.

Cardiovascular Disease

Some studies show that getting enough calcium might decrease the risk of heart disease and stroke. Other studies find that high amounts of calcium, particularly from supplements, might increase the risk of heart disease. But when all the studies are considered together, scientists have concluded that as long as intakes are not above the upper limit, calcium from food or supplements will not increase or decrease the risk of having a heart attack or stroke.

High Blood Pressure

Some studies have found that getting recommended intakes of calcium can reduce the risk of developing high blood pressure (hypertension). One large study, in particular, found that eating a diet high in fat-free and low-fat dairy products, vegetables, and fruits lowered blood pressure.

Preeclampsia

Preeclampsia is a serious medical condition in which a pregnant woman develops high blood pressure and kidney problems that cause protein to spill into the urine. It is a leading cause of sickness and death in pregnant women and their newborn babies. For women who get less than about 900 mg of calcium a day, taking calcium supplements during pregnancy (1,000 mg a day or more) reduces the risk of preeclampsia. But most women in the United States who become pregnant get enough calcium from their diets.

Kidney Stones

Most kidney stones are rich in calcium oxalate. Some studies have found that higher intakes of calcium from dietary supplements are linked to a greater risk of kidney stones, especially among older adults. But calcium from foods does not appear to cause kidney stones. For most people, other factors (such as not drinking enough fluids) probably have a larger effect on the risk of kidney stones than calcium intake.

Weight Loss

Although several studies have shown that getting more calcium helps lower body weight or reduce weight gain over time, most studies have found that calcium—from foods or dietary supplements—has little if any effect on body weight and amount of body fat.

Can Calcium Be Harmful?

Getting too much calcium can cause constipation. It might also interfere with the body's ability to absorb iron and zinc, but this effect is not well established. In adults, too much calcium (from dietary supplements but not food) might increase the risk of kidney stones. Some studies show that people who consume high amounts of calcium might have increased risks of prostate cancer and heart disease, but more research is needed to understand these possible links.

The upper limits for calcium are listed below. Most people do not get amounts above the upper limits from food alone; excess intakes usually come from the use of calcium supplements. Surveys show that some older women in the United States probably get amounts somewhat above the upper limit since the use of calcium supplements is common among these women.

Table 4.2. Upper Limit for Calcium Supplements

Life Stage	Upper Limit
Birth to 6 months	1,000 mg
Infants 7–12 months	1,500 mg
Children 1–8 years	2,500 mg
Children 9–18 years	3,000 mg
Adults 19–50 years	2,500 mg
Adults 51 years and older	2,000 mg
Pregnant and breastfeeding teens	3,000 mg
Pregnant and breastfeeding adults	2,500 mg

Are There Any Interactions with Calcium That I Should Know About?

Calcium dietary supplements can interact or interfere with certain medicines that you take, and some medicines can lower or raise calcium levels in the body. Here are some examples:

- Calcium can reduce the absorption of these drugs when taken together:

  - Bisphosphonates (to treat osteoporosis)

  - Antibiotics of the fluoroquinolone and tetracycline families

  - Levothyroxine (to treat low thyroid activity)

  - Phenytoin (an anticonvulsant)

  - Tiludronate disodium (to treat Paget disease (PD))

- Diuretics differ in their effects. Thiazide-type diuretics (such as Diuril® and Lozol®) reduce calcium excretion by the kidneys which in turn can raise blood calcium levels too high. But loop diuretics (such as Lasix® and Bumex®) increase calcium excretion and thereby lower blood calcium levels.

- Antacids containing aluminum or magnesium increase calcium loss in the urine.

- Mineral oil and stimulant laxatives reduce calcium absorption.

- Glucocorticoids (such as prednisone) can cause calcium depletion and eventually osteoporosis when people use them for months at a time.

Tell your doctor, pharmacist, and other healthcare providers about any dietary supplements and medicines you take. They can tell you if those dietary supplements might interact or interfere with your prescription or over-the-counter (OTC) medicines or if the medicines might interfere with how your body absorbs, uses, or breaks down nutrients.

Calcium and Healthful Eating

People should get most of their nutrients from food, advises the federal government's *Dietary Guidelines for Americans* (DGA). Foods contain vitamins, minerals, dietary fiber, and other substances that benefit health. In some cases, fortified foods and dietary supplements may provide nutrients that otherwise may be consumed in less-than-recommended amounts.

Section 4.2

Role of Vitamin D in Bone Health

This section includes text excerpted from "Vitamin D Fact Sheet for Consumers," Office of Dietary Supplements (ODS), National Institutes of Health (NIH), February 17, 2016.

What Is Vitamin D and What Does It Do?

Vitamin D is a nutrient found in some foods that is needed for health and to maintain strong bones. It does so by helping the body absorb calcium (one of bone's main building blocks) from food and supplements. People who get too little vitamin D may develop soft, thin, and brittle bones, a condition known as rickets in children and osteomalacia in adults.

Vitamin D is important to the body in many other ways as well. Muscles need it to move, for example, nerves need it to carry messages between the brain and every body part, and the immune system needs vitamin D to fight off invading bacteria and viruses. Together with calcium, vitamin D also helps protect older adults from osteoporosis. Vitamin D is found in cells throughout the body.

How Much Vitamin D Do I Need?

The amount of vitamin D you need each day depends on your age. Average daily recommended amounts from the Food and Nutrition Board (FNB) (a national group of experts) for different ages are listed below in International Units (IU):

Table 4.3. Vitamin D International Units

Life Stage	Recommended Amount
Birth to 12 months	400 IU
Children 1–13 years	600 IU
Teens 14–18 years	600 IU
Adults 19–70 years	600 IU
Adults 71 years and older	800 IU
Pregnant and breastfeeding women	600 IU

What Foods Provide Vitamin D

Very few foods naturally have vitamin D. Fortified foods provide most of the vitamin D in American diets.

- Fatty fish such as salmon, tuna, and mackerel are among the best sources

- Beef liver, cheese, and egg yolks provide small amounts

- Mushrooms provide some vitamin D. In some mushrooms that are newly available in stores, the vitamin D content is being boosted by exposing these mushrooms to ultraviolet light.

- Almost all of the U.S. milk supply is fortified with 400 IU of vitamin D per quart. But foods made from milk, like cheese and ice cream, are usually not fortified.

- Vitamin D is added to many breakfast cereals and to some brands of orange juice, yogurt, margarine, and soy beverages; check the labels.

Can I Get Vitamin D from the Sun?

The body makes vitamin D when skin is directly exposed to the sun, and most people meet at least some of their vitamin D needs this way. Skin exposed to sunshine indoors through a window will not produce vitamin D. Cloudy days, shade, and having dark-colored skin also cut down on the amount of vitamin D the skin makes.

However, despite the importance of the sun to vitamin D synthesis, it is prudent to limit exposure of skin to sunlight in order to lower the risk for skin cancer. When out in the sun for more than a few minutes, wear protective clothing and apply sunscreen with an SPF (sun protection factor) of eight or more. Tanning beds also cause the skin to make vitamin D, but pose similar risks for skin cancer.

People who avoid the sun or who cover their bodies with sunscreen or clothing should include good sources of vitamin D in their diets or take a supplement. Recommended intakes of vitamin D are set on the assumption of little sun exposure.

What Kinds of Vitamin D Dietary Supplements Are Available?

Vitamin D is found in supplements (and fortified foods) in two different forms: D2 (ergocalciferol) and D3 (cholecalciferol). Both increase vitamin D in the blood.

Am I Getting Enough Vitamin D?

Because vitamin D can come from sun, food, and supplements, the best measure of one's vitamin D status is blood levels of a form known as 25-hydroxyvitamin D. Levels are described in either nanomoles per liter (nmol/L) or nanograms per milliliter (ng/mL), where 1 nmol/L = 0.4 ng/mL.

In general, levels below 30 nmol/L (12 ng/mL) are too low for bone or overall health, and levels above 125 nmol/L (50 ng/mL) are probably too high. Levels of 50 nmol/L or above (20 ng/mL or above) are sufficient for most people.

By these measures, some Americans are vitamin D deficient and almost no one has levels that are too high. In general, young people have higher blood levels of 25-hydroxyvitamin D than older people and males have higher levels than females. By race, non-Hispanic blacks tend to have the lowest levels and non-Hispanic whites the highest. The majority of Americans have blood levels lower than 75 nmol/L (30 ng/mL).

Certain other groups may not get enough vitamin D:

- Breastfed infants, because human milk is a poor source of the nutrient. Breastfed infants should be given a supplement of 400 IU of vitamin D each day

- Older adults, because their skin doesn't make vitamin D when exposed to sunlight as efficiently as when they were young, and their kidneys are less able to convert vitamin D to its active form

- People with dark skin, because their skin has less ability to produce vitamin D from the sun

- People with disorders such as Crohn disease or celiac disease who don't handle fat properly, because vitamin D needs fat to be absorbed

- Obese people, because their body fat binds to some vitamin D and prevents it from getting into the blood

What Happens If I Don't Get Enough Vitamin D

People can become deficient in vitamin D because they don't consume enough or absorb enough from food, their exposure to sunlight is limited, or their kidneys cannot convert vitamin D to its active form in the body. In children, vitamin D deficiency causes rickets, a condition in which the bones become soft and bend. It's a rare disease but still occurs, especially among African American infants and children. In adults, vitamin D deficiency leads to osteomalacia, causing bone pain and muscle weakness.

What Are Some Effects of Vitamin D on Health?

Vitamin D is being studied for its possible connections to several diseases and medical problems, including diabetes, hypertension, and autoimmune conditions such as multiple sclerosis. Two of them discussed below are bone disorders and some types of cancer.

Bone Disorders

As they get older, millions of people (mostly women, but men too) develop, or are at risk of, osteoporosis, condition in which bones become fragile and may fracture if one falls. It is one consequence of not getting enough calcium and vitamin D over the longterm. Supplements of both vitamin D3 (at 700 to 800 IU/day) and calcium (500 to 1,200 mg/day) have been shown to reduce the risk of bone loss and fractures in elderly people aged 62 to 85 years. Men and women should talk with their healthcare providers about their needs for vitamin D (and calcium) as part of an overall plan to prevent or treat osteoporosis.

Cancer

Some studies suggest that vitamin D may protect against colon cancer and perhaps even cancers of the prostate and breast. But higher levels of vitamin D in the blood have also been linked to higher rates of pancreatic cancer. At this time, it's too early to say whether low vitamin D status increases cancer risk and whether higher levels protect or even increase risk in some people.

Can Vitamin D Be Harmful?

Yes, when amounts in the blood become too high. Signs of toxicity include nausea, vomiting, poor appetite, constipation, weakness, and weight loss. And by raising blood levels of calcium, too much vitamin D can cause confusion, disorientation, and problems with heart rhythm. Excess vitamin D can also damage the kidneys.

The upper limit for vitamin D is 1,000 to 1,500 IU/day for infants, 2,500 to 3,000 IU/day for children 1 to 8 years, and 4,000 IU/day for children nine years and older, adults, and pregnant and lactating teens and women. Vitamin D toxicity almost always occurs from overuse of supplements. Excessive sun exposure doesn't cause vitamin D poisoning because the body limits the amount of this vitamin it produces.

Are There Any Interactions with Vitamin D That I Should Know About?

Like most dietary supplements, vitamin D may interact or interfere with other medicines or supplements you might be taking. Here are several examples:

- Prednisone and other corticosteroid medicines to reduce inflammation impair how the body handles vitamin D, which leads to lower calcium absorption and loss of bone over time

- Both the weight-loss drug orlistat (brand names Xenical® and Alli®) and the cholesterol-lowering drug cholestyramine (brand names Questran®, LoCholest®, and Prevalite®) can reduce the absorption of vitamin D and other fat-soluble vitamins (A, E, and K)

- Both phenobarbital and phenytoin (brand name Dilantin®), used to prevent and control epileptic seizures, increase the breakdown of vitamin D and reduce calcium absorption

Tell your doctor, pharmacist, and other healthcare providers about any dietary supplements and medicines you take. They can tell you if those dietary supplements might interact or interfere with your prescription or over-the-counter (OTC) medicines, or if the medicines might interfere with how your body absorbs, uses, or breaks down nutrients.

Vitamin D and Healthful Eating

People should get most of their nutrients from food, advises the federal government's *Dietary Guidelines for Americans* (DGA). Foods contain vitamins, minerals, dietary fiber, and other substances that benefit health. In some cases, fortified foods and dietary supplements may provide nutrients that otherwise may be consumed in less-than-recommended amounts.

Chapter 5

Osteoporosis and Arthritis: Two Common but Different Conditions

Osteoporosis

Osteoporosis is a condition in which the bones become less dense and more likely to fracture. In the United States, more than 53 million people either already have osteoporosis or are at high risk due to low bone mass. In osteoporosis, there is a loss of bone tissue that leaves bones less dense and more likely to fracture. It can result in a loss of height, severe back pain, and change in one's posture. Osteoporosis can impair a person's ability to walk and can cause prolonged or permanent disability.

Risk factors for developing osteoporosis include:

- Thinness or small frame

- Family history of the disease

- Being postmenopausal and particularly having had early menopause

---

This chapter includes text excerpted from "Osteoporosis and Arthritis: Two Common but Different Conditions," NIH Osteoporosis and Related Bone Diseases—National Resource Center (NIH ORBD—NRC), May 2016.

- Abnormal absence of menstrual periods (amenorrhea)

- Prolonged use of certain medications, such as those used to treat lupus, asthma, thyroid deficiencies, and seizures

- Low calcium intake

- Lack of physical activity

- Smoking

- Excessive alcohol intake

Osteoporosis is known as a silent disease because it can progress undetected for many years without symptoms until a fracture occurs. Osteoporosis is diagnosed by a bone mineral density test, which is a safe and painless way to detect low bone density.

Although there is no cure for the disease, the U.S. Food and Drug Administration (FDA) has approved several medications to prevent and treat osteoporosis. In addition, a diet rich in calcium and vitamin D, regular weight-bearing exercise, and a healthy lifestyle can prevent or lessen the effects of the disease.

Arthritis

Arthritis is a general term for conditions that affect the joints and surrounding tissues. Joints are places in the body where bones come together, such as the knees, wrists, fingers, toes, and hips. Two common types of arthritis are osteoarthritis and rheumatoid arthritis.

- **Osteoarthritis (OA)** is a painful, degenerative joint disease that often involves the hips, knees, neck, lower back, or small joints of the hands. OA usually develops in joints that are injured by repeated overuse from performing a particular task or playing a favorite sport or from carrying around excess body weight. Eventually this injury or repeated impact thins or wears away the cartilage that cushions the ends of the bones in the joint. As a result, the bones rub together, causing a grating sensation. Joint flexibility is reduced, bony spurs develop, and the joint swells. Usually, the first symptom of OA is pain that worsens following exercise or immobility. Treatment usually includes analgesics, topical creams, or nonsteroidal anti-inflammatory drugs (NSAIDs), appropriate exercises or physical therapy; joint splinting; or joint replacement surgery for seriously damaged larger joints, such as the knee or hip.

- **Rheumatoid arthritis (RA)** is an autoimmune inflammatory disease that usually involves various joints in the fingers, thumbs, wrists, elbows, shoulders, knees, feet, and ankles. An autoimmune disease is one in which the body releases enzymes that attack its own healthy tissues. In rheumatoid arthritis, these enzymes destroy the linings of joints. This causes pain, swelling, stiffness, malformation, and reduced movement and function. People with RA also may have systemic symptoms, such as fatigue, fever, weight loss, eye inflammation, anemia, subcutaneous nodules (bumps under the skin), or pleurisy (a lung inflammation).

Although osteoporosis and osteoarthritis are two very different medical conditions with little in common, the similarity of their names causes great confusion. These conditions develop differently, have different symptoms, are diagnosed differently, and are treated differently.

Osteoporosis and arthritis do share many coping strategies. With either or both of these conditions, many people benefit from exercise programs that may include physical therapy and rehabilitation. In general, exercises that emphasize stretching, strengthening, posture, and range of motion are appropriate. Examples include low-impact aerobics, swimming, tai chi, and low-stress yoga.

However, people with osteoporosis must take care to avoid activities that include bending forward from the waist, twisting the spine, or lifting heavy weights. People with arthritis must compensate for limited movement in affected joints. Always check with your doctor to determine whether a certain exercise or exercise program is safe for your specific medical situation.

Most people with arthritis will use pain management strategies at some time. This is not always true for people with osteoporosis. Usually, people with osteoporosis need pain relief when they are recovering from a fracture. In cases of severe osteoporosis with multiple spine fractures, pain control also may become part of daily life. Regardless of the cause, pain management strategies are similar for people with osteoporosis, OA, and RA.

Chapter 6

The Importance and Impact of Osteoporosis

Osteoporosis, or porous bone (see figure 6.1), is a disease characterized by low bone mass and structural deterioration of bone tissue, leading to bone fragility and an increased risk of fractures of the hip, spine, and wrist. It is often called a "silent" disease because it has no discernable symptoms until there is a bone fracture. Like other tissues in the body, bone tissue is in a state of constant flux—remodeling and rebuilding. There are many influences on bone mass and strength, such as genetics, hormones, physical exercise, and diet (especially intake of calcium, phosphate, vitamin D, and other nutrients). Osteoporosis occurs when there are problems with these factors, resulting in more bone loss than bone rebuilding. Osteoporosis can strike at any age and affects both men and women. In the United States today, more than 40 million people either already have osteoporosis or are at high risk for fractures due to low bone mass.

Yesterday

- Relatively little was known or could be done about osteoporosis; both the disease and the fractures that go along with it were

This chapter includes text excerpted from "Osteoporosis," Research Portfolio Online Reporting Tools (RePORT), National Institutes of Health (NIH), June 30, 2018.

thought of as an inevitable part of old age. Few risk factors other than the menopause had been identified.

- A limited number of effective diagnostic tools were available to assist healthcare providers in identifying and treating individuals at risk for osteoporosis.

- Osteoporosis was viewed solely as a "woman's disease." Men did not recognize the disease as a significant threat to their mobility and independence.

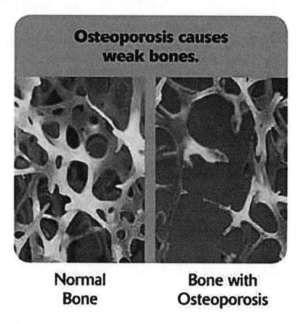

Figure 6.1. *Normal Bone versus Bone with Osteoporosis* (Source: "The Surgeon General's Report on Bone Health and Osteoporosis: What It Means to You," NIH Osteoporosis and Related Bone Diseases—National Resource Center (NIH ORBD—NRC).)

Today

- The devastating consequences of low bone mass—that is, broken bones—can often be prevented. For example, simple changes to a person's home (e.g., adding more lights, removing clutter) can prevent falls. A balanced diet and modest exercise enhance bone strength. And, medications can slow disease progression.

- Enhancing bone health is important at any age. National Institutes of Health (NIH), in partnership with other federal agencies and nongovernmental organizations, are implementing programs to help young people adopt bone-healthy behaviors that will last a lifetime. Furthermore, NIH-supported clinical studies in nutrition and physical activity interventions provide strong evidence that fractures can be prevented and bone loss reduced even in older individuals, providing evidence that osteoporosis does not need to be a natural consequence of aging.

- Identification of risk factors for osteoporosis is providing clinicians with important information about who is at most risk for this debilitating disease and who would benefit from treatment. Major contributions from the Study of Osteoporotic Fractures (SOF), which began over 20 years ago, and its counterpart for men (Mr. OS), revealed that bone mineral density of the hip is one of the best predictors of fracture. These studies, and others, also showed that body weight, diet, physical activity, family history, and medication use are important risk factors.

- Researchers have dispelled the myth that some fractures in older people are "earned" and, therefore, do not necessarily signal osteoporosis. SOF, Mr. OS, and other studies have shown that older people who have a fracture should be tested for osteoporosis—even if the fracture occurred because of a fall.

- Dual-energy X-ray absorptiometry (DXA) has become one of the most commonly used methods of assessing bone mineral density. Mr. OS is generating data that the U.S. Preventive Services Task Force (USPSTF) can incorporate into guidance on using bone mineral density to assess fracture risk. Mr. OS data also will be useful when developing guidelines for diagnosing osteoporosis in men.

- New classes of drugs have been developed that significantly reduce the risk of fractures in individuals with bone disease. Federal support for unique clinical intervention studies of combination therapies for osteoporosis has played an important role in determining the best therapeutic practices associated with these drugs, potentially minimizing drug use and cost.

- These advances—along with other efforts to improve osteoporosis prevention, diagnosis, and treatment—are having a positive effect on bone health. Between 1995 and 2005, the age-adjusted hospitalization rate for hip fractures among older Americans decreased. For women aged 65 years or more, the rate decreased 24.5 percent. For men in the same age range, the rate decreased 19.2 percent.

Tomorrow

- Advances in scientific knowledge have ushered in a new era in bone health, one in which bone fractures can be prevented in the vast majority of individuals, and identified early and treated effectively in those who do get them.

- Although bone mineral density is one of the best measures for assessing osteoporosis and fracture risk, there are some limitations to using bone mineral density as a single predictive measure of fracture risk. Cutting edge imaging, identification of clinical risk factors, as well as biomarker research, will continue to provide insight into the other characteristics of bone that may inform studies of skeletal health.

- Results from additional long-term studies in the elderly, minority populations, and women and men will assist researchers and clinicians in designing and prescribing targeted therapies and prevention strategies based on the individual characteristics of patients.

- Genetics can account for up to 75 percent of a person's bone mineral density. Now, researchers are determining which genes and bone formation pathways are involved in bone remodeling, in hopes that their discoveries will lead to the development of better strategies to treat or prevent osteoporosis.

Chapter 7

Fast Facts on Osteoporosis

What Is Osteoporosis?

Osteoporosis is a disease in which the bones become weak and are more likely to break. People with osteoporosis most often break bones in the hip, spine, and wrist.

Who Gets Osteoporosis

In the United States, millions of people either already have osteoporosis or are at high risk due to low bone mass. Osteoporosis can occur in both men and women and at any age, but it is most common in older women.

What Causes Osteoporosis

Many risk factors can lead to bone loss and osteoporosis. Some of these things you cannot change and others you can.

Risk factors you cannot change include:

- **Gender.** Women get osteoporosis more often than men.

- **Age.** The older you are, the greater your risk of osteoporosis.

- **Body size.** Small, thin women are at greater risk.

This chapter includes text excerpted from "What Is Osteoporosis?" NIH Osteoporosis and Related Bone Diseases—National Resource Center (NIH ORBD—NRC), November 2014. Reviewed January 2019.

- **Ethnicity.** White and Asian women are at highest risk. Black and Hispanic women have a lower risk.

- **Family history.** Osteoporosis tends to run in families. If a family member has osteoporosis or breaks a bone, there is a greater chance that you will too.

Other risk factors are:

- **Sex hormones.** Low estrogen levels due to missing menstrual periods or to menopause can cause osteoporosis in women. Low testosterone levels can bring on osteoporosis in men.

- **Anorexia nervosa.** This eating disorder can lead to osteoporosis.

- **Calcium and vitamin D intake.** A diet low in calcium and vitamin D makes you more prone to bone loss.

- **Medication use.** Some medicines increase the risk of osteoporosis.

- **Activity level.** Lack of exercise or long-term bed rest can cause weak bones.

- **Smoking.** Cigarettes are bad for bones, and the heart, and lungs, too.

- **Drinking alcohol.** Too much alcohol can cause bone loss and broken bones.

Can Osteoporosis Be Prevented?

There are many steps you can take to help keep your bones healthy. To help keep your bones strong and slow down bone loss, you can:

- Eat a diet rich in calcium and vitamin D

- Exercise

- Do not smoke or drink to excess

Nutrition

A healthy diet with enough calcium and vitamin D helps make your bones strong. Many people get less than half the calcium they need. Good sources of calcium are:

- Low-fat milk, yogurt, and cheese

- Foods with added calcium such as orange juice, cereals, and breads

Vitamin D is also needed for strong bones. Some people may need to take vitamin D pills. The chart on this page shows the amount of calcium and vitamin D you should get each day.

Table 7.1. Recommended Calcium and Vitamin D Intakes

Life-Stage Group	Calcium (mg/day)	Vitamin D (IU/day)
Infants 0 to 6 months	200	400
Infants 6 to 12 months	260	400
1 to 3 years old	700	600
4 to 8 years old	1000	600
9 to 13 years old	1300	600
14 to 18 years old	1300	600
19 to 30 years old	1000	600
31 to 50 years old	1000	600
51- to 70-year-old males	1000	600
51- to 70-year-old females	1200	600
>70 years old	1200	800
14 to 18 years old, pregnant/lactating	1300	600
19 to 50 years old, pregnant/lactating	1000	600

Definitions: mg = milligrams; IU = International Units
(Source: Food and Nutrition Board (FNB), Institute of Medicine (IOM), National Academy of Sciences (NAS), 2010.)

Exercise

Exercise helps your bones grow stronger. To increase bone strength, you can:

- Walk
- Hike
- Jog
- Climb stairs
- Lift weights

- Play tennis
- Dance

Healthy Lifestyle

Smoking is bad for bones as well as the heart and lungs. Also, people who drink a lot of alcohol are more prone to bone loss and broken bones due to poor diet and risk of falling.

What Are the Symptoms of Osteoporosis?

Osteoporosis is called the "silent disease" because bone is lost with no signs. You may not know that you have osteoporosis until a strain, bump, or fall causes a bone to break.

How Is Osteoporosis Diagnosed?

A bone mineral density test is the best way to check your bone health. This test can:

- Diagnose osteoporosis and tell you whether you are likely to break a bone
- Check bone strength
- See if treatments are making the bones stronger

How Is Osteoporosis Treated?

Treatment for osteoporosis includes:

- A balanced diet rich in calcium and vitamin D
- An exercise plan
- A healthy lifestyle
- Medications, if needed

How Can I Prevent Falls?

Men and women with osteoporosis need to take care not to fall down. Falls can break bones. Some reasons people fall are:

- Poor vision
- Poor balance

- Certain diseases that affect how you walk
- Some types of medicine, such as sleeping pills

Some tips to help prevent falls outdoors are:

- Use a cane or walker
- Wear rubber-soled shoes so you don't slip
- Walk on grass when sidewalks are slippery
- In winter, put salt or kitty litter on icy sidewalks

Some ways to help prevent falls indoors are:

- Keep rooms free of clutter, especially on floors.
- Use plastic or carpet runners on slippery floors.
- Wear low-heeled shoes that provide good support.
- Do not walk in socks, stockings, or slippers.
- Be sure carpets and area rugs have skid-proof backs or are tacked to the floor.
- Be sure stairs are well lit and have rails on both sides.
- Put grab bars on bathroom walls near tub, shower, and toilet.
- Use a rubber bath mat in the shower or tub.
- Keep a flashlight next to your bed.
- Use a sturdy step stool with a handrail and wide steps.
- Add more lights in rooms.
- Buy a cordless phone to keep with you so that you don't have to rush to the phone when it rings and so that you can call for help if you fall.

Chapter 8

Osteoporosis and Related Skeletal Challenges in the Elderly

Key Findings

Data from the National Health and Nutrition Examination Survey (NHANES), 2005–2008:

- Nine percent of adults aged 50 years and over had osteoporosis, as defined by the World Health Organization (WHO), at either the femur neck or lumbar spine. About one-half had low bone mass at either site, while 48 percent had normal bone mass at both sites.

- Estimates of poor skeletal status at the femur neck or lumbar spine, when considered alone, were not the same as estimates based on the two skeletal sites together because some individuals had the condition at one site but not the other.

- The prevalence of osteoporosis or low bone mass at either the femur neck or lumbar spine differed by age, sex, and race and ethnicity. The prevalence was higher in women and increased

This chapter includes text excerpted from "Osteoporosis or Low Bone Mass at the Femur Neck or Lumbar Spine in Older Adults: United States, 2005–2008," Centers for Disease Control and Prevention (CDC), November 6, 2015. Reviewed January 2019.

with age. Differences between racial and ethnic groups varied by sex and skeletal status category.

Many clinical guidelines recommend that assessment of osteoporosis or low bone mass, as defined by the WHO, be based on bone mineral density at either the femur neck region of the proximal femur (hip) or the lumbar spine. This data brief presents the national data on osteoporosis or low bone mass at either the femur neck or lumbar spine among older adults in the United States population based on these WHO categories. Results are presented by age, sex, and race and ethnicity.

In 2005–2008, What Was the Skeletal Status of the Noninstitutionalized U.S. Population Aged 50 Years and over Based on Bone Mineral Density at Either the Femur Neck or Lumbar Spine?

Nine percent of persons aged 50 years and over had osteoporosis at either the femur neck or lumbar spine in 2005–2008 (Figure 8.1). Roughly one-half of older adults in the population had low bone mass at either the femur neck or lumbar spine. Forty-eight percent of older adults in the United States had normal bone density at both the femur neck and lumbar spine.

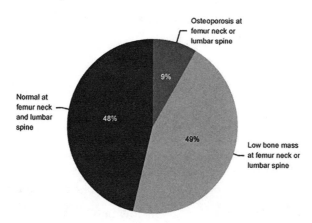

Figure 8.1. *Skeletal Status of Persons Aged 50 Years and Over: United States, 2005–2008.* (Source: Centers for Disease Control and Prevention (CDC)/National Center for Health Statistics (NCHS), National Health and Nutrition Examination Survey (NHANES), 2005–2008.)

The percentages shown will not add up to 100% due to double counting among those with osteoporosis at either skeletal site or low bone mass at either skeletal site.

What Is the Prevalence of Osteoporosis or Low Bone Mass at the Femur Neck or the Lumbar Spine When Considered Separately?

The prevalence of osteoporosis at the femur neck is 5 percent and the prevalence of osteoporosis at the lumbar spine is 6 percent. The prevalence estimates of low bone mass at the femur neck or lumbar spine when considered separately are 39 percent and 27 percent, respectively. These prevalence estimates are not the same as the prevalence of osteoporosis or low bone mass at either the femur neck or lumbar spine when considered together. This occurs because the prevalence of osteoporosis or low bone mass at either the femur neck or lumbar spine includes some individuals who have the condition at one of the two skeletal sites but not the other.

In specific, the prevalence of osteoporosis at either the femur neck or lumbar spine is 9 percent, which consists of 4 percent with osteoporosis at the lumbar spine only, 3 percent with osteoporosis at the femur neck only, and 2 percent with osteoporosis at both the lumbar spine and femur neck. The prevalence of low bone mass at either skeletal site is 49 percent, which consists of 10 percent with low bone mass at the lumbar spine, 22 percent with low bone mass at the femur neck, and 17 percent with low bone mass at both the lumbar spine and femur neck.

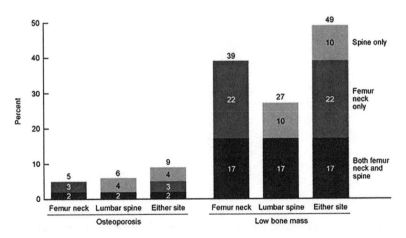

Figure 8.2. *Osteoporosis or Low Bone Mass at the Femur Neck Only, Lumbar Spine Only, or Either Site in Adults Aged 50 Years and Over.* (Source: Centers for Disease Control and Prevention (CDC)/National Center for Health Statistics (NCHS), National Health and Nutrition Examination Survey (NHANES), 2005–2008.)

What Is the Prevalence of Osteoporosis or Low Bone Mass at Either the Femur Neck or Lumbar Spine by Age?

The prevalence of osteoporosis at either skeletal site by age ranged from 3 to 10 percent in men and 7 to 35 percent in women. In men, the prevalence of osteoporosis did not increase with age until aged 80 years and over, but in women, it increased for each decade after age 50 years. The prevalence of low bone mass at either skeletal site by age ranged from 32 to 60 percent in men and 54 to 67 percent in women. In men, the prevalence of low bone mass did not increase with age until aged 70 years, after which it increased progressively. In women, the prevalence of low bone mass increased until age 70 years, after which it remained stable.

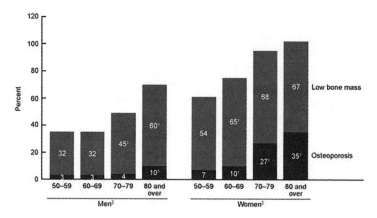

Figure 8.3. *Osteoporosis or Low Bone Mass at the Femur Neck or Lumbar Spine, by Age in Adults Aged 50 Years and Over.* (Source: Centers for Disease Control and Prevention (CDC)/National Center for Health Statistics (NCHS), National Health and Nutrition Examination Survey (NHANES), 2005–2008.)

[1] *p < 0.05 compared with preceding age group within sex and skeletal status category.*
[2] *p < 0.05 for trend by age group within sex for both osteoporosis and low bone mass.*

Does the Prevalence of Osteoporosis or Low Bone Mass at Either the Femur Neck or Lumbar Spine Differ by Sex?

The prevalence of osteoporosis or low bone mass at either the femur neck or lumbar spine is higher in women than men in each decade or when compared overall for aged 50 years and over after adjusting for age differences between the two sexes. The age-adjusted prevalence of osteoporosis at either skeletal site was 16 percent in women compared with 4 percent in men. The age-adjusted prevalence of low bone mass at either skeletal site was 61 percent in women compared with 38 percent in men.

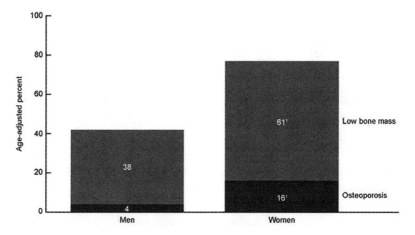

Figure 8.4. *Osteoporosis or Low Bone Mass at the Femur Neck or Lumbar Spine, by Sex in Adults Aged 50 Years or Over.* (Source: Centers for Disease Control and Prevention (CDC)/National Center for Health Statistics (NCHS), National Health and Nutrition Examination Survey (NHANES), 2005–2008.)

[1]p < 0.05 compared with men within skeletal status category.

Does the Prevalence of Osteoporosis or Low Bone Mass at the Femur Neck or Lumbar Spine Differ by Race and Ethnicity in Men?

The prevalence of osteoporosis or low bone mass at either skeletal site differ by race and ethnicity in men after adjusting for age differences between the racial and ethnic groups. The age-adjusted prevalence of osteoporosis at either skeletal site in men of other races (9%) was higher than the prevalence in non-Hispanic white men (4%). The age-adjusted prevalence of low bone mass at either skeletal site was lower in non-Hispanic black men (24%) compared with non-Hispanic white men (39%).

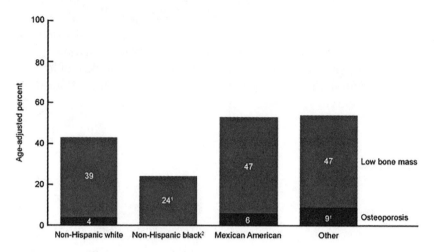

Figure 8.5. *Osteoporosis or Low Bone Mass at the Femur Neck or Lumbar Spine, by Race and Ethnicity in Men Aged 50 Years and Over.* (Source: Centers for Disease Control and Prevention (CDC)/National Center for Health Statistics (NCHS), National Health and Nutrition Examination Survey (NHANES), 2005–2008.)

[1]*p < 0.05 compared with non-Hispanic white men within skeletal status category.*
[2]*Prevalence of osteoporosis in non-Hispanic black men not shown because the standard error divided by the percentage exceeded 40 percent.*

Does the Prevalence of Osteoporosis or Low Bone Mass at the Femur Neck or Lumbar Spine Differ by Race and Ethnicity in Women?

The prevalence of osteoporosis or low bone mass at either the femur neck or lumbar spine differ by race and ethnicity in women after adjusting for age differences between the racial and ethnic groups. When compared with the age-adjusted prevalence of osteoporosis in non-Hispanic white women (15%), the age-adjusted prevalence of osteoporosis at either skeletal site is higher in Mexican American women (26%) and lower in non-Hispanic black women (9%). When compared with the age-adjusted prevalence in non-Hispanic white women (62%), the age-adjusted prevalence of low bone mass at either skeletal site is higher in women of other races (72%) and lower in non-Hispanic black women (44%).

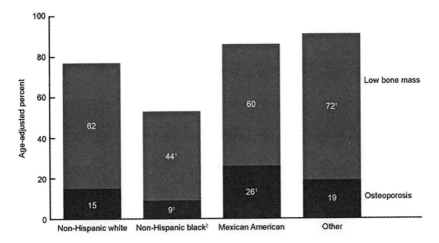

Figure 8.6. *Osteoporosis or Low Bone Mass at the Femur Neck or Lumbar Spine, by Race and Ethnicity in Women Aged 50 Years and Over.* (Source: Centers for Disease Control and Prevention (CDC)/National Center for Health Statistics (NCHS), National Health and Nutrition Examination Survey (NHANES), 2005–2008.)

[1]*p < 0.05 compared with non-Hispanic white women within skeletal status category.*

Part Two

Osteoporosis in Women, Children, Men, and Older Adults

Chapter 9

Osteoporosis in Women

Chapter Contents

Section 9.1

Bone Health in Girls/Young Women

This section includes text excerpted from "Eating for
Strong Bones," girlshealth.gov, Office on Women's
Health (OWH), September 13, 2018.

Why Should Girls Think about Bone Health?

Girls build most of their bone mass during their childhood and teen
years. (Bone mass is the amount of strength inside your bones.) If you
do not build strong bones now, you face a greater risk of osteoporosis
later in life. Osteoporosis is a disease that weakens bones to the point
where they break easily. More than half of women over age 65 have
osteoporosis. Although it doesn't usually happen, you also can get
osteoporosis when you're young.

What Nutrients Do Girls Need to Protect Their Bones?

To build bones and keep them strong, your body needs calcium and
vitamin D.

- Calcium helps bones develop properly and grow strong. Calcium
  is also needed for many other activities in your body. If your
  body doesn't get enough calcium from foods and drinks, it takes
  the calcium from bones, which can weaken your bones.

- Your body needs vitamin D to help it use calcium.

How Much Calcium and Vitamin D Do Girls Need?

It is very important that girls age 9 to 18 get 1,300 milligrams of
calcium and 600 International Units (15 micrograms) of vitamin D
per day.

How Can Girls Get Calcium and Vitamin D?

Calcium is in foods such as milk and other dairy products, leafy
green vegetables, cereals fortified with calcium, and almonds.

Vitamin D is in milk and some other foods, such as certain breakfast
cereals, salmon, and tuna. You can read the Nutrition Facts labels on
packages to see how much calcium and vitamin D foods have.

Can Girls Who Don't Drink Milk Get Enough Calcium and Vitamin D?

Some girls don't drink milk because they have lactose intolerance or a milk allergy, which means they can get stomach aches and other problems from dairy products. Some girls are vegans, which means they don't eat any animal products, including dairy.

If you have lactose intolerance, look for milk and other dairy products that are labeled "lactose-free" or "lactose-reduced." You can also talk to your doctor about pills or drops that make it easier to digest dairy.

If you don't eat dairy, it is harder to get enough calcium. Try to eat more foods with calcium, like calcium-fortified cereals. If you can't get enough calcium from food, ask your doctor if a calcium supplement is right for you.

You can get vitamin D from foods other than dairy products, but it can be very hard to get enough. Some foods, like cereal, have vitamin D added, so read package labels. If you don't eat or drink any dairy products, you may need to take a vitamin D supplement pill.

Are Dairy Products Fattening?

If you are concerned about your weight, try low-fat and fat-free dairy products. These have the same amount of calcium and fewer calories than regular dairy products.

How Does Physical Activity Help Build Bones?

Physical activity causes new bone to form. All girls should do bone-strengthening activities, such as walking, running, or jumping rope. If exercising outdoors is a problem for you, try climbing stairs, dancing, or marching in place while watching TV.

What Kinds of Activities Can Girls with Physical Disabilities Do to Keep Their Bones Strong?

Here are some examples of bone-strengthening exercises for girls in wheelchairs.

- Wheelchair aerobics focused on upper-body movements
- Arm cycling, which is a bicycling motion using one's arms
- Wheeling a wheelchair forward, using the arms or legs, over an extended distance

- Resistance training using wide elastic bands

- Sports that are adapted for girls with physical disabilities, such as wheelchair tennis

What Else Can Girls Do to Promote Their Bone Health?

It is important for girls to not drink alcohol or smoke. Those behaviors can hurt bone health (and overall health, of course).

It is also important to have a healthy diet with enough nutrients, including calcium and vitamin D. That's why girls with eating disorders face an extra risk of developing weaker bones.

Also, try not to drink a lot of colas and other sodas. Studies suggest that teen girls who drink a lot of soda, especially colas, have more bone problems. This may be because they are choosing sodas instead of milk, so they aren't getting all the calcium they need to build strong bones.

Try not to eat a lot of sodium. Too much sodium can make your body lose calcium. It can lead to other health problems too, such as high blood pressure.

Section 9.2

Osteoporosis and African American Women

This section includes text excerpted from "Osteoporosis and African American Women," NIH Osteoporosis and Related Bone Diseases—National Resource Center (NIH ORBD—NRC), June 2015. Reviewed January 2019.

Although African American women tend to have higher bone mineral density (BMD) than white women throughout life, they are still at significant risk of developing osteoporosis. The misperception that osteoporosis is only a concern for white women can delay prevention and treatment in African American women who do not believe they are at risk for the disease.

What Is Osteoporosis?

Osteoporosis is a metabolic bone disease characterized by low bone mass, which makes bones fragile and susceptible to fracture. Osteoporosis is known as a silent disease because symptoms and pain do not appear until a fracture occurs. Without prevention or treatment, osteoporosis can progress painlessly until a bone breaks, typically in the hip, spine, or wrist. A hip fracture can limit mobility and lead to a loss of independence, and vertebral fractures can result in a loss of height, stooped posture, and chronic pain.

What Are the Risk Factors for Osteoporosis?

Risk factors for developing osteoporosis include:

- A thin, small-boned frame

- Previous fracture or family history of osteoporotic fracture

- Estrogen deficiency resulting from early menopause (before age 45), either naturally, from surgical removal of the ovaries, or as a result of prolonged amenorrhea (abnormal absence of menstruation) in younger women

- Advanced age

- A diet low in calcium

- White and Asian ancestry (African American and Hispanic women are at lower but significant risk)

- Cigarette smoking

- Excessive use of alcohol

- Prolonged use of certain medications, such as those used to treat lupus, asthma, thyroid deficiencies, and seizures

Are There Special Issues for African American Women Regarding Bone Health?

Many scientific studies highlight the risk that African American women face with regard to developing osteoporosis and fracture.

- Many African American women are at increased risk for osteoporosis because they consume less calcium than the Recommended Dietary Allowance.

- African Americans are more prone to lactose intolerance than are other groups. Lactose intolerance can hinder optimal calcium intake. People with lactose intolerance often may avoid milk and other dairy products that are excellent sources of calcium because they have trouble digesting lactose, the primary sugar in milk.

How Can Osteoporosis Be Prevented?

Osteoporosis prevention begins in childhood. The recommendations listed below should be followed throughout life to lower your risk of osteoporosis.

- Eat a well-balanced diet adequate in calcium and vitamin D.

- Exercise regularly, with an emphasis on weight-bearing activities such as walking, jogging, dancing, and weight training.

- Live a healthy lifestyle. Avoid smoking and, if you drink alcohol, do so in moderation.

Talk to your doctor if you have a family history of osteoporosis or other risk factors that may put you at increased risk for the disease. Your doctor may suggest that you have your bone density measured to determine your risk for fractures (broken bones) and measure your response to osteoporosis treatment. The most widely recognized bone mineral density test is called a dual-energy X-ray absorptiometry, or DXA test. It is safe and painless, a bit like having an X-ray, but with much less exposure to radiation. This test can measure bone density at your hip and spine.

What Treatments Are Available

Although there is no cure for osteoporosis, several medications are available for the prevention and/or treatment of the disease, including: bisphosphonates; estrogen agonists/antagonists (also called selective estrogen receptor modulators or SERMS); calcitonin; parathyroid hormone; estrogen therapy; hormone therapy; and a recently approved receptor activator of nuclear factor kappa-β ligand (RANKL) inhibitor.

Section 9.3

Osteoporosis and Asian American Women

This section includes text excerpted from "Osteoporosis
and Asian American Women," NIH Osteoporosis and Related
Bone Diseases—National Resource Center (NIH ORBD—NRC),
June 2015. Reviewed January 2019.

Asian American women are at high risk for developing osteoporosis
(porous bones), a disease that is preventable and treatable. Studies
show that Asian Americans share many of the risk factors that apply
to white women. As an Asian American woman, it is important that
you understand what osteoporosis is and what steps you can take to
prevent or treat it.

What Is Osteoporosis?

Osteoporosis is a condition in which the bones become less dense
and more likely to fracture. If not prevented or if left untreated, bone
loss can progress painlessly until a bone breaks, typically in the hip,
spine, or wrist. A hip fracture can limit mobility and lead to a loss of
independence, and vertebral fractures can result in a loss of height,
stooped posture, and chronic pain.

What Are the Risk Factors for Osteoporosis?

Several risk factors increase your chances of developing osteoporosis, including:

- A thin, small-boned frame

- Previous fracture or family history of osteoporotic fracture

- Estrogen deficiency resulting from early menopause (before
  age 45), either naturally, from surgical removal of the ovaries,
  or as a result of prolonged amenorrhea (abnormal absence of
  menstruation) in younger women

- Advanced age

- A diet low in calcium

- White and Asian ancestry (African American and Hispanic
  women are at lower but significant risk)

- Cigarette smoking

- Excessive use of alcohol

- Prolonged use of certain medications

Are There Any Special Issues for Asian Women Regarding Bone Health?

Some studies indicate a number of facts that highlight the risk that Asian American women face with regard to developing osteoporosis:

- Compared with white women, Asian women have been found to consume less calcium. One reason for this may be that Asian Americans are more prone to lactose intolerance than are other groups. Therefore, they may avoid dairy products, the primary source of calcium in the diet. Calcium is essential for building and maintaining a healthy skeleton.

- Asian women generally have lower hip fracture rates than white women, although the prevalence of vertebral fractures among Asians seems to be as high as that in whites.

- Slender women have less bone mass than heavy or obese women and, therefore, are at greater risk for osteoporotic bone fractures.

How Can Osteoporosis Be Prevented?

Building strong bones, especially before the age of 20, can be the best defense against developing osteoporosis. A healthy lifestyle can be critically important for keeping bones strong. To help prevent osteoporosis:

- Eat a well-balanced diet rich in calcium and vitamin D.

- Exercise regularly, with an emphasis on weight-bearing activities such as walking, jogging, dancing, and weight training.

- Don't smoke, and limit alcohol intake.

Talk to your doctor if you have a family history of osteoporosis or other factors that may put you at increased risk for the disease. Your doctor may suggest that you have your bone density measured through a safe test that can determine your risk for fractures (broken bones) and measure your response to osteoporosis treatment. The most widely recognized bone mineral density (BMD) test is called a dual-energy X-ray absorptiometry, or DXA test. The BMD test is painless, a bit like having an X-ray, but with much less exposure to radiation. It can measure bone density at your hip and spine.

What Treatments Are Available

Although there is no cure for osteoporosis, several medications are available for the prevention and/or treatment of osteoporosis, including: bisphosphonates; estrogen agonists/antagonists (also called selective estrogen receptor modulators or SERMS); calcitonin; parathyroid hormone; estrogen therapy; hormone therapy; and a recently approved receptor activator of nuclear factor kappa-β ligand (RANKL) inhibitor.

Section 9.4

Osteoporosis and Hispanic Women

This section includes text excerpted from "Osteoporosis and Hispanic Women," NIH Osteoporosis and Related Bone Diseases—National Resource Center (NIH ORBD—NRC), June 2015. Reviewed January 2019.

It is a common misconception that osteoporosis only affects white women. But, according to the *Surgeon General's Report on Bone Health and Osteoporosis*, in the United States, the prevalence of osteoporosis in Hispanic women is similar to that in white women. Fortunately, osteoporosis is preventable and treatable. As a Hispanic woman, it is important that you understand your risk for osteoporosis, the steps you can take to protect your bones, and, if you have the disease, the options for treating it.

What Is Osteoporosis?

Osteoporosis is a condition in which the bones become less dense and more likely to fracture. If not prevented or if left untreated, bone loss can progress painlessly until a bone breaks, typically in the hip, spine, or wrist. A hip fracture can limit mobility and lead to a loss of independence, and vertebral fractures can result in a loss of height, stooped posture, and chronic pain.

What Are the Risk Factors for Osteoporosis?

Several risk factors increase your chances of developing osteoporosis, including:

- A thin, small-boned frame

- Previous fracture or family history of osteoporotic fracture

- Estrogen deficiency resulting from early menopause (before age 45), either naturally, from surgical removal of the ovaries, or as a result of prolonged amenorrhea (abnormal absence of menstruation) in younger women

- Advanced age

- A diet low in calcium

- White and Asian ancestry (African American and Hispanic women are at lower but significant risk)

- Cigarette smoking

- Excessive use of alcohol

- Prolonged use of certain medications, such as those used to treat lupus, asthma, thyroid deficiencies, and seizures.

Are There Any Special Issues for Hispanic Women Regarding Bone Health?

Several studies indicate a number of facts that highlight the risk that Hispanic women face with regard to developing osteoporosis:

- Hispanics are more prone to lactose intolerance than are other groups.

- Studies have shown that Hispanic women consume less calcium than the Recommended Dietary Allowance in all age groups.

- Hispanic women are more likely than white women to develop diabetes, which may increase their risk for osteoporosis.

How Can Osteoporosis Be Prevented?

Osteoporosis prevention begins in childhood. Building strong bones, especially before the age of 20, can be the best defense against developing bone loss. A healthy lifestyle can be critically important for keeping bones strong. The recommendations listed below should be followed throughout life to help lower your risk of osteoporosis.

- Eat a well-balanced diet rich in calcium and vitamin D.

- Exercise regularly, with an emphasis on weight-bearing activities such as walking, jogging, dancing, and weight training.

- Don't smoke, and, if you drink alcohol, do so in moderation.

Talk to your doctor if you have a family history of osteoporosis or other factors that may put you at increased risk for the disease. Your doctor may suggest that you have your bone density measured through a safe and painless test that can determine your risk for fractures (broken bones), and measure your response to osteoporosis treatment. The most widely recognized bone mineral density (BMD) test is called a dual-energy X-ray absorptiometry, or DXA test. The BMD test is painless—a bit like having an X-ray, but with much less exposure to radiation. It can measure bone density at your hip and spine.

What Treatments Are Available

Although there is no cure for osteoporosis, several medications are available for the prevention and/or treatment of osteoporosis, including: bisphosphonates; estrogen agonists/antagonists (also called selective estrogen receptor modulators or SERMS); calcitonin; parathyroid hormone; estrogen therapy; hormone therapy; and a recently approved receptor activator of nuclear factor kappa-β ligand (RANKL) inhibitor.

Section 9.5

How Often Should Women Have Bone Tests?

This section includes text excerpted from "How Often Should Women Have Bone Tests?" National Institutes of Health (NIH), January 30, 2012. Reviewed January 2019.

Experts recommend that older women have regular bone density tests to screen for osteoporosis. But it's been unclear how often to repeat the tests. A study of nearly 5,000 women now reports that patients with healthy bone density on their first test might safely wait 15 years before getting rescreened.

Osteoporosis is a disorder marked by weakened bones and an increased risk of fractures. More than 40 million people nationwide either have osteoporosis or are at increased risk for broken bones because of low bone mineral density (osteopenia).

Osteoporosis is often called a "silent disease" because it usually progresses slowly and without symptoms until a fracture occurs. When low bone density is identified early through screening, lifestyle changes and therapies can help protect bone health and reduce the risk of fractures. That's why the U.S. Preventive Services Task Force (USPSTF) recommends routine screening of bone mineral density for women ages 65 and older.

To help doctors decide how often to repeat bone density tests in women who don't have osteoporosis at their initial screening, a research team led by Dr. Margaret Gourlay of the University of North Carolina (UNC) at Chapel Hill analyzed data on nearly 5,000 women, age 67 or older. The women were participants in the Study of Osteoporotic Fractures, a long-term nationwide study supported by National Institutes of Health's (NIH) National Institute of Arthritis and Musculoskeletal and Skin Diseases (NIAMS), National Institute on Aging (NIA) and National Center for Research Resources (NCRR).

Researchers divided the women divided into 4 groups based on initial bone density tests that were either normal or showed mild, moderate or advanced osteopenia. They were given 2 to 5 bone density tests at varying intervals during the 15-year study period.

As reported in the January 19, 2012, issue of the *New England Journal of Medicine (NEJM)*, the scientists found that less than 1 percent of women who initially had normal bone mineral density went on to develop osteoporosis during the study. Only 5 percent of those with mildly low bone density at the start made the transition to osteoporosis. Overall, the data suggest that women in these 2 categories might safely wait about 15 years before being rescreened for osteoporosis.

The scientists also found that about 1 in 10 women with moderate osteopenia at baseline developed osteoporosis within 5 years. For those with advanced osteopenia at the start, about 10 percent had developed osteoporosis within a year, suggesting that 1-year screening intervals might be advisable for this group.

"If a woman's bone density at age 67 is very good, then she doesn't need to be rescreened in 2 years or 3 years, because we're not likely to see much change," Gourlay says. "Our study found it would take about

15 years for 10 percent of women in the highest bone density ranges to develop osteoporosis. That was longer than we expected, and it's great news for this group of women."

These findings can help guide doctors in their bone screening recommendations. Other risk factors, such age, medications or specific diseases, would also influence screening frequency.

Chapter 10

Osteoporosis in Children and Young Adults

Chapter Contents

Section 10.1

Kids and Their Bones

This section includes text excerpted from "Kids and Their
Bones: A Guide for Parents," NIH Osteoporosis and Related Bone
Diseases—National Resource Center (NIH ORBD—NRC),
March 2015. Reviewed January 2019.

Typically, when parents think about their children's health, they
don't think about their bones. But building healthy bones by adopting
healthy nutritional and lifestyle habits in childhood is important to
help prevent osteoporosis and fractures later in life.

Osteoporosis, the disease that causes bones to become less dense
and more prone to fractures, has been called "a pediatric disease with
geriatric consequences," because the bone mass attained in childhood
and adolescence is an important determinant of lifelong skeletal
health. The health habits your kids are forming now can make, or
literally break, their bones as they age.

Why Is Childhood Such an Important Time for Bone Development?

Bones are the framework for your child's growing body. Bone is living tissue that changes constantly, with bits of old bone being removed
and replaced by new bone. You can think of bone as a bank account,
where (with your help) your kids make "deposits" and "withdrawals"
of bone tissue. During childhood and adolescence, much more bone
is deposited than withdrawn as the skeleton grows in both size and
density.

For most people, the amount of bone tissue in the skeleton (known
as bone mass) peaks by their late twenties. At that point, bones have
reached their maximum strength and density. Up to 90 percent of peak
bone mass is acquired by age 18 in girls and age 20 in boys, which
makes youth the best time for your kids to "invest" in their bone health.

What Is Osteoporosis? Isn't It Something Old People Get?

Osteoporosis is a disease that causes bones to become fragile and
break easily. When someone has osteoporosis, it means her or his
"bank account" of bone tissue has dropped to a low level. If there is

significant bone loss, even sneezing or bending over to tie a shoe can cause a bone in the spine to break. Hips, ribs, and wrist bones also break easily. The fractures from osteoporosis can be painful and disfiguring. There is no cure for the disease.

Osteoporosis is most common in older people but can also occur in young and middle-aged adults. Optimizing peak bone mass and developing lifelong healthy bone behaviors during youth are important ways to help prevent or minimize osteoporosis risk as an adult.

Factors Affecting Peak Bone Mass

Peak bone mass is influenced by a variety of factors: some that you can't change, like gender and race, and some that you can, like nutrition and physical activity.

Gender: Bone mass or density is generally higher in men than in women. Before puberty, boys and girls develop bone mass at similar rates. After puberty, however, boys tend to acquire greater bone mass than girls.

Race: For reasons still not well understood, African American girls tend to achieve higher peak bone mass than white girls, and African American women are at lower risk for osteoporosis later in life. More research is needed to understand the differences in bone density between the various racial and ethnic groups. However, because all women, regardless of race, are at significant risk for osteoporosis, girls of all races need to build as much bone as possible to protect them against this disease.

Hormonal factors: Sex hormones, including estrogen and testosterone, are essential for the development of bone mass. Girls who start to menstruate at an early age typically have greater bone density. Those who frequently miss their menstrual periods sometimes have lower bone density.

Nutritional status: Calcium is an essential nutrient for bone health. A well-balanced diet including adequate amounts of vitamins and minerals such as magnesium, zinc, and vitamin D is also important.

Physical activity: Physical activity is important for building healthy bones, and provides benefits that are most pronounced in the areas of the skeleton that bear the most weight. These areas include the hips during walking and running and the arms during gymnastics and weightlifting.

How Can I Help Keep My Kids' Bones Healthy?

The same healthy habits that keep your kids going and growing will also benefit their bones. One of the best ways to encourage healthy habits in your children is to be a good role model yourself. Believe it or not, your kids are watching, and your habits, both good and bad, have a strong influence on theirs.

The two most important lifelong bone health habits to encourage now are proper nutrition and plenty of physical activity.

Eating for healthy bones means getting plenty of foods that are rich in calcium and vitamin D. Most kids do not get enough calcium in their diets to help ensure optimal peak bone mass. Are your kids getting enough calcium?

Table 10.1. Recommended Calcium Intakes

Age	Amount of Calcium (Milligrams)
Infants	
Birth to 6 months	200
6 months to 1 year	260
Children/Young Adults	
1 to 3 years	700
4 to 8 years	1,000
9 to 18 years	1,300
Adult Women and Men	
19 to 50 years old	1,000
51 to 70 years males	1,000
51 to 70 years females	1,200
70+ years	1,200
Pregnant or Lactating Women	
14 to 18 years	1,300
19 to 50 years	1,000

(Source: Food and Nutrition Board (FNB), Institute of Medicine (IOM), National Academy of Sciences (NAS), 2010.)

Calcium is found in many foods, but the most common source is milk and other dairy products. Drinking one 8-oz glass of milk provides

300 milligrams (mg) of calcium, which is about one-third of the recommended intake for younger children and about one-fourth of the recommended intake for teens. In addition, milk supplies other minerals and vitamins needed by the body. The chart on the next page lists the calcium content for several high-calcium foods and beverages. Your kids need several servings of these foods each day to meet their need for calcium.

How Can I Persuade My Daughter to Drink Milk Instead of Diet Soda? She Thinks Milk Will Make Her Fat.

Soft drinks tend to displace calcium-rich beverages in the diets of many children and adolescents. In fact, research has shown that girls who drink soft drinks consume much less calcium than those who do not.

It's important for your daughter to know that good sources of calcium don't have to be fattening. Skim milk, low-fat cheeses and yogurt, calcium-fortified juices and cereals, and green leafy vegetables can all fit easily into a healthy, low-fat diet. Replacing even one soda each day with milk or a milk-based fruit smoothie can significantly increase her calcium intake.

Table 10.2. Selected Food Sources of Calcium

Food	Calcium (mg)	Daily Value (%)
Sardines, canned in oil, with bones, 3 oz.	324	32
Cheddar cheese, 1½ oz., shredded	306	31
Milk, nonfat, 8 fluid oz.	302	30
Yogurt, plain, low fat, 8 oz.	300	30
Milk, reduced fat (2% milk fat), no solids, 8 fluid oz.	297	30
Milk, whole (3.25% milk fat), 8 fluid oz.	291	29
Milk, buttermilk, 8 fluid oz.	285	29
Milk, lactose reduced, 8 fluid oz. (content varies slightly according to fat content; average = 300 mg)	285 to 302	29 to 30
Cottage cheese, 1% milk fat, 2 cups unpacked	276	28
Mozzarella, part skim, 1½ oz.	275	28

Table 10.2. Continued

Food	Calcium (mg)	Daily Value (%)
Tofu, firm, with calcium, ½ cup*	204	20
Orange juice, calcium-fortified, 6 fluid oz.	200 to 260	20 to 26
Salmon, pink, canned, solids with bone, 3 oz.	181	18
Pudding, chocolate, instant, made with 2% milk, ½ cup	153	15
Tofu, soft, with calcium, ½ cup*	138	14
Breakfast drink, orange flavor, powder prepared with water, 8 fluid oz.	133	13
Frozen yogurt, vanilla, soft serve, ½ cup	103	10
Ready to eat cereal, calcium-fortified, 1 cup	100 to 1000	10 to 100
Turnip greens, boiled, ½ cup	99	10
Kale, raw, 1 cup	90	9
Kale, cooked, 1 cup	94	9
Ice cream, vanilla, ½ cup	85	8.5
Soy beverage, calcium-fortified, 8 fluid oz.	80 to 500	8 to 50
Chinese cabbage, raw, 1 cup	74	7
Tortilla, corn, ready to bake/fry, 1 medium	42	4
Tortilla, flour, ready to bake/fry, one 6" diameter	37	4
Sour cream, reduced fat, cultured, 2 tbsp	32	3
Bread, white, 1 oz.	31	3
Broccoli, raw, ½ cup	21	2
Bread, whole wheat, 1 slice	20	2
Cheese, cream, regular, 1 tbsp	12	1

* Calcium values are only for tofu processed with a calcium salt. Tofu processed with a noncalcium salt will not contain significant amounts of calcium.

But My Kids Don't like Milk

Drinking milk isn't the only way to enjoy its benefits. For example, try making soup and oatmeal or other hot cereals with milk instead of water. Pour milk over cold cereal for breakfast or a snack. Incorporate milk into a fruit smoothie or milkshake. Chocolate milk and cocoa made with milk are also ways to increase the milk in your child's diet.

Sources of calcium also might include an ounce or two of cheese on pizza or a cheeseburger, a cup of calcium-enriched orange juice, or a small carton of yogurt. Your kids can also get calcium from dark green, leafy vegetables such as kale or bok choy, or foods such as broccoli, almonds, tortillas, or tofu made with calcium. Many popular foods such as cereals, breads, and juices now have calcium added too. Check the Nutrition Facts label on the package to be sure.

My Teenage Son Loves Milk, but It Seems to Upset His Stomach. Could He Have Lactose Intolerance?

People with lactose intolerance have trouble digesting lactose, the sugar found in milk and dairy foods. Lactose intolerance is not common among infants and young children, but can occur in older children, adolescents, and adults. It is more common among people of African American, Hispanic, Asian, and American Indian descent.

Most kids with lactose intolerance are able to digest milk when it is served in small amounts, and combined with other foods such as cereal. They may tolerate other dairy products such as cheese or yogurt even if milk is a problem. Lactose-free milk products are now available in most stores, and there are pills and drops you can add to milk and dairy products that make them easier to digest.

Be sure to include plenty of foods with calcium in the meals and snacks you plan for your kids. Almonds, calcium-fortified orange juice, tortillas, fortified cereals, soy beverages, and broccoli with dip are a few great choices. Although it's best to get calcium from food, calcium supplements can also be helpful.

How to Read a Food Label for Calcium

The food label, called Nutrition Facts, shows you how much one serving of that food contributes to the total amount of calcium, as well as other nutrients, you need every day. This is expressed as a percentage of the daily value (%DV) of calcium that is recommended. For labeling purposes, this is based on the daily calcium recommendation of 1,000 milligrams for people 19 to 50 years old. Since children and teens 9 to 18 years old require more calcium, their %DV target is higher, as indicated below:

Table 10.3. Daily Calcium Recommendation

Age	Recommended Calcium Intake	%DV Target
9 to 18	1,300 mg	130%DV
19 to 50	1,000 mg	100%DV

Here is an easy rule of thumb for evaluating the calcium content of a food: 20%DV or more is high for calcium. That means it is a high-calcium food and contributes a lot of calcium to the diet. A food with a calcium content of 5%DV or lower contributes little calcium to the diet and is a low source.

If you want to convert the %DV for calcium into milligrams, you can multiply by 10. For example, if a single-serving container of yogurt lists 30%DV for calcium, it contains 300 mg of calcium (30 × 10).

Getting plenty of high-calcium foods every day is important. To meet their calcium needs, children 9 to 18 years old need about four servings of foods with a 30%DV for calcium (300 mg each) or 6 to 7 servings of foods with a 20%DV for calcium (200 mg each) every day. Foods with a lower %DV for calcium are also important to fill gaps and help ensure that your children get all the calcium they need.

Section 10.2

Parents Concerns about Kids' Bone Health

This section includes text excerpted from "Kids and Their Bones: A Guide for Parents," NIH Osteoporosis and Related Bone Diseases—National Resource Center (NIH ORBD—NRC), March 2015. Reviewed January 2019.

My Daughter Is Constantly Dieting. Should I Be Concerned?

Maintaining proper weight is important to overall health, but so is good nutrition. If your daughter is avoiding all milk and dairy products and severely restricting her food intake, she is probably not getting enough calcium. She needs a more balanced diet that includes low-fat milk products and other calcium-rich foods. Calcium supplements may also be helpful to ensure that she gets enough of this essential nutrient.

You should discuss your concerns with your daughter's doctor. If your daughter is one of up to three percent of American girls and young women with eating disorders, the problem is even more serious. Eating disorders, especially anorexia nervosa, can lead to missed or irregular menstrual periods or the complete absence of periods, known as amen-orrhea. These are signs of low estrogen, a hormone that is essential for developing bone density and reaching peak bone mass. Girls with anorexia nervosa will often have fractures as a first sign of the dis-ease. Furthermore, reduction in estrogen production in adolescence can increase your daughter's risk of osteoporosis and fracture later in life. In severe cases, girls with eating disorders may even develop osteoporosis in their twenties, and they may find the damage to their bones cannot be reversed later in life.

Look for the following signs and see your daughter's physician if you think your daughter has, or is at risk of developing, an eating disorder:

- Missed menstrual periods after having had them regularly for at least several months
- Extreme and/or unhealthy-looking thinness
- Extreme or rapid weight loss
- Frequent dieting practices such as:
  - Eating very little
  - Not eating in front of others
  - Trips to the bathroom following meals
  - Preoccupation with thinness
  - Focus on low-calorie and diet foods
  - Overtraining or excessive exercise

Should I Give My Kids Calcium Supplements?

Experts believe calcium should come from food sources whenever possible. However, if you think your children are not getting ade-quate calcium from their diet, you may want to consider a calcium supplement.

How Does Physical Activity Help My Kids' Bones?

Maintaining proper weight is important to overall health, but so is good nutrition. If your daughter is avoiding all milk and dairy products and severely restricting her food intake, she is probably not getting enough calcium. She needs a more balanced diet that includes low-fat milk products and other calcium-rich foods. Calcium supplements may also be helpful to ensure that she gets enough of this essential nutrient.

You should discuss your concerns with your daughter's doctor. If your daughter is one of up to three percent of American girls and young women with eating disorders, the problem is even more serious. Eating disorders, especially anorexia nervosa, can lead to missed or irregular menstrual periods or the complete absence of periods, known as amenorrhea. These are signs of low estrogen, a hormone that is essential for developing bone density and reaching peak bone mass. Girls with anorexia nervosa will often have fractures as a first sign of the disease. Furthermore, reduction in estrogen production in adolescence can increase your daughter's risk of osteoporosis and fracture later in life. In severe cases, girls with eating disorders may even develop osteoporosis in their twenties, and they may find the damage to their bones cannot be reversed later in life.

Look for the following signs and see your daughter's physician if you think your daughter has, or is at risk of developing, an eating disorder:

- Walking

- Tennis

- Running

- Volleyball

- Hiking

- Ice hockey/field hockey

- Dancing

- Skiing

- Soccer

- Skateboarding

- Gymnastics

- In-line skating

- Basketball

- Lifting weights

- Jumping rope

- Aerobics

Is It Possible to Get Too Much Exercise?

For most people, including children and teens, the challenge is to get enough physical activity. However, excessive exercise and over-training, often coupled with restrictive eating, can be a problem, especially for some female athletes and dancers, as well as girls who become obsessive about weight loss. Overtraining, like eating disorders, can result in decreased estrogen and eventually lead to thin bones that break easily.

Years ago, it was not unusual for coaches and trainers to encourage athletes to be as thin as possible for many sports, including dancing, gymnastics, figure skating, running, and diving. Fortunately, many coaches now realize that being too thin is unhealthy and can negatively affect performance, as well as lifelong health.

What Else Can My Kids Do besides Eating Calcium-Rich Foods and Getting Plenty of Weight-Bearing Exercise to Keep Their Bones Healthy?

They should avoid smoking. You probably know that smoking is bad for the heart and lungs, but you may not know that it's harmful to bone tissue. Smoking may harm your bones both directly and indirectly. Several studies have linked smoking to higher risk of fracture. The many dangers associated with smoking make it a habit to be avoided.

You may think it's too early to worry about smoking, but the habit typically starts during childhood or adolescence. In fact, most people who use tobacco products start before they finish high school. The good news? If your kids finish high school as nonsmokers, they will probably stay that way for life.

My Son Has Asthma and Takes a Steroid Medication to Control It. His Doctor Said This Might Affect His Bones. Is There Anything We Can Do about This?

Asthma itself does not pose a threat to bone health, but some medications used to treat the disease can have a negative effect on bones when taken for a long time. Corticosteroids, a type of anti-inflammatory medication, are often prescribed for asthma. These medications can decrease calcium absorbed from food, increase calcium loss from the kidneys, and shrink a child's bone bank account.

95

Kids with asthma need to take special care of their bones, making sure to get enough calcium and weight-bearing exercise. Some health-care providers recommend extra calcium each day. Many people think milk and dairy products—great sources of calcium and vitamin D— trigger asthma attacks, but this is probably true only if your child is allergic to dairy foods. Unfortunately, this misconception often results in an unnecessary avoidance of dairy products, which is concerning, especially during the bone-building years.

Because exercise can often trigger an asthma attack, many people with asthma avoid weight-bearing physical activities that strengthen bone. Kids with asthma may be able to exercise more comfortably in an air-conditioned place, such as a school gym or health club.

My 8-Year-Old Son Is a Daredevil and Has Already Broken Several Bones. Could He Have a Problem like Osteoporosis at This Young Age?

Osteoporosis is rare among children and adolescents. When it occurs, it is usually caused by an underlying medical disorder or by medications used to treat such disorders. This is called secondary osteoporosis. It may also be the result of a genetic disorder such as osteogenesis imperfecta, in which bones break easily from little or no apparent cause. Sometimes there is no identifiable cause of juvenile osteoporosis. This is known as idiopathic juvenile osteo-porosis. Two or more low-impact fractures may be a sign of one of these disorders.

If you are concerned about your son's frequent fractures, talk to his doctor.

How Can I Get through to My Kids? They Sure Don't Think about Their Bones.

You are absolutely right. Research has shown that children and adolescents do not tend to think much about their health. Their decisions about diet and exercise, for example, are rarely made based on "what's good for them." But we also know that you have a much greater influence on your kids' decisions and behaviors than you may believe. For example, many teenagers, when asked who has been the greatest influence in their life, name parents before friends, siblings, grandparents, and romantic partners.

The best way to help your kids develop healthy habits for life is to be a good role model. Research suggests that active children have active parents. If you make physical activity a priority and try hard to maintain a healthy diet, including plenty of calcium, chances are your positive lifestyle will "rub off" on them along the way. Here are some things you can do:

- Be a role model. Drink milk with meals, eat calcium-rich snacks, and get plenty of weight-bearing exercise. Don't smoke.

- Incorporate calcium-rich foods into family meals.

- Serve fat-free or low-fat milk with meals and snacks.

- Stock up on calcium-rich snacks that are easy for hungry children to find, such as:

  - Single-serving puddings

  - Yogurt and frozen yogurt

  - Cereal with low-fat milk

  - Broccoli with yogurt dip

  - Calcium-fortified orange juice

  - Individual cheese pizzas

  - Calcium-fortified tortillas

  - Almonds

- Limit access to soft drinks and other snacks that don't provide calcium by not keeping them in the house.

- Help your kids to find a variety of physical activities or sports they enjoy participating in.

- Establish a firm time limit for sedentary activities such as TV, computers, and video games.

- Teach your kids to never start smoking, as it is highly addictive and toxic.

- Look for signs of eating disorders and overtraining, especially in preteen and teenage girls, and address these problems right away.

- Talk to your children's pediatrician about their bone health. If your child has a special medical condition that may interfere with bone mass development, ask the doctor for ways to minimize the problem and protect your child's bone health.

- Talk to your children about their bone health, and let them know it is a priority for you. Your kids may not think much about health, but they are probably attracted to such health benefits as energy, confidence, good looks, and strength.

Section 10.3

Juvenile Osteoporosis

This section includes text excerpted from "Juvenile Osteoporosis," NIH Osteoporosis and Related Bone Diseases—National Resource Center (NIH ORBD—NRC), June 2015. Reviewed January 2019.

Osteoporosis literally means "porous bone." This disease is characterized by too little bone formation, excessive bone loss, or a combination of both. People with osteoporosis have an increased risk of fractures. It is most common in older people, especially older women.

Osteoporosis is rare in children and adolescents. When it does occur, it is usually caused by an underlying medical disorder or by medications used to treat the disorder. This is called secondary osteoporosis. Sometimes, however, there is no identifiable cause of osteoporosis in a child. This is known as idiopathic osteoporosis.

No matter what causes it, juvenile osteoporosis can be a significant problem because it occurs during the child's prime bone-building years. From birth through young adulthood, children steadily accumulate bone mass, which peaks sometime before age 30. The greater their peak bone mass, the lower their risk for osteoporosis later in life. After people reach their mid-thirties, bone mass typically begins to decline—very slowly at first but increasing in their fifties and sixties. Both heredity and lifestyle choices—especially the amount of calcium in the diet and the level of physical activity influence the development of peak bone mass and the rate at which bone is lost later in life.

Secondary Osteoporosis

Secondary osteoporosis, which can affect both adults and children, results from another primary disorder or therapy. Some examples are included in the box below.

As the primary condition, juvenile idiopathic arthritis (JIA) (also known as juvenile rheumatoid arthritis) provides a good illustration of the possible causes of secondary osteoporosis. In some cases, the disease process itself can cause osteoporosis. For example, some studies have found that children with juvenile idiopathic arthritis have bone mass that is lower than expected, especially near the joints affected by arthritis. In other cases, medication used to treat the primary disorder may reduce bone mass. For example, drugs such as prednisone, used to treat severe cases of juvenile idiopathic arthritis, negatively affect bone mass. Finally, some behaviors associated with the primary disorder may lead to bone loss or reduction in bone formation. For example, a child with juvenile idiopathic arthritis may avoid physical activity, which is necessary for building and maintaining bone mass, because it may aggravate his or her condition or cause pain.

*Disorders, Medications, and Behaviors That May Affect Bone Mass**
Primary Disorders

- Juvenile rheumatoid arthritis

- Diabetes

- Osteogenesis imperfecta

- Hyperthyroidism

- Hyperparathyroidism

- Cushing syndrome

- Malabsorption syndromes

- Anorexia nervosa

- Kidney disease

* This is not a complete list. The cause of a child's osteoporosis can best be determined with the help of his or her doctor.

Medications

- Anticonvulsants (e.g., for epilepsy)

- Corticosteroids (e.g., for rheumatoid arthritis (RA) and asthma)

- Immunosuppressive agents (e.g., for cancer)

Behaviors

- Prolonged inactivity or immobility

- Inadequate nutrition (especially lack of calcium and vitamin D)

- Excessive exercise leading to amenorrhea (absence of menstrual periods)

- Smoking

- Alcohol abuse

For children secondary osteoporosis, the best course of action is to identify and treat the underlying disorder. In the case of medication-induced juvenile osteoporosis, it is best to treat the primary disorder with the lowest effective dose of the osteoporosis-inducing medication. If an alternative medication is available and effective, the child's doctor may consider prescribing it. Like all children, those with secondary osteoporosis also need a diet rich in calcium and vitamin D and as much physical activity as possible given the limitations of the primary disorder.

Idiopathic Juvenile Osteoporosis

Idiopathic juvenile osteoporosis (IJO) is a primary condition with no known cause. It is diagnosed after the doctor has excluded other causes of juvenile osteoporosis, including primary diseases or medical therapies known to cause bone loss.

This rare form of osteoporosis typically occurs just before the onset of puberty in previously healthy children. The average age at onset is 7 years, with a range of 1 to 13 years. The good news is that most children experience complete recovery of bone.

Clinical features. The first sign of IJO is usually pain in the lower back, hips, and feet, often accompanied by difficulty walking. Knee and ankle pain and fractures of the lower extremities also may occur.

Physical malformations include abnormal curvature of the upper spine (kyphosis), loss of height, a sunken chest, or a limp. These physical malformations are sometimes reversible after IJO has run its course.

X-rays of children with IJO often show low bone density, fractures of weight-bearing bones, and collapsed or misshapen vertebrae. However, conventional X-rays may not be able to detect osteoporosis until significant bone mass already has been lost. Newer methods such as dual-energy X-ray absorptiometry (DXA), dual photon absorptiometry (DPA), and quantitative computed tomography (CAT scans) allow for earlier and more accurate diagnosis of low bone mass. These noninvasive, painless tests are a bit like X-rays.

Treatment. There is no established medical or surgical therapy for juvenile osteoporosis. In some cases, no treatment may be needed because the condition usually goes away spontaneously. However, early diagnosis of juvenile osteoporosis is important so that steps can be taken to protect the child's spine and other bones from fracture until remission occurs. These steps may include physical therapy, using crutches, avoiding unsafe weight-bearing activities, and other supportive care. A well-balanced diet rich in calcium and vitamin D is also important. In severe, long-lasting cases of juvenile osteoporosis, some medications called bisphosphonates, approved by the U.S. Food and Drug Administration (FDA) for the treatment of osteoporosis in adults, have been given to children experimentally.

Prognosis. Most children with IJO experience a complete recovery of bone tissue. Although growth may be somewhat impaired during the acute phase of the disorder, normal growth resumes—and catch-up growth often occurs—afterward. Unfortunately, in some cases, IJO can result in permanent disability such as curvature of the upper spine (kyphoscoliosis) or collapse of the rib cage.

Distinguishing Juvenile Osteoporosis from Osteogenesis Imperfecta

Osteogenesis imperfecta (OI) is a rare genetic disorder that, like juvenile osteoporosis, is characterized by bones that break easily, often from little or no apparent cause. However, OI is caused by a problem with the quantity or quality of bone collagen resulting from a genetic defect.

Because most children with OI never attain normal bone mass, they suffer from secondary osteoporosis as well. There are several distinct forms of OI, representing extreme variations in severity. For example, a person with OI may have as few as 10 or as many as several hundred fractures in a lifetime. Although the number of people affected with OI in the United States is unknown, the best estimate suggests a minimum of 20,000 and possibly as many as 50,000. The clinical features of OI and their severity vary greatly from person to person. Many individuals with OI have some, but not all, of the clinical features. Children with milder OI, in particular, may have few obvious clinical symptoms. The most common features of OI include:

- Bones that fracture easily

- Ligament laxity (hypermobile joints) and low muscle strength

- Family history of OI (present in about 65 percent of cases)

- Small stature in moderate and severe types

- Sclera ("whites" of the eyes) tinted blue, purple, or gray in about 50 percent of cases

- Possible hearing loss in late childhood or early adulthood

- Possible brittle teeth (known as dentinogenesis imperfecta)

The features that most often distinguish OI from juvenile osteoporosis are the family history of the disease and the blue, purple, or gray sclera commonly found in patients with OI. Distinguishing between OI and IJO may require genetic testing or, in some cases, bone biopsy.

Chapter 11

Osteoporosis in Men

Osteoporosis is a disease that causes the skeleton to weaken and the bones to break. It poses a significant threat to millions of men in the United States.

Despite these compelling figures, surveys suggest that a majority of American men view osteoporosis solely as a "woman's disease." Moreover, among men whose lifestyle habits put them at increased risk, few recognize the disease as a significant threat to their mobility and independence.

Osteoporosis is called a "silent disease" because it progresses without symptoms until a fracture occurs. It develops less often in men than in women because men have larger skeletons, their bone loss starts later and progresses more slowly, and they have no period of rapid hormonal change and bone loss. However, in the past few years the problem of osteoporosis in men has been recognized as an important public health issue, particularly in light of estimates that the number of men above the age of 70 will continue to increase as life expectancy continues to rise.

What Causes Osteoporosis

Bone is constantly changing—that is, old bone is removed and replaced by new bone. During childhood, more bone is produced than

This chapter includes text excerpted from "Osteoporosis in Men," NIH Osteoporosis and Related Bone Diseases—National Resource Center (NIH ORBD—NRC), June 2015. Reviewed January 2019.

removed, so the skeleton grows in both size and strength. For most people, bone mass peaks during the third decade of life. By this age, men typically have accumulated more bone mass than women. After this point, the amount of bone in the skeleton typically begins to decline slowly as removal of old bone exceeds formation of new bone.

Men in their fifties do not experience the rapid loss of bone mass that women do in the years following menopause. By age 65 or 70, however, men and women are losing bone mass at the same rate, and the absorption of calcium, an essential nutrient for bone health throughout life, decreases in both sexes. Excessive bone loss causes bone to become fragile and more likely to fracture.

Fractures resulting from osteoporosis most commonly occur in the hip, spine, and wrist, and can be permanently disabling. Hip fractures are especially dangerous. Perhaps because such fractures tend to occur at older ages in men than in women, men who sustain hip fractures are more likely than women to die from complications.

Causes of Secondary Osteoporosis in Men

- Glucocorticoid medications

- Other immunosuppressive drugs

- Hypogonadism (low testosterone levels)

- Excessive alcohol consumption

- Smoking

- Chronic obstructive pulmonary disease and asthma

- Cystic fibrosis

- Gastrointestinal disease

- Hypercalciuria

- Anticonvulsant medications

- Thyrotoxicosis

- Hyperparathyroidism

- Immobilization

- Osteogenesis imperfecta

- Homocystinuria

- Neoplastic disease

- Ankylosing spondylitis and rheumatoid arthritis
- Systemic mastocytosis

Primary and Secondary Osteoporosis

There are two main types of osteoporosis: primary and secondary. In cases of primary osteoporosis, either the condition is caused by age-related bone loss (sometimes called senile osteoporosis) or the cause is unknown (idiopathic osteoporosis). The term "idiopathic osteoporosis" is typically used only for men younger than 70 years old; in older men, age-related bone loss is assumed to be the cause.

The majority of men with osteoporosis have at least one (sometimes more than one) secondary cause. In cases of secondary osteoporosis, the loss of bone mass is caused by certain lifestyle behaviors, diseases, or medications. The most common causes of secondary osteoporosis in men include exposure to glucocorticoid medications, hypogonadism (low levels of testosterone), alcohol abuse, smoking, gastrointestinal disease, hypercalciuria, and immobilization.

Glucocorticoid medications: Glucocorticoids are steroid medications used to treat diseases such as asthma and rheumatoid arthritis. Bone loss is a very common side effect of these medications. The bone loss these medications cause may be due to their direct effect on bone, muscle weakness or immobility, reduced intestinal absorption of calcium, a decrease in testosterone levels, or, most likely, a combination of these factors.

When glucocorticoid medications are used on an ongoing basis, bone mass often decreases quickly and continuously, with most of the bone loss in the ribs and vertebrae. Therefore, people taking these medications should talk to their doctor about having a bone mineral density (BMD) test. Men should also be tested to monitor testosterone levels, as glucocorticoids often reduce testosterone in the blood.

A treatment plan to minimize loss of bone during long-term glucocorticoid therapy may include using the minimal effective dose, and discontinuing the drug or administering it through the skin, if possible. Adequate calcium and vitamin D intake is important, as these nutrients help reduce the impact of glucocorticoids on the bones. Other possible treatments include testosterone replacement and osteoporosis medication.

Hypogonadism: Hypogonadism refers to abnormally low levels of sex hormones. It is well known that loss of estrogen causes osteoporosis in women. In men, reduced levels of sex hormones may also cause osteoporosis.

Although it is natural for testosterone levels to decrease with age, there should not be a sudden drop in this hormone that is comparable to the drop in estrogen experienced by women at menopause. However, medications such as glucocorticoids (discussed above), cancer treatments (especially for prostate cancer), and many other factors can affect testosterone levels. Testosterone replacement therapy may be helpful in preventing or slowing bone loss. Its success depends on factors such as age and how long testosterone levels have been reduced. Also, it is not yet clear how long any beneficial effect of testosterone replacement will last. Therefore, doctors usually treat the osteoporosis directly, using medications approved for this purpose.

Research suggests that estrogen deficiency may also be a cause of osteoporosis in men. For example, estrogen levels are low in men with hypogonadism and may play a part in bone loss. Osteoporosis has been found in some men who have rare disorders involving estrogen. Therefore, the role of estrogen in men is under active investigation.

Alcohol abuse: There is a wealth of evidence that alcohol abuse may decrease bone density and lead to an increase in fractures. Low bone mass is common in men who seek medical help for alcohol abuse.

In cases where bone loss is linked to alcohol abuse, the first goal of treatment is to help the patient stop, or at least reduce, consumption of alcohol. More research is needed to determine whether bone lost to alcohol abuse will rebuild once drinking stops, or even whether further damage will be prevented. It is clear, though, that alcohol abuse causes many other health and social problems, so quitting is ideal. A treatment plan may also include a balanced diet with lots of calcium- and vitamin D-rich foods, a program of physical exercise, and smoking cessation.

Smoking: Bone loss is more rapid, and rates of hip and vertebral fracture are higher, among men who smoke, although more research is needed to determine exactly how smoking damages bone. Tobacco, nicotine, and other chemicals found in cigarettes may be directly toxic to bone, or they may inhibit absorption of calcium and other nutrients needed for bone health. Quitting is the ideal approach, as smoking is harmful in so many ways. As with alcohol, it is not known whether quitting smoking leads to reduced rates of bone loss or to a gain in bone mass.

Gastrointestinal disorders: Several nutrients, including amino acids, calcium, magnesium, phosphorous, and vitamins D and K, are important for bone health. Diseases of the stomach and intestines can lead to bone disease when they impair absorption of these nutrients. In such cases, treatment for bone loss may include taking supplements to replenish these nutrients.

Hypercalciuria: Hypercalciuria is a disorder that causes too much calcium to be lost through the urine, which makes the calcium unavailable for building bone. Patients with hypercalciuria should talk to their doctor about having a BMD test and, if bone density is low, discuss treatment options.

Immobilization: Weight-bearing exercise is essential for maintaining healthy bones. Without it, bone density may decline rapidly. Prolonged bed rest (following fractures, surgery, spinal cord injuries, or illness) or immobilization of some part of the body often results in significant bone loss. It is crucial to resume weight-bearing exercise (such as walking, jogging, dancing, and lifting weights) as soon as possible after a period of prolonged bed rest. If this is not possible, you should work with your doctor to minimize other risk factors for osteoporosis.

How Is Osteoporosis Diagnosed in Men?

Osteoporosis can be effectively treated if it is detected before significant bone loss has occurred. A medical workup to diagnose osteoporosis will include a complete medical history, X-rays, and urine and blood tests. The doctor may also order a bone mineral density test. This test can identify osteoporosis, determine your risk for fractures (broken bones), and measure your response to osteoporosis treatment. The most widely recognized BMD test is called a central dual-energy X-ray absorptiometry, or central dual-energy X-ray absorptiometry (DXA) test. It is painless a bit like having an X-ray, but with much less exposure to radiation. It can measure bone density at your hip and spine.

It is increasingly common for women to be diagnosed with osteoporosis or low bone mass using a BMD test, often at midlife when doctors begin to watch for signs of bone loss. In men, however, the diagnosis is often not made until a fracture occurs or a man complains of back pain and sees his doctor. This makes it especially important for men to inform their doctors about risk factors for developing osteoporosis, loss of height or change in posture, a fracture, or sudden back pain.

What Are the Risk Factors for Men?

Several risk factors have been linked to osteoporosis in men:

- Chronic diseases that affect the kidneys, lungs, stomach, and intestines or alter hormone levels

- Regular use of certain medications, such as glucocorticoids

- Undiagnosed low levels of the sex hormone testosterone

- Unhealthy lifestyle habits: smoking, excessive alcohol use, low calcium intake, and inadequate physical exercise

- Age. The older you are, the greater your risk.

- Race. White men appear to be at particularly high risk, but all men can develop this disease.

What Treatments Are Available

Once a man has been diagnosed with osteoporosis, his doctor may prescribe one of the medications approved by the U.S. Food and Drug Administration (FDA) for this disease. The treatment plan will also likely include the nutrition, exercise, and lifestyle guidelines for preventing bone loss.

If bone loss is due to glucocorticoid use, the doctor may prescribe a medication approved to prevent or treat glucocorticoid-induced osteoporosis, monitor bone density and testosterone levels, and suggest using the minimum effective dose of glucocorticoid.

Other possible prevention or treatment approaches include calcium and/or vitamin D supplements and regular physical activity.

If osteoporosis is the result of another condition (such as testosterone deficiency) or exposure to certain other medications, the doctor may design a treatment plan to address the underlying cause.

How Can Osteoporosis Be Prevented?

There have been fewer research studies on osteoporosis in men than in women. However, experts agree that all people should take the following steps to preserve their bone health:

- Avoid smoking, reduce alcohol intake, and increase your level of physical activity. Ensure a daily calcium intake that is adequate for your age.

- Ensure an adequate intake of vitamin D.

- Dietary vitamin D intake should be 600 IU (International Units) per day up to age 70. Men over age 70 should increase their uptake to 800 IU daily (see table below). The amount of vitamin D found in 1 quart of fortified milk and most multivitamins is 400 IU.

- Engage in a regular regimen of weight-bearing exercises in which bones and muscles work against gravity. This might include walking, jogging, racquet sports, climbing stairs, team sports, weight training, and using resistance machines. A doctor should evaluate the exercise program of anyone already diagnosed with osteoporosis to determine if twisting motions and impact activities, such as those used in golf, tennis, or basketball, need to be curtailed.

- Discuss with your doctor the use of medications that are known to cause bone loss, such as glucocorticoids.

- Recognize and seek treatment for any underlying medical conditions that affect bone health.

Table 11.1. Recommended Calcium and Vitamin D Intakes

Life-Stage Group	Calcium (mg/day)	Vitamin D (IU/day)
Infants 0 to 6 months	200	400
Infants 6 to 12 months	260	400
1 to 3 years old	700	600
4 to 8 years old	1,000	600
9 to 13 years old	1,300	600
14 to 18 years old	1,300	600
19 to 30 years old	1,000	600
31 to 50 years old	1,000	600
51- to 70-year-old males	1,000	600
51- to 70-year-old females	1,200	600
70 years old	1,200	800
14 to 18 years old, pregnant/lactating	1,300	600
19 to 50 years old, pregnant/lactating	1,000	600

(Source: Food and Nutrition Board (FNB), Institute of Medicine (IOM), National Academy of Sciences (NAS), 2010.)

Chapter 12

Osteoporosis in Older Adults

Chapter Contents

Section 12.1

Mechanisms of Age-Related Bone Loss

This section includes text excerpted from "Mechanisms
of Age-Related Bone Loss," National Institutes of
Health (NIH), October 17, 2017.

Bone is comprised of a mineral and protein scaffold filled with bone cells. This structure is continually broken down and renewed. When the rate of bone loss outpaces the rate of replacement, bones weaken, eventually leading to a condition known as osteoporosis. Many factors can contribute to osteoporosis, including aging, certain medications, and hormonal changes.

Osteoblasts, the cells that build bone, are derived from mesenchymal stem cells in the bone marrow. These skeletal stem cells can also give rise to other types of cells, including fat cells. The bone marrow of older adults has fewer bone-building osteoblasts and more fat cells than that of younger people. The mechanisms responsible for these changes, however, are unknown.

A research team led by Drs. Yi-Ping Li and Wei Chen at the University of Alabama at Birmingham has been studying the signals that determine whether marrow mesenchymal stem cells develop, or "differentiate," into osteoblasts or fat cells. In past work, the team found that a protein called Core Binding Factor β (Cbfβ) is involved in osteoblast differentiation. Cbfβ is also involved in skeletal development and fracture healing.

In the current study, the team explored how Cbfβ affects marrow stem cell differentiation in mice. They deleted the Cbfβ gene at three different stages of osteoblast development: in mesenchymal stem cells, an intermediate stage, and early osteoblasts. The work was funded by National Institutes of Health's (NIH) National Institute of Arthritis and Musculoskeletal and Skin Diseases (NIAMS) and National Institute of Dental and Craniofacial Research (NIDCR). Results appeared in Proceedings of the National Academy of Sciences (NAS) on September 19, 2017.

Cbfβ deficiency at all three stages of differentiation reduced bone density in the mice and dramatically increased their bone marrow fat content. Further testing confirmed that there were more fat cells in the bone marrow of the Cbfβ-deficient mice than the control mice. The bones of the Cbfβ-deficient mice resembled that of aged control mice. Cbfβ levels were also dramatically lower in the aged control mice than in younger control mice. These results suggest that a drop in Cbfβ could contribute to the age-related shift from osteoblast to fat cell production.

A series of lab experiments confirmed that, without Cbfβ, cells at any stage of osteoblast differentiation could switch to form fat cells. Cbfβ inhibits fat cell formation through an important cell signaling pathway called Wnt/β-catenin. It also inhibits expression of a gene that regulates adipose cell formation called c/ebpα. The team showed that Cbfβ plays a critical role in maintaining osteoblast lineage through both these mechanisms.

"Our data detail the underlying pathways that cause progenitor cells and early osteoblasts to create fat cells instead of bone-producing cells," Li says. "They also suggest that maintaining Cbfβ might be an effective way to prevent age-associated osteoporosis in people." However, this idea still needs to be tested in humans.

Section 12.2

Osteoporosis in Aging

This section includes text excerpted from "Osteoporosis in Aging," *NIH News in Health*, National Institutes of Health (NIH), January 2015. Reviewed January 2019.

Bones feel solid, but the inside of a bone is actually filled with holes like a honeycomb. Bone tissues are broken down and rebuilt all the time. While some cells build new bone tissue, others dissolve bone and release the minerals inside.

As we get older, we begin to lose more bone than we build. The tiny holes within bones get bigger, and the solid outer layer becomes thinner. In other words, our bones get less dense. Hard bones turn spongy, and spongy bones turn spongier. If this loss of bone density goes too far, it's called osteoporosis. Over 10 million people nationwide are estimated to have osteoporosis.

It's normal for bones to break in bad accidents. But if your bones are dense enough, they should be able to stand up to most falls. Bones weakened by osteoporosis, though, are more likely to break.

"It's just like any other engineering material," says Dr. Joan McGowan, an National Institutes of Health (NIH) expert on osteoporosis. If you fall and slam your weight onto a fragile bone, "it reaches a point where the structures aren't adequate to support the weight you're putting on them." If the bone breaks, it's a major hint that an older person has osteoporosis.

Broken bones can lead to serious problems for seniors. The hip is a common site for osteoporosis, and hip fractures can lead to a downward spiral of disability and loss of independence. Osteoporosis is also common in the wrist and the spine.

The hormone estrogen helps to make and rebuild bones. A woman's estrogen levels drop after menopause, and bone loss speeds up. That's why osteoporosis is most common among older women. But men get osteoporosis, too.

"A third of all hip fractures occur in men, yet the problem of osteoporosis in men is frequently downplayed or ignored," says Dr. Eric Orwoll, a physician-researcher who studies osteoporosis at Oregon Health and Science University (OHSU). Men tend to do worse than women after a hip fracture, Orwoll says.

Experts suggest that women start getting screened for osteoporosis at age 65. Women younger than age 65 who are at high risk for fractures should also be screened. Men should discuss screening recommendations with their healthcare providers.

Screening is done with a bone mineral density test at the hip and spine. The most common test is known as dual-energy X-ray absorptiometry (DXA). It's painless, like having an X-ray. Your results are often reported as a T-score, which compares your bone density to that of a healthy young woman. A T-score of –2.5 or lower indicates osteoporosis.

Protect Your Bones with Exercise

There's a lot you can do to lower your risk of osteoporosis. Getting plenty of calcium, vitamin D, and exercise is a good start, Orwoll says.

Calcium is a mineral that helps bones stay strong. It can come from the foods you eat—including milk and milk products, dark green leafy vegetables like kale and collard greens—or from dietary supplements. Women over age 50 need 1,200 mg of calcium a day. Men need 1,000 mg a day from ages 51 to 70 and 1,200 mg a day after that.

Vitamin D helps your body absorb calcium. As you grow older, your body needs more vitamin D, which is made by your skin when you're in the sun. You can also get vitamin D from dietary supplements and from certain foods, such as milk, eggs, fatty fish, and fortified cereals. Talk with your healthcare provider to make sure you're getting a healthy amount of vitamin D. Problems can arise if you're getting too little or too much.

Exercise, especially weight-bearing exercise, helps bones, too. Weight-bearing exercises include jogging, walking, tennis, and dancing. The pull of muscles is a reminder to the cells in your bones that they need to keep the tissue dense.

Smoking, in contrast, weakens bones. Heavy drinking does too— and makes people more likely to fall. Certain drugs may also increase the risk of osteoporosis. Having family members with osteoporosis can raise your risk for the condition as well.

The good news is, even if you already have osteoporosis, it's not too late to start taking care of your bones. Since your bones are rebuilding themselves all the time, you can help push the balance toward more bone growth by giving them exercise, calcium, and vitamin D.

Several medications can also help fight bone loss. The most widely used are bisphosphonates. These drugs are generally prescribed to people diagnosed with osteoporosis after a DXA test, or to those who've had a fracture that suggests their bones are too weak. Bisphosphonates have been tested more thoroughly in women, but are approved for men too.

Researchers are trying to develop drugs that increase bone growth. For now, there's only one available: parathyroid hormone. It's effective at building bone and is approved for women and men with osteoporosis who are at high risk for having a fracture.

Another important way to avoid broken bones is to prevent falling and occasions for fracture in the first place. Unfortunately, more than 2 million so-called fragility fractures (which wouldn't have happened if the bones had been stronger) occur nationwide each year. "To reduce the societal burden of fracture, it's going to take a combined approach of not only focusing on the skeleton but focusing on fall prevention," says Dr. Kristine Ensrud, a physician-researcher who studies aging-related disorders at the University of Minnesota and Minneapolis VA healthcare system.

Many things can affect the risk for a fall, such as how good a person's balance is and how many trip hazards are in the environment. The kind of fall matters, too. Wrist fractures often occur when a person falls forward or backward. "It's the active older person who trips and puts her hand out," McGowan says. Hip fractures often arise when a person falls to the side. Your hip may be strong enough to handle weight that goes up and down, but not an impact from another direction.

"That's why exercise that builds balance and confidence is very good at preventing fractures," McGowan says. For example, she says, tai chi won't provide the loads needed to build bone mass, but it can increase balance and coordination—and make you more likely to catch yourself before you topple.

NIH-funded researchers are looking for better ways to tell how strong your bones are, and how high your chances are of breaking a bone. For now, though, the DXA test is the best measure, and many seniors, even older women, don't get it, Ensrud says. If you're concerned about your bone health, she adds, "Ask your healthcare provider about the possibility of a bone density test."

Section 12.3

Prostate Cancer and Osteoporosis

This section includes text excerpted from "What Prostate Cancer Survivors Need to Know about Osteoporosis," NIH Osteoporosis and Related Bone Diseases—National Resource Center (NIH ORBD—NRC), April 2016.

The Impact of Prostate Cancer

The National Cancer Institute (NCI) reports that next to skin cancer, prostate cancer is the most common type of cancer among American men. The cancer usually grows very slowly, however, and most men who are diagnosed with prostate cancer live for many years. Still, prostate cancer can be serious and, in some cases, life-threatening.

All men are at risk for prostate cancer, but most men diagnosed with it are age 65 or older. And as men get older, their risk for developing another disease, osteoporosis, increases. Osteoporosis is of particular concern for men with prostate cancer. Research has found a strong link between hormone deprivation therapy, which is one of the treatments for prostate cancer, and osteoporosis. Hormone-deprivation therapy is also called "androgen-deprivation therapy" because it deprives cancer cells of the male hormones (called androgens) that the cancer needs to grow.

Facts about Osteoporosis

Osteoporosis is a condition in which bones become weaker, less dense, and more likely to break. Many people—even some doctors—think of osteoporosis as a women's disease, but millions of men develop it, too. Men who break bones are less likely than women to be treated for bone disease, even though treatment can help prevent broken bones in the future.

Besides taking hormone deprivation therapy for prostate cancer, other risk factors for developing osteoporosis include:

- Being thin or having a small frame

- Having a family history of the disease

- Using certain medications, such as glucocorticoids

- Not getting enough calcium

- Not getting enough physical activity

- Smoking

- Drinking too much alcohol

Osteoporosis is a silent disease because it can weaken bones over the years without causing symptoms. For men coping with prostate cancer, weak bones may not seem very important. But weak bones can cause problems because they break easily, and broken bones often initiate a downward health spiral. But it is never too late to improve your bone health: osteoporosis can be treated and prevented.

The Link between Prostate Cancer and Osteoporosis

Studies show that men who receive hormone-deprivation therapy for prostate cancer have an increased risk of developing osteoporosis and broken bones. Hormones such as testosterone protect against bone loss. So, once these hormones are blocked, bone becomes less dense and can break more easily.

Osteoporosis Management Strategies

Several strategies can reduce a man's risk for osteoporosis, or lessen its effects if he already has it.

Nutrition. A well-balanced diet rich in calcium and vitamin D is important for bone health. Good sources of calcium include low-fat dairy products; dark green, leafy vegetables; and calcium-fortified foods and beverages. Taking dietary supplements or multivitamins also can help ensure that you meet your body's daily calcium requirement.

However, some evidence suggests that high calcium intake might be associated with the development of prostate cancer. But the studies that produced these findings are not definitive. In fact, other studies have shown a weak relationship, no relationship at all, or the opposite relationship between calcium and prostate cancer. At this point, researchers can only say that the relationship between calcium and prostate cancer risk remains unclear. It is recommended that men age 19 to 70 consume 1,000 mg (milligrams) of calcium per day, and those over age 70 consume 1,200 mg per day.

Vitamin D plays an important role in calcium absorption and bone health. Some individuals may require vitamin D supplements to achieve the recommended intake of 600 to 800 IU (International Units) each day.

Exercise. Like muscle, bone is living tissue that responds to exercise by becoming stronger. The best exercise for bones is weight-bearing exercise that forces you to work against gravity. Some examples include walking, climbing stairs, dancing, and weight training. Regular exercise, such as walking, may help prevent bone loss and provide many other health benefits, such as reducing pain, relieving stress, and making cancer treatment easier to handle.

Healthy lifestyle. Smoking is toxic to bones as well as the heart and lungs. In addition, smokers may absorb less calcium from their diets. Studies also have found that heavy drinking hurts your overall health, weakens your bones, and increases your risk of broken bones. Moderate drinking—for most men, this means not more than two alcoholic drinks per day—has not been shown to hurt your bones.

Bone mineral density test. A bone mineral density (BMD) test is the best way to determine your bone health. BMD tests can identify osteoporosis, determine your risk for fractures (broken bones), and measure your response to osteoporosis treatment. The most widely recognized BMD test is called a central dual-energy X-ray absorptiometry (DXA) test. The test is painless—a bit like having an X-ray, but with much less exposure to radiation—and can measure bone density at your hip and spine.

Men being treated for prostate cancer with hormone-deprivation therapy should discuss with their doctor whether BMD testing is a good idea. Don't wait for your doctor to bring up your bone health with you. A study shows that many men on hormone-deprivation therapy for prostate cancer are not being screened or treated for osteoporosis, even when they have other risk factors for the condition.

Medication. There is no cure for osteoporosis, but medications are approved by the U.S. Food and Drug Administration (FDA) for men with the disease. Although no medications have been approved specifically to treat men with bone problems caused by hormone-deprivation therapy for prostate cancer, studies of several medications are underway for this purpose.

Part Three

Osteoporosis and Related Conditions

Chapter 13

Dripping Candle Wax Bone Disease (Melorheostosis)

Melorheostosis is a rare bone disease. It causes the abnormal growth of new bone tissue on the surface of existing bones. The new bone has a characteristic appearance on X-rays, often described as "flowing" or like dripping candle wax. The excess bone growth typically occurs on the bones in one arm or leg, although it can also affect the pelvis, breastbone (sternum), ribs, or other bones. (The term "melorheostosis" is derived from the Greek words "melos," which means limb; "rheos," which means flow; and "ostosis," which refers to bone formation.) The abnormal bone growth associated with melorheostosis is noncancerous (benign), and it does not spread from one bone to another.

Another rare disease, Buschke-Ollendorff syndrome, can include melorheostosis. Buschke-Ollendorff syndrome is characterized by skin growths called connective tissue nevi and areas of increased bone density called osteopoikilosis. A small percentage of affected individuals also have melorheostosis or other bone abnormalities. Scientists

This chapter contains text excerpted from the following sources: Text in this chapter begins with excerpts from "Melorheostosis," Genetics Home Reference (GHR), National Institutes of Health (NIH), January 22, 2019; Text under the heading "NIH Researchers Crack Mystery behind Rare Bone Disorder" is excerpted from "NIH Researchers Crack Mystery behind Rare Bone Disorder," National Institute of Arthritis and Musculoskeletal and Skin Diseases (NIAMS), April 11, 2018.

originally speculated that melorheostosis that occurs without the other features of Buschke-Ollendorff syndrome might have the same genetic cause as that syndrome. However, it has since been determined that Buschke-Ollendorff syndrome and melorheostosis that occurs alone are caused by mutations in different genes, and the two conditions are considered separate disorders.

Signs and Symptoms

The signs and symptoms of melorheostosis usually appear in childhood or adolescence. The condition can cause long-lasting (chronic) pain, permanent joint deformities (contractures), and a limited range of motion of the affected body part. In some people, the limb may appear thickened or enlarged, and the skin overlying the affected area can become red, thick, and shiny.

Frequency

Melorheostosis affects about 1 in 1 million people. Approximately 400 cases have been reported worldwide.

Causes

Mutations in the *MAP2K1* gene are estimated to cause about half of all cases of melorheostosis. The *MAP2K1* gene provides instructions for making a protein called MEK1 protein kinase. This protein is active in many kinds of cells, including bone cells. It is part of a signaling pathway called RAS/MAPK. This signaling pathway helps control the growth and division (proliferation) of cells, the process by which cells mature to carry out specific functions (differentiation), and cell movement (migration). RAS/MAPK signaling is critical for normal development, including the formation of bones.

The *MAP2K1* gene mutations that cause melorheostosis are somatic, which means that they occur during a person's lifetime and are present only in certain cells, in this case, bone cells in a particular area of the body. The mutations lead to the production of a version of MEK1 protein kinase that is overactive, which increases RAS/MAPK signaling in bone tissue. The increased signaling disrupts the regulation of bone cell proliferation, allowing new bone to grow abnormally. Studies suggest that increased RAS/MAPK signaling also stimulates excess bone remodeling, a normal process in which old bone is broken down and new bone is created to replace it. These changes in bone growth and turnover underlie the bone abnormalities characteristic of melorheostosis.

In cases of melorheostosis without an identified mutation in the *MAP2K1* gene, the cause of the condition is usually unknown. Studies suggest that somatic mutations in other genes, particularly genes related to the RAS/MAPK signaling pathway, may also cause the disorder.

Inheritance Pattern

This condition is not inherited from a parent, and it cannot be passed down to children. It arises from somatic mutations in bone cells that occur during an individual's lifetime.

Study Finds Gene Mutations That Cause "Dripping Candle Wax" Bone Disease

Researchers at the National Institutes of Health (NIH) worked with 15 patients from around the world to uncover a genetic basis for "dripping candle wax" bone disease. The rare disorder, known as melorheostosis, causes excess bone formation that resembles dripping candle wax on X-rays. The results, appearing in *Nature Communications*, offer potential treatment targets for this rare disease, provide important clues about bone development, and may lead to insights about fracture healing and osteoporosis.

Though there are only about 400 known cases of this disorder worldwide, 15 unrelated adults with the condition from around the globe volunteered to come to the NIH Clinical Center to undergo biopsies of both affected and unaffected bones. The condition causes pain and bone deformity, which can limit the function of bones.

"Scientists previously assumed that the genetic mutations responsible for melorheostosis occurred in all cells of a person with the disorder," said co-senior author Timothy Bhattacharyya, M.D., head of the Clinical and Investigative Orthopaedics Surgery Unit at the National Institute of Arthritis and Musculoskeletal and Skin Diseases (NIAMS) at NIH. "Our team hypothesized that mutations might only occur in the affected bone tissue."

Researchers compared samples of healthy and affected bone from each participant to look for differences in the exome, the portion of the genome that codes for proteins. Comparing genetic information from both samples in each patient allowed the team to pinpoint even low levels of the mutations. Experts from NIAMS and the *Eunice Kennedy*

Shriver National Institute of Child Health and Human Development (NICHD) worked together on this study.

The analysis revealed that 8 of the 15 participants had mutations in the *MAP2K1* gene in the affected bone only. *MAP2K1* produces the protein MEK1. The gene *MAP2K1* has previously been linked to some types of cancerous growths as well as to conditions that lead to abnormal blood vessel formation in the head, face, or neck.

In melorheostosis, all the identified *MAP2K1* mutations affect a region of the MEK1 protein that normally suppresses its activity, thus they cause MEK1 to become overactive. The bone growth is considered benign and does not spread to other parts of the body.

"This is an exciting study of a very rare bone disorder that not only identified the responsible mutation in half of the patients, but uncovered fundamental information about the role of a cancer-related gene in the metabolic pathways of normal bone," said study co-senior author Joan Marini, Ph.D., M.D., of NICHD. "When we started, we had no preconceived causative pathways, but the participation of the patients has really changed the scientific landscape on this topic. Further studies on how this pathway works in both normal and mutant bone cells may have broad implications that could benefit a wider population."

"Most adults have the problem of weakening bones as they grow older. These patients have the opposite problem as some of their bones are rock hard and still growing," said Bhattacharyya. "The prospect that we could somehow harness this pathway in the future is so exciting."

Chapter 14

Fibrous Dysplasia

What Is Fibrous Dysplasia?

Fibrous dysplasia happens when healthy bone is replaced with other types of tissue. Bones may become weak, oddly shaped, or even break. You may also feel pain.

The disease can affect any bone in the body. The most common bones affected are in the skull and face, leg bones, upper arm, pelvis, and ribs. Affected bones are often found on one side of the body, although the disease does not spread from one bone to another.

Who Gets Fibrous Dysplasia

Fibrous dysplasia is not common, although anyone can get it. It usually starts in children and young adults. Once a person has the condition, they will have it for the rest of their life.

What Are the Symptoms of Fibrous Dysplasia?

The most common symptoms of fibrous dysplasia include:

- Pain

- Bones that are oddly shaped

This chapter includes text excerpted from "Fibrous Dysplasia," National Institute of Arthritis and Musculoskeletal and Skin Diseases (NIAMS), June 30, 2015. Reviewed January 2019.

- Broken bones, which are more common between the ages of 6 and 10

Other symptoms depend on the bones that are affected and can include:

- Legs of different lengths, leading to a limp
- Sinus problems
- In very rare cases, vision loss or cancer

What Causes Fibrous Dysplasia

Fibrous dysplasia is caused by a problem with a gene that forms bone and other affected tissues. This gene is not inherited from your parents, and you will not pass the disease to your children.

Is There a Test for Fibrous Dysplasia?

To diagnose you with fibrous dysplasia, your doctor may use one or more of the following tests:

- X-rays of your bones
- Magnetic resonance imaging (MRI) or computed tomography (CT)
- Small bone sample

It's not clear whether testing for the problem gene is useful.

How Is Fibrous Dysplasia Treated?

There is no cure for fibrous dysplasia. Doctors will treat the symptoms with treatments such as:

- Casts for broken bones
- Surgery to:
  - Repair broken bones
  - Prevent fracture
  - Correct the shape of a bone
  - Relieve bone pain
- Medications, such as bisphosphonates, that can reduce pain associated with the disease

Living with Fibrous Dysplasia

Besides seeing your doctor, there are a few things you can do to keep your bones healthy:

- **Exercise:** talk to your doctor before beginning an exercise program.

- **Diet:** you should eat foods that are high in calcium, phosphorus, and vitamin D.

Chapter 15

Gaucher Disease

Gaucher disease is an inherited disorder that affects many of the body's organs and tissues. The signs and symptoms of this condition vary widely among affected individuals. Researchers have described several types of Gaucher disease based on their characteristic features.

Types of Gaucher Disease

Type 1 Gaucher disease is the most common form of this condition. Type 1 is also called nonneuronopathic Gaucher disease because the brain and spinal cord (the central nervous system) are usually not affected. The features of this condition range from mild to severe and may appear anytime from childhood to adulthood. Major signs and symptoms include enlargement of the liver and spleen (hepatospleno-megaly), a low number of red blood cells (anemia), easy bruising caused by a decrease in blood platelets (thrombocytopenia), lung disease, and bone abnormalities such as bone pain, fractures, and arthritis.

Types 2 and 3 Gaucher disease are known as neuronopathic forms of the disorder because they are characterized by problems that affect the central nervous system. In addition to the signs and symptoms described above, these conditions can cause abnormal eye movements,

This chapter contains text excerpted from the following sources: Text in this chapter begins with excerpts from "Gaucher Disease," Genetics Home Reference (GHR), National Institutes of Health (NIH), January 22, 2019; Text beginning with the heading "Symptoms" is excerpted from "Gaucher Disease Information Page," National Institute of Neurological Disorders and Stroke (NINDS), September 17, 2018.

seizures, and brain damage. Type 2 Gaucher disease usually causes life-threatening medical problems beginning in infancy. Type 3 Gaucher disease also affects the nervous system, but it tends to worsen more slowly than type 2.

The most severe type of Gaucher disease is called the perinatal lethal form. This condition causes severe or life-threatening complications starting before birth or in infancy. Features of the perinatal lethal form can include extensive swelling caused by fluid accumulation before birth (hydrops fetalis); dry, scaly skin (ichthyosis) or other skin abnormalities; hepatosplenomegaly; distinctive facial features; and serious neurological problems. As its name indicates, most infants with the perinatal lethal form of Gaucher disease survive for only a few days after birth.

Another form of Gaucher disease is known as the cardiovascular type because it primarily affects the heart, causing the heart valves to harden (calcify). People with the cardiovascular form of Gaucher disease may also have eye abnormalities, bone disease, and mild enlargement of the spleen (splenomegaly).

Frequency

Gaucher disease occurs in 1 in 50,000 to 100,000 people in the general population. Type 1 is the most common form of the disorder; it occurs more frequently in people of Ashkenazi (eastern and central European) Jewish heritage than in those with other backgrounds. This form of the condition affects 1 in 500 to 1,000 people of Ashkenazi Jewish heritage. The other forms of Gaucher disease are uncommon and do not occur more frequently in people of Ashkenazi Jewish descent.

Inheritance Pattern

This condition is inherited in an autosomal recessive pattern, which means both copies of the gene in each cell have mutations. The parents of an individual with an autosomal recessive condition each carry one copy of the mutated gene, but they typically do not show signs and symptoms of the condition.

Causes

Mutations in the GBA gene cause Gaucher disease. The GBA gene provides instructions for making an enzyme called beta-glucocerebrosidase. This enzyme breaks down a fatty substance called glucocerebroside into a sugar (glucose) and a simpler fat molecule (ceramide). Mutations in the GBA gene greatly reduce or eliminate the activity of beta-glucocerebrosidase. Without enough of this enzyme, glucocerebroside and related substances can build up to toxic levels within cells. Tissues and organs are damaged by the abnormal accumulation and storage of these substances, causing the characteristic features of Gaucher disease.

Symptoms

General symptoms may begin in early life or adulthood and include skeletal disorders and bone lesions that may cause pain and fractures, enlarged spleen and liver, liver malfunction, anemia, and yellow spots in the eyes.

Treatment

Treatment can prevent or lessen some symptoms of the disease. Enzyme-replacement therapy is available for most people with types one and three Gaucher disease. Given intravenously every two weeks, this therapy decreases liver and spleen size, reduces skeletal abnormalities, and reverses other symptoms of the disorder. The U.S. Food and Drug Administration (FDA) has approved eliglustat tartrate for Gaucher treatment, which works by administering small molecules that reduce the action of the enzyme that catalyzes glucose to ceramide. Surgery to remove part of or the whole spleen may be required on rare occasions, and blood transfusions may benefit some anemic individuals. Other individuals may require joint replacement surgery to improve mobility and quality of life (QOL). There is no effective treatment for the severe brain damage that may occur in persons with types two and three Gaucher disease.

Prognosis

Enzyme-replacement therapy is very beneficial for type one and most type three individuals with this condition. Successful bone-marrow transplantation can reverse the nonneurological effects of the disease, but the procedure carries a high risk and is rarely performed in individuals with Gaucher disease. People with Gaucher disease type one are at increased risk for Parkinson disease and Lewy body dementia. Gaucher disease type two is usually fatal by age two. People with Gaucher type three may have a shortened life expectancy.

Chapter 16

Otosclerosis

What Is Otosclerosis?

"Otosclerosis" is a term derived from "oto," meaning "of the ear," and "sclerosis," meaning "abnormal hardening of body tissue." The condition is caused by abnormal bone remodeling in the middle ear. Bone remodeling is a lifelong process in which bone tissue renews itself by replacing old tissue with new. In otosclerosis, abnormal remodeling disrupts the ability of sound to travel from the middle ear to the inner ear. Otosclerosis affects more than three million Americans. Many cases of otosclerosis are thought to be inherited. White, middle-aged women are most at risk.

How Do We Hear?

Healthy hearing relies on a series of events that change sound waves in the air into electrochemical signals within the ear. The auditory nerve then carries these signals to the brain.

First, sound waves enter the outer ear and travel through a narrow passageway called the ear canal, which leads to the eardrum.

The incoming sound waves make the eardrum vibrate, and the vibrations travel to three tiny bones in the middle ear called the malleus, incus, and stapes—the Latin names for hammer, anvil, and stirrup.

This chapter includes text excerpted from "Otosclerosis," National Institute on Deafness and Other Communication Disorders (NIDCD), July 17, 2018.

The middle-ear bones amplify the sound vibrations and send them to the cochlea, a fluid-filled structure shaped like a snail, in the inner ear. The upper and lower parts of the cochlea are separated by an elastic, "basilar" membrane that serves as the base, or ground floor, upon which key hearing structures sit.

Incoming sound vibrations cause the fluid inside the cochlea to ripple, and a traveling wave forms along the basilar membrane. Hair cells that sit on top of the membrane "ride" this wave and move up and down with it.

The bristly structures of the hair cells then bump up against an overlying membrane, which causes the bristles to tilt to one side and open pore-like channels. Certain chemicals then rush in, creating an electrical signal that is carried by the auditory nerve to the brain. The end result is a recognizable sound.

Hair cells near the base of the cochlea detect higher-pitched sounds, such as a cell phone ringing. Those nearer the middle detect lower-pitched sounds, such as a large dog barking.

What Causes Otosclerosis

Otosclerosis is most often caused when one of the bones in the middle ear, the stapes, becomes stuck in place. When this bone is unable to vibrate, the sound is unable to travel through the ear and hearing becomes impaired.

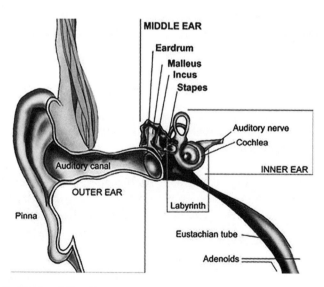

Figure 16.1. *Parts of the Ear*

Why this happens is still unclear, but scientists think it could be related to previous measles infection, stress fractures to the bony tissue surrounding the inner ear, or immune disorders. Otosclerosis also tends to run in families.

It may also have to do with the interaction among three different immune-system cells known as "cytokines." Researchers believe that the proper balance of these three substances is necessary for healthy bone remodeling and that an imbalance in their levels could cause the kind of abnormal remodeling that occurs in otosclerosis.

What Are the Symptoms of Otosclerosis?

Hearing loss, the most frequently reported symptom of otosclerosis, usually starts in one ear and then moves to the other. This loss may appear very gradually. Many people with otosclerosis first notice that they are unable to hear low-pitched sounds or can't hear a whisper. Some people may also experience dizziness, balance problems, or tinnitus. Tinnitus is a ringing, roaring, buzzing, or hissing in the ears or head that sometimes occurs with hearing loss.

How Is Otosclerosis Diagnosed?

Otosclerosis is diagnosed by healthcare providers who specialize in hearing. These include an otolaryngologist (commonly called an ear, nose and throat (ENT) specialist, because they are doctors who specialize in diseases of the ears, nose, throat, and neck), an otologist (a doctor who specializes in diseases of the ears), or an audiologist (a healthcare professional trained to identify, measure, and treat hearing disorders). The first step in diagnosis is to rule out other diseases or health problems that can cause the same symptoms as otosclerosis. Next steps include hearing tests that measure hearing sensitivity (audiogram) and middle-ear sound conduction (tympanogram). Sometimes, imaging tests—such as a computerized tomography (CT) scan—are also used to diagnose otosclerosis.

How Is Otosclerosis Treated?

Currently, there is no effective drug treatment for otosclerosis, although there is hope that continued bone-remodeling research could identify potential new therapies. Mild otosclerosis can be treated with a hearing aid that amplifies sound, but surgery is often required. In a procedure known as a "stapedectomy," a surgeon inserts a prosthetic device into the middle ear to bypass the abnormal bone and permit sound waves to travel to the inner ear and restore hearing.

It is important to discuss any surgical procedure with an ear specialist to clarify the potential risks and limitations of the operation. For example, some hearing loss may persist after stapedectomy, and in rare cases, surgery can actually worsen hearing loss.

Chapter 17

Hypercalcemia

Calcium is one of the essential minerals that gets stored in the hard part of the bones. Our body needs calcium to grow, as well as to strengthen the bones. It also maintains hormone levels, and optimizes nerve function and muscle contraction. However, too much of calcium in your blood will interfere with the way your heart and brain function, create stones in the kidneys, and also weaken your bones. Extremely high levels can be dangerous.

Calcium exists in blood in three forms and the third form mentioned below is the only active form, which our body utilizes for various functions.

- Bound to proteins (such as albumin). It is physiologically inactive.

- Bound to anions (such as phosphate and citrate)

- Unbound (free-ionized calcium). It is physiologically inactive.

Usually, our body regulates the calcium level on its own and the normal level of calcium has been estimated and termed as "normal reference range."

Calcium—Normal Reference Range

Table 17.1. Calcium Reference Range

mmol/L	mg/dL	mg/dL
2.1 to 2.6	8.8 to 10.7	8.8 to 10.7

Two major medical conditions are classified based on the abnormality of calcium level:

- Hypercalcemia–high levels of calcium in the blood

- Hypocalcemia–low levels of calcium in the blood

How Does Our Body Regulate Calcium?

Four small parathyroid glands that are located behind the neck secrete a hormone called "parathyroid hormone" (PTH). This PTH regulates:

- Calcium absorption from our dietary intake along with vitamin D

- Calcium secretion by our kidneys

- Calcium storage in our bones

What Exactly Is Hypercalcemia?

Hypercalcemia is a condition of having a high concentration of calcium in blood as a result of the use of certain medication or other health conditions. Untreated hypercalcemia that persists for a long time leads to complications such as fractures, bone loss, osteoporosis (thinning of the bones), kidney failure, hypertension, and bradycardia (slowed heart rate). These complications were commonly found in the past due to missing or late diagnosis. Nowadays, hypercalcemia is being diagnosed very early by healthcare providers with the help of routine blood work, which is a part of the patient's annual exam.

What Causes Hypercalcemia?

More than 25 separate diseases contribute to the cause of hypercalcemia, but hyperparathyroidism accounts for the greatest percentage. Other factors include certain medications, various types of cancers, and dehydration.

Some of the more common causes include:

- **Hyperparathyroidism**—The previously mentioned parathyroid glands produce PTH, which helps the kidneys, intestines, and skeleton regulate and maintain calcium. Sometimes, these glands become enlarged and overactive, and produces excess hormones, which, in turn, cause elevation of calcium in the blood.

- **Medication side effects**—Certain medications such as thiazide diuretics (prescribed for hypertension and edema: e.g., hydrochlorothiazide, lithium, etc.) cause hypercalcemia.

- **Dietary supplements**—Increased intake of calcium, vitamin D (obtained primarily when skin is exposed to sunlight and also from dietary sources), or vitamin A supplements can also cause hypercalcemia.

- **Over-the-counter (OTC) medications**—Taking a large amount of calcium carbonate in the form of Tums® or Rolaids® is also a major cause of hypercalcemia.

- **Hereditary factors**—Familial hypocalciuric hypercalcemia is a rare genetic disorder causing high levels of calcium in the blood due to faulty calcium receptors, and this condition does not cause any symptoms or complications of hypercalcemia.

Some of the less common causes include:

- Hyperthyroidism (overactive thyroid)

- Kidney failure

- Multiple myelomas

- Paget disease of bone

- Lung diseases such as sarcoidosis and tuberculosis

- Being bed-bound or immobilized for a relatively short period

What Are Signs and Symptoms of Hypercalcemia?

One might not observe any signs or symptoms if the hypercalcemia is mild, only moderate-to-severe cases experience symptoms. When blood containing high calcium concentration is supplied to organs such as the brain, heart, kidney, and so on., it interferes with the way the organ works, which in turn causes the following symptoms.

- **Brain**—Confusion, lethargy, fatigue, memory loss, or irritability, and even depression in some cases

- **Heart**—Fainting, palpitations, bradycardia (slowed heart beat), cardiac arrhythmia, and other heart problems

- **Digestive system**—Nausea, vomiting, a decrease in appetite, stomach upset, and constipation

- **Kidney**—Difficulty in filtering the excess calcium in the blood leading to polydipsia (excessive thirst) and polyuria (frequent urination)

- **Bones and muscles**—When PTH demands calcium, a high amount of calcium is supplied to the blood from the bones, which leads to osteoporosis—which in turn can cause weakness and pain in the bones and muscles

How Is Hypercalcemia Diagnosed?

- To determine if you have hypercalcemia, your healthcare provider will order a blood test and urinalysis (analyzing the presence of calcium in the urine). These recommended lab orders include:

  - Serum calcium

  - Serum PTH

  - Serum PTHrP (PTH-related protein)

  - Serum vitamin D level

  - Urine calcium

- If your result shows elevated calcium, the physician will often conduct a physical exam, review your medical history and medications, and then sometimes ask you to see an endocrinologist (a doctor who specializes in treating hormonal disorders) for further evaluation and testing.

- To determine if your parathyroid hormone (PTH) level is high, indicating hyperparathyroidism (which is one of the main causes of hypercalcemia), your endocrinologist may order a blood test.

- To determine if your hypercalcemia is secondary to other medical conditions such as cancer or sarcoidosis, your healthcare provider may recommend imaging tests of your bones, as well as lungs.

How Hypercalcemia Is Treated?

As with other medical conditions, treatment of hypercalcemia depends on the cause and severity of the condition. If you have a mild elevation of calcium, your healthcare provider may suggest that you:

- Keep yourself hydrated
- Switch to a nonthiazide blood-pressure medicine or diuretic
- Discontinue over-the-counter (OTC) calcium supplements
- Discontinue calcium-rich antacid tablets

If your calcium elevation is found to be secondary to hyperparathyroidism, your healthcare provider may suggest:

- Ordering blood tests at regular intervals to closely monitor your calcium levels
- That a referral be made for surgical removal of the overactive thyroid gland
- Medication trials with cinacalcet (Sensipar®), diuretics such as frusemide and steroids such as glucocorticoids

If your hypercalcemia is secondary to cancer, your healthcare provider may suggest:

- Intravenous bisphosphonates and osteoporosis drug trials
- If you do not respond to bisphosphonates, bone-strengthening drugs such as denosumab (XGEVA®) can be used to achieve some amount of calcemic control

If you become symptomatic with severe hypercalcemia, your healthcare provider may suggest:

- Immediate hospitalization for intravenous (IV) fluids
- Dialysis if kidney damage is involved

How Can You Prepare for Your Appointment?

Make a list of the following, which can help with diagnosing your condition appropriately.

143

- Your symptoms, and when they began, (e.g., bone pain, unexplained weight loss, fatigue, and so on)

- Key stressors, which include recent major life changes, past and present medical illnesses (e.g., a history of kidney stones, bone fractures, or previous diagnosis of osteoporosis), and your family medical history, especially the history of hypercalcemia or kidney stones in any family members

- Medication intake with dosage amounts (and be sure to note any recent supplementary and dietary changes)

What Questions You Can Ask Your Doctor?

- What tests do I need?

- What could be the most likely cause of my symptoms?

- What are the available treatment options?

- What would be your recommend if I test positive?

- What are the possible side effects I can expect from the treatment?

- Is there an alternative approach?

- How can I best manage this along with my other health conditions?

How Can You Prevent Hypercalcemia?

- Do not take any OTC calcium/vitamin D supplements

- Check with your family physician or healthcare provider and make sure that you are taking correct doses of vitamin D and calcium supplements

- Women above age 60 should have their calcium levels checked regularly to make sure they are not developing hypercalcemia or hypocalcemia, which can also help them to monitor their bone health

With all that being said, most of the causes of hypercalcemia cannot be prevented. So once you experience symptoms, contact your physician for further evaluation—and the sooner the better.

References

1. "Hypercalcemia Discharge," U.S. National Library of Medicine (NLM), January 7, 2019.

2. "Health Encyclopedia," FloridaHealthFinder.gov, February 3, 2016.

3. "Hypercalcemia," Cleveland Clinic, July 2, 2018.

4. "Hypercalcemia," Mayo Clinic, March 6, 2018.

Chapter 18

Hypocalcemia

Autosomal dominant hypocalcemia is characterized by low levels of calcium in the blood (hypocalcemia). Affected individuals can have an imbalance of other molecules in the blood as well, including too much phosphate (hyperphosphatemia) or too little magnesium (hypomagnesemia). Some people with autosomal dominant hypocalcemia also have low levels of a hormone called parathyroid hormone (hypoparathyroidism). This hormone is involved in the regulation of calcium levels in the blood. Abnormal levels of calcium and other molecules in the body can lead to a variety of signs and symptoms, although about half of affected individuals have no associated health problems.

The most common features of autosomal dominant hypocalcemia include muscle spasms in the hands and feet (carpopedal spasms) and muscle cramping, prickling or tingling sensations (paresthesias), or twitching of the nerves and muscles (neuromuscular irritability) in various parts of the body. More severely affected individuals develop seizures, usually in infancy or childhood. Sometimes, these symptoms occur only during episodes of illness or fever.

Some people with autosomal dominant hypocalcemia have high levels of calcium in their urine (hypercalciuria), which can lead to

This chapter contains text excerpted from the following sources: Text in this chapter begins with excerpts from "Autosomal Dominant Hypocalcemia," Genetics Home Reference (GHR), National Institutes of Health (NIH), January 22, 2019; Text under the heading "Management and Treatment" is excerpted from " Hypocalcemia, Autosomal Dominant," Genetic and Rare Diseases Information Center (GARD), National Center for Advancing Translational Sciences (NCATS), May 13, 2014. Reviewed January 2019.

deposits of calcium in the kidneys (nephrocalcinosis) or the formation of kidney stones (nephrolithiasis). These conditions can damage the kidneys and impair their function. Sometimes, abnormal deposits of calcium form in the brain, typically in structures called basal ganglia, which help control movement.

A small percentage of severely affected individuals have features of a kidney disorder called Bartter syndrome in addition to hypocalcemia. These features can include a shortage of potassium (hypokalemia) and magnesium and a buildup of the hormone aldosterone (hyper-aldosteronism) in the blood. The abnormal balance of molecules can raise the pH of the blood, which is known as metabolic alkalosis. The combination of features of these two conditions is sometimes referred to as autosomal dominant hypocalcemia with Bartter syndrome or Bartter syndrome type V.

There are two types of autosomal dominant hypocalcemia distinguished by their genetic cause. The signs and symptoms of the two types are generally the same.

Frequency

The prevalence of autosomal dominant hypocalcemia is unknown. The condition is likely underdiagnosed because it often causes no signs or symptoms.

Causes

Autosomal dominant hypocalcemia is primarily caused by mutations in the *CASR* gene; these cases are known as type 1. A small percentage of cases, known as type 2, are caused by mutations in the *GNA11* gene. The proteins produced from these genes work together to regulate the amount of calcium in the blood.

The *CASR* gene provides instructions for making a protein called the calcium-sensing receptor (CaSR). Calcium molecules attach (bind) to the CaSR protein, which allows this protein to monitor and regulate the amount of calcium in the blood. $G\alpha_{11}$, which is produced from the *GNA11* gene, is one component of a signaling protein that works in conjunction with CaSR. When a certain concentration of calcium is reached, CaSR stimulates $G\alpha_{11}$ to send signals to block processes that increase the amount of calcium in the blood.

Mutations in the CASR or GNA11 gene lead to overactivity of the respective protein. The altered CaSR protein is more sensitive to calcium, meaning even low levels of calcium can trigger it to stimulate

$G\alpha_{11}$ signaling. Similarly, the altered $G\alpha_{11}$ protein continues to send signals to prevent calcium increases, even when levels in the blood are very low. As a result, calcium levels in the blood remain low, causing hypocalcemia. Calcium plays an important role in the control of muscle movement, and a shortage of this molecule can lead to cramping or twitching of the muscles. Impairment of the processes that increase calcium can also disrupt the normal regulation of other molecules, such as phosphate and magnesium, leading to other signs of autosomal dominant hypocalcemia. Studies show that the lower the amount of calcium in the blood, the more severe the symptoms of the condition are.

Inheritance Pattern

This condition is inherited in an autosomal dominant pattern, which means one copy of the altered gene in each cell is sufficient to cause the disorder.

In most cases, an affected person inherits the mutation from one affected parent. A small number of cases result from new mutations in the gene and occur in people with no history of the disorder in their family.

Management and Treatment

Treatment to normalize calcemia levels should be considered with caution, as any increase in calcium levels (even within the normal range) will be perceived by renal cells as hypercalcemia and lead to increased urinary calcium excretion, and possibly to nephrocalcinosis and renal failure. Treatment should aim towards finding a balance between the clinical signs of hypocalcemia and maintenance of calcium homeostasis, without being iatrogenic. Urine calcium levels should be monitored in order to avoid hypercalciuria rather than adapting treatment towards hypocalcemia. In asymptomatic and mildly symptomatic patients, treatment may not be necessary. Special care must be given to children as chronic hypocalcemia has deleterious effects on intellectual development. Treatment is based on administration of 1-alpha hydroxylated vitamin D (doses ranging from 0.5 to 1.5 micrograms/day in adults; higher doses are sometimes required in children). Careful monitoring of calciuria and regular kidney ultrasound are required. In cases where calcium homeostasis is difficult to achieve, exogenous parathyroid hormone (PTH) administered by infusion pump can be proposed.

Chapter 19

Hyperparathyroidism

What Is Primary Hyperparathyroidism?

Primary hyperparathyroidism is a disorder of the parathyroid glands, also called "parathyroids." "Primary" means this disorder originates in the parathyroid glands. In primary hyperparathyroidism, one or more of the parathyroid glands are overactive. As a result, the gland releases too much parathyroid hormone (PTH). The disorder includes the problems that occur in the rest of the body as a result of too much PTH—for example, loss of calcium from bones. In the United States, about 100,000 people develop primary hyperparathyroidism each year. The disorder is diagnosed most often in people between age 50 and 60, and women are affected about three times as often as men.

Secondary, or reactive, hyperparathyroidism can occur if a problem such as kidney failure causes the parathyroid glands to be overactive.

What Are the Parathyroid Glands?

The parathyroid glands are four pea-sized glands located on or near the thyroid gland in the neck. Occasionally, a person is born with one or more of the parathyroid glands in another location. For example, a gland may be embedded in the thyroid, in the thymus—an immune

This chapter includes text excerpted from "Primary Hyperparathyroidism," National Institute of Diabetes and Digestive and Kidney Diseases (NIDDK), August 2012. Reviewed January 2019.

system organ located in the chest—or elsewhere around this area. In most such cases, however, the parathyroid glands function normally.

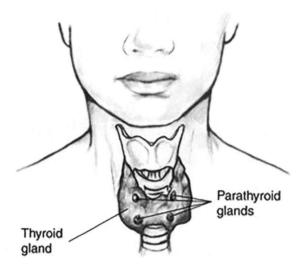

Figure 19.1. *Thyroid and Parathyroid Glands*

The parathyroid glands are located on or near the thyroid gland in the neck.

The parathyroid glands are part of the body's endocrine system. Endocrine glands produce, store, and release hormones, which travel in the bloodstream to target cells elsewhere in the body and direct the cells' activity.

Though their names are similar, the thyroid and parathyroid glands are entirely different glands, each producing distinct hormones with specific functions. The parathyroid glands produce PTH, a hormone that helps maintain the correct balance of calcium in the body. PTH regulates the level of calcium in the blood, release of calcium from bone, absorption of calcium in the small intestine, and excretion of calcium in the urine.

When the level of calcium in the blood falls too low, normal parathyroid glands release just enough PTH to restore the blood calcium level.

What Are the Effects of High Parathyroid-Hormone Levels?

High PTH levels trigger the bones to release increased amounts of calcium into the blood, causing blood calcium levels to rise above normal. The loss of calcium from bones may weaken the bones. Also, the small intestine may absorb more calcium from food, adding to the excess calcium in the blood. In response to high blood calcium levels, the kidneys excrete more calcium in the urine, which can lead to kidney stones.

High blood calcium levels might contribute to other problems, such as heart disease, high blood pressure, and difficulty with concentration. However, more research is needed to better understand how primary hyperparathyroidism affects the cardiovascular system—the heart and blood vessels—and the central nervous system—the brain and spinal cord.

Why Is Calcium Important?

Calcium is essential for good health. Calcium plays an important role in bone and tooth development and, combined with phosphorus, strengthens bones and teeth. Calcium also helps muscles contract and nerves transmit signals.

What Causes Primary Hyperparathyroidism

In about 80 percent of people with primary hyperparathyroidism, a benign, or noncancerous, tumor called an "adenoma" forms in one of the parathyroid glands. The tumor causes the gland to become overactive. In most other cases, the excess hormone comes from two or more overactive parathyroid glands, a condition called "multiple tumors" or "hyperplasia." Rarely, primary hyperparathyroidism is caused by cancer of a parathyroid gland.

In most cases, healthcare providers don't know why adenoma or multiple tumors occur in the parathyroid glands. Most people with primary hyperparathyroidism have no family history of the disorder, but some cases can be linked to an inherited problem. For example, familial multiple endocrine neoplasia type one is a rare, inherited syndrome that causes multiple tumors in the parathyroid glands as well as in the pancreas and the pituitary gland. Another rare genetic disorder, familial hypocalciuric hypercalcemia (FHH), causes a kind of hyperparathyroidism that is atypical, in part because it does not respond to standard parathyroid surgery.

What Are the Symptoms of Primary Hyperparathyroidism?

Most people with primary hyperparathyroidism have no symptoms. When symptoms appear, they are often mild and nonspecific, such as:

- Muscle weakness
- Fatigue and an increased need for sleep
- Feelings of depression
- Aches and pains in bones and joints

People with more severe disease may have:

- Loss of appetite
- Nausea
- Vomiting
- Constipation
- Confusion or impaired thinking and memory
- Increased thirst and urination

These symptoms are mainly due to the high blood calcium levels that result from excessive PTH.

How Is Primary Hyperparathyroidism Diagnosed?

Healthcare providers diagnose primary hyperparathyroidism when a person has high blood calcium and PTH levels. High blood calcium is usually the first sign that leads healthcare providers to suspect parathyroid gland overactivity. Other diseases can cause high blood calcium levels, but only in primary hyperparathyroidism is the elevated calcium the result of too much PTH.

Routine blood tests that screen for a wide range of conditions, including high blood calcium levels, are helping healthcare providers diagnose primary hyperparathyroidism in people who have mild forms of the disorder and are symptom-free. For a blood test, blood is drawn at a healthcare provider's office or commercial facility and sent to a lab for analysis.

What Tests May Be Done to Check for Possible Complications?

Once the diagnosis of primary hyperparathyroidism is established, other tests may be done to assess complications:

- **Bone mineral density (BMD) test.** Dual-energy X-ray absorptiometry (DXA), sometimes called a "DXA" or "DEXA" scan uses low-dose X-rays to measure bone density. During the test, a person lies on a padded table while a technician moves the scanner over the person's body. DXA scans are performed in a healthcare provider's office, outpatient center, or hospital by a specially trained technician and may be interpreted by a metabolic bone disease expert or radiologist—a doctor who specializes in medical imaging—or other specialists; anesthesia is not needed. The test can help assess bone loss and risk of fractures.

- **Ultrasound.** Ultrasound uses a device, called a "transducer," that bounces safe, painless sound waves off organs to create an image of their structure. The procedure is performed in a healthcare provider's office, outpatient center, or hospital by a specially trained technician, and the images are interpreted by a radiologist; anesthesia is not needed. The images can show the presence of kidney stones.

- **Computerized tomography (CT) scan.** CT scans use a combination of X-rays and computer technology to create three-dimensional (3-D) images. A CT scan may include the injection of a special dye, called "contrast medium." CT scans require the person to lie on a table that slides into a tunnel-shaped device where the X-rays are taken. The procedure is performed in an outpatient center or hospital by an X-ray technician, and the images are interpreted by a radiologist; anesthesia is not needed. CT scans can show the presence of kidney stones.

- **Urine collection.** A 24-hour urine collection may be done to measure selected chemicals, such as calcium and creatinine, which is a waste product healthy kidneys remove. The person collects urine over a 24-hour period, and the urine is sent to a laboratory for analysis. The urine collection may provide information on kidney damage, the risk of kidney stone formation, and the risk of familial hypocalciuric hypercalcemia.

- **25-hydroxyvitamin D blood test.** This test is recommended because vitamin D deficiency is common in people with primary hyperparathyroidism.

How Is Primary Hyperparathyroidism Treated?
Surgery

Surgery to remove the overactive parathyroid gland or glands is the only definitive treatment for the disorder, particularly if the patient has a very high blood calcium level or has had a fracture or a kidney stone. In patients without any symptoms, guidelines are used to identify who might benefit from parathyroid surgery.

When performed by experienced endocrine surgeons, surgery cures primary hyperparathyroidism in more than 95 percent of operations.

Surgeons often use imaging tests before surgery to locate the overactive gland to be removed. The most commonly used tests are sestamibi and ultrasound scans. In a sestamibi scan, the patient receives an injection of a small amount of radioactive dye that is absorbed by overactive parathyroid glands. The overactive glands can then be viewed using a special camera. Surgeons use two main strategies to remove the overactive gland or glands:

- **Minimally invasive parathyroidectomy (MIP).** This type of surgery, which can be done on an outpatient basis, may be used when only one of the parathyroid glands is likely to be overactive. Guided by a tumor-imaging test, the surgeon makes a small incision in the neck to remove the gland. The small incision means that patients typically have less pain and a quicker recovery than with more invasive surgery. Local or general anesthesia may be used for this type of surgery.

- **Standard neck exploration.** This type of surgery involves a larger incision that allows the surgeon to access and examine all four parathyroid glands and remove the overactive ones. This type of surgery is more extensive and typically requires a hospital stay of one to two days. Surgeons use this approach if they plan to inspect more than one gland. General anesthesia is used for this type of surgery.

Almost all people with primary hyperparathyroidism who have symptoms can benefit from surgery. Experts believe that those without symptoms but who meet guidelines for surgery will also benefit from surgery. Surgery can lead to improved bone density and fewer fractures and can reduce the chance of forming kidney stones. Other potential benefits are being studied by researchers.

Surgery for primary hyperparathyroidism has a complication rate of one to three percent when performed by experienced endocrine surgeons. Rarely, patients undergoing surgery experience damage to the nerves controlling the vocal cords, which can affect speech. A small number of patients lose all their healthy parathyroid tissue and thus develop chronic low calcium levels, requiring lifelong treatment with calcium and some form of vitamin D. This complication is called "hypoparathyroidism." The complication rate is slightly higher for operations on multiple tumors than for a single adenoma because more extensive surgery is needed.

People with primary hyperparathyroidism due to familial hypocalciuric hypercalcemia should not have surgery.

Monitoring

Some people who have mild primary hyperparathyroidism may not need immediate or even any surgery and can be safely monitored. People may wish to talk with their healthcare provider about long-term monitoring if they:

- Are symptom-free

- Have only slightly elevated blood calcium levels

- Have normal kidneys and bone density

Long-term monitoring should include periodic clinical evaluations, annual serum calcium measurements, annual serum creatinine measurements to check kidney function, and bone density measurements every one to two years.

Vitamin D deficiency should be corrected if present. Patients who are monitored need not restrict calcium in their diets.

If the patient and healthcare provider choose long-term monitoring, the patient should:

- Drink plenty of water

- Exercise regularly

- Avoid certain diuretics, such as thiazides

Either immobilization—the inability to move due to illness or injury—or gastrointestinal illness with vomiting or diarrhea that leads to dehydration can cause blood calcium levels to rise further in someone with primary hyperparathyroidism. People with primary hyperparathyroidism should seek medical attention if they find themselves immobilized or dehydrated due to vomiting or diarrhea.

Medications

Calcimimetics are a new class of medications that decrease parathyroid gland secretion of PTH. The calcimimetic cinacalcet (Sensipar), has been approved by the U.S. Food and Drug Administration (FDA) for the treatment of secondary hyperparathyroidism caused by dialysis—a blood-filtering treatment for kidney failure—and primary hyperparathyroidism caused by parathyroid cancer. Cinacalcet has also been approved for the management of hypercalcemia associated with primary hyperparathyroidism.

A number of other medications are being studied to learn whether they may be helpful in treating primary hyperparathyroidism. These medications include bisphosphonates and selective estrogen receptor modulators (SERMs).

Which Healthcare Providers Specialize in Treating Primary Hyperparathyroidism

Primary hyperparathyroidism is treated by endocrinologists—doctors who specialize in hormonal problems—and nephrologists—doctors who specialize in kidney disorders. Surgery for primary hyperparathyroidism is generally performed by endocrine surgeons; head and neck surgeons; and ear, nose, and throat (ENT) surgeons. Organizations that help people with primary hyperparathyroidism may have additional information to assist in finding a qualified healthcare provider nearby.

Eating, Diet, and Nutrition

Eating, diet, and nutrition have not been shown to play a role in causing or preventing primary hyperparathyroidism.

Vitamin D. Experts suggest correcting vitamin D deficiency in people with primary hyperparathyroidism to achieve a serum level of 25-hydroxyvitamin D greater than 20 nanograms per deciliter (50 nanomoles per liter). Research is ongoing to determine optimal doses and regimens of vitamin D supplementation for people with primary hyperparathyroidism. For the healthy public, the Institute of Medicine (IOM) guidelines for vitamin D intake are:

- People ages 1 to 70 years may require 600 International Units (IUs)

- People age 71 and older may require as much as 800 IUs

The IOM also recommends that no more than 4,000 IUs of vitamin D be taken per day.

Calcium. People with primary hyperparathyroidism without symptoms who are being monitored do not need to restrict calcium in their diet. People with low calcium levels due to loss of all parathyroid tissue from surgery will need to take calcium supplements for the rest of their life. To help ensure coordinated and safe care, people should discuss their use of complementary and alternative medicine practices, including their use of dietary supplements, with their healthcare provider. Tips for talking with healthcare providers are available through the National Center for Complementary and Integrative Health (NCCIH).

Chapter 20

Hypophosphatasia

Hypophosphatasia (HPP) is a genetic condition that causes abnormal development of the bones and teeth. The severity of HPP can vary widely, from fetal death to fractures that don't begin until adulthood. Signs and symptoms may include poor feeding and respiratory problems in infancy; short stature; weak and soft bones; short limbs; other skeletal abnormalities; and hypercalcemia. Complications can be life-threatening.

The mildest form of the condition, called "odontohypophosphatasia" (odonto-HPP), only affects the teeth. HPP is caused by mutations in the *ALPL* (Alkaline Phosphatase, Liver/Bone/Kidney) gene. Perinatal (onset before birth) and infantile HPP are inherited in an autosomal recessive manner. The milder forms, especially adult forms and odontohypophosphatasia, may be inherited in an autosomal recessive or autosomal dominant manner. While treatment has always been symptomatic and supportive, recently enzyme-replacement therapy (ERT) called "asfotase alfa" has been shown to improve bone manifestations in people with childhood-onset HPP and has been approved by the U.S. Food and Drug Administration (FDA).

Signs and Symptoms

The signs and symptoms of hypophosphatasia vary widely and can appear anywhere from before birth to adulthood. The most severe

This chapter includes text excerpted from "Hypophosphatasia," Genetic and Rare Diseases Information Center (GARD), National Center for Advancing Translational Sciences (NCATS), February 1, 2016.

forms of the disorder tend to occur before birth and in early infancy. Hypophosphatasia weakens and softens the bones, causing skeletal abnormalities similar to another childhood bone disorder called "rickets." Affected infants are born with short limbs, an abnormally shaped chest, and soft skull bones. Additional complications in infancy include poor feeding and a failure to gain weight, respiratory problems, and high levels of calcium in the blood (hypercalcemia), which can lead to recurrent vomiting and kidney problems. These complications are life-threatening in some cases.

The forms of hypophosphatasia that appear in childhood or adulthood are typically less severe than those that appear in infancy. Early loss of primary (baby) teeth is one of the first signs of the condition in children. Affected children may have short stature with bowed legs or knock knees, enlarged wrist and ankle joints, and an abnormal skull shape. Adult forms of hypophosphatasia are characterized by a softening of the bones known as "osteomalacia." In adults, recurrent fractures in the foot and thigh bones can lead to chronic pain. Affected adults may lose their secondary (adult) teeth prematurely and are at increased risk for joint pain and inflammation.

The mildest form of this condition, called "odontohypophosphatasia," only affects the teeth. People with this disorder typically experience abnormal tooth development and premature tooth loss, but do not have the skeletal abnormalities seen in other forms of hypophosphatasia.

The below table lists symptoms that people with this disease may have. For most diseases, symptoms will vary from person to person. People with the same disease may not have all the symptoms listed. This information comes from a database called the "Human Phenotype Ontology" (HPO). The HPO collects information on symptoms that have been described in medical resources. The HPO is updated regularly. Use the HPO ID to access more in-depth information about a symptom.

Table 20.1. Signs and Symptoms of Hypophosphatasia

Medical Terms	Other Names
80 to 99% of people have these symptoms	
Abnormality of the dentition	Abnormal dentition; abnormal teeth; dental abnormalities; dental abnormality
Abnormality of the metaphysis	Abnormality of the wide portion of a long bone

Table 20.1. Continued

Medical Terms	Other Names
80 to 99% of people have these symptoms	
Abnormality of the ribs	Rib abnormalities
Bowing of the long bones	Bowed long bones; bowing of long bones
Craniosynostosis	
Emphysema	
Failure to thrive in infancy	Faltering weight in infancy; weight faltering in infancy
Feeding difficulties in infancy	
Large fontanelles	Wide fontanelles
Narrow chest	Low chest circumference; narrow shoulders
Short stature	Decreased body height; small stature
Skin dimple over apex of long bone angulation	
30 to 79% of people have these symptoms	
Anemia	Low number of red blood cells or hemoglobin
Hypercalcemia	High blood calcium levels; increased calcium in blood
Irritability	Irritable
Muscular hypotonia	Low or weak muscle tone
Recurrent fractures	Increased fracture rate; increased fractures; multiple fractures; multiple spontaneous fractures; varying degree of multiple fractures
Respiratory insufficiency	Respiratory impairment
Seizures	Seizure

Cause

Hypophosphatasia is a genetic condition caused by mutations in the *ALPL* gene. This gene gives the body instructions to make an enzyme called "alkaline phosphatase" (ALP), which is needed for mineralization of the bones and teeth. Mutations in this gene lead to an abnormal version of the enzyme, thus affecting the mineralization process. A shortage of the enzyme also causes other substances to build up in the body. These abnormalities lead to the features of HPP.

ALPL mutations that almost completely eliminate alkaline phosphatase activity generally cause the more severe forms of HPP, while mutations that reduce activity to a lesser extent often cause the milder forms of HPP.

Inheritance

Perinatal (onset before birth) and infantile hypophosphatasia are inherited in an autosomal recessive manner. This means that to be affected, a person must have a mutation in both copies of the responsible gene (*ALPL*) in each cell. Affected people inherit one mutated copy of the gene from each parent, who is referred to as a carrier. Carriers of an autosomal recessive condition typically do not have any signs or symptoms (i.e., they are unaffected). When two carriers of an autosomal recessive condition have children, each child has a:

- 25 percent (1 in 4) chance to be affected

- 50 percent (1 in 2) chance to be an unaffected carrier like each parent

- 25 percent chance to be unaffected and not be a carrier

The milder forms, especially adult HPP and odontohypophosphatasia, may be inherited in an autosomal recessive or autosomal dominant manner—depending on the effect the *ALPL* mutation has on enzyme activity. In autosomal dominant inheritance, having a mutation in only one copy of the *ALPL* gene in each cell is enough to cause features of the condition. When a person with a mutation that causes an autosomal dominant HPP has children, each child has a 50 percent (1 in 2) chance to inherit that mutation.

Most people with autosomal dominant HPP have inherited the mutation from a parent who may or may not have symptoms. Not all people with a mutation that causes autosomal dominant HPP develop symptoms of the condition. While it is possible to have autosomal dominant HPP due to a new mutation that was not inherited, this has never been reported in HPP.

Treatment

Until recently, management of hypophosphatasia has mostly been aimed at addressing symptoms of the condition. For example:

- Hydration, restriction of dietary calcium, vitamin D, and sometimes thiazide diuretics for hypercalcemia

- Ventilatory support for severely affected infants, some of which need a tracheostomy, which can lead to problems with speech and language development and tolerance of oral feeds

- Physiotherapy, occupational therapy, and chronic-pain management for pain and motor difficulty

- Surgery for fractures that fail to heal

More recently, research has shown positive effects of human recombinant enzyme replacement therapy (ERT), called asfotase alfa, on people who began having symptoms before six months of age. There reportedly have been significant improvements in the X-ray appearances of bone tissue, along with improvements in growth, respiratory function, motor development, and calcium homeostasis after 6 to 12 months of treatment. The children in the original study have now received more than three years of treatment, without apparent major side effects, and with continuing improvement in affected systems. Asfotase alfa appears to be a valuable emerging therapy for the treatment of bone manifestations in people with pediatric-onset HPP. In October 2015, the FDA approved asfotase alfa, sold as Strensiq.

Bone-marrow and stem-cell transplantation in infancy and childhood have improved the severity of the disease, but have not provided long-term improvement.

Related Diseases

Related diseases are conditions that have similar signs and symptoms. A healthcare provider may consider these conditions when making a diagnosis.

Chapter 21

Inflammatory Bowel Disease

What Is Inflammatory Bowel Disease?

Inflammatory bowel disease (IBD) is the name for a group of conditions that cause the digestive system to become inflamed (red, swollen, and sometimes painful). The most common types of IBD are ulcerative colitis and Crohn disease. These cause similar symptoms, including diarrhea, abdominal pain, and fever. IBD affects women in unique ways. IBD symptoms can get worse during your menstrual period and can cause problems getting pregnant.

Your digestive system runs from your mouth to your anus. If your digestive system is healthy, food moves smoothly through your digestive system and out of your body. Your body absorbs the nutrients it needs from food. The rest passes through your body and leaves as urine (pee) or stool (poop).

If you have IBD, part of your digestive system is inflamed. Over time, the inflammation can cause severe pain, diarrhea, and sometimes bloody stool. IBD symptoms come and go in episodes or flares. Because of the inflammation in your digestive system from IBD, your body cannot absorb all of the nutrients it needs. This can lead to

This chapter includes text excerpted from "Inflammatory Bowel Disease," Office on Women's Health (OWH), U.S. Department of Health and Human Services (HHS), November 21, 2018.

malnutrition, other symptoms of IBD, or other health problems, such as anemia.

What Are the Different Types of Inflammatory Bowel Disease?

The most common types of IBD are ulcerative colitis and Crohn disease. The diseases are similar but affect different parts of the digestive system.

- Ulcerative colitis (UC) affects the large intestine and rectum. The disease causes swelling and tiny open sores, or ulcers, on the surface of the lining of the large intestine or rectum. The ulcers can bleed and produce pus. With ulcerative colitis, there is a continuous area of damage along the large intestine and rectum rather than patches of damage.

- Crohn disease can affect any part of the digestive system, from the mouth to the anus. Inflammation in Crohn disease often happens in patches on digestive organs such as the stomach or intestines. With Crohn disease, there is normal tissue next to an inflamed area, or patches of damage.

Who Gets Inflammatory Bowel Disease

More than three million people in the United States have IBD. IBD is more common in people who are over age 45.

Are You at Risk of Inflammatory Bowel Disease?

Yes. Your risk of IBD is higher if you:

- Are Hispanic or non-Hispanic white. In the past, studies have shown that non-Hispanic black people have the lowest rates, although recent studies have found that IBD is increasing in people who are African-American or Hispanic.

- Are Jewish of European descent (Ashkenazi)

- Smoke. If you smoke, you are more likely to get Crohn disease.

- Have a family member with IBD. Researchers think certain genes you inherit from family members may cause the immune systems in people with IBD to overreact and may cause pain and inflammation.

What Are the Symptoms of Inflammatory Bowel Disease

The symptoms of IBD are often similar for ulcerative colitis and Crohn disease. Symptoms include:

- Diarrhea (often loose and watery with Crohn disease or bloody with ulcerative colitis)
- Severe or chronic cramping pain in the abdomen
- Loss of appetite, leading to weight loss
- Fatigue
- Fever
- Rectal bleeding
- Joint pain
- Skin problems, such as rashes

Symptoms can range from mild to severe. Your symptoms can sometimes go away for months or even years (called "remission") before coming back (called a "flare-up").

What Causes Inflammatory Bowel Disease

Researchers do not know exactly what causes IBD. The body's immune (defense) system may trigger IBD. Usually, the immune system protects the body from infections caused by viruses or bacteria (germs). Once the infection is gone, that part of the immune system "shuts off" until it is needed again.

But in people with IBD, the immune system may overreact to normal bacteria in the digestive system. Once the immune system starts, it does not shut off when it should. Over time, this leads to inflammation, which damages the digestive system.

While researchers do not know why IBD starts, some studies suggest that the risk of developing IBD may be higher for women who take antibiotics, birth control pills, or nonsteroidal anti-inflammatories (NSAIDs), such as aspirin or ibuprofen.

Stress does not cause IBD. But it may make IBD symptoms worse.

How Is Inflammatory Bowel Disease Diagnosed?

If you think you have inflammatory bowel disease (IBD), talk to your doctor or nurse. Your doctor will ask you questions about your symptoms and do tests to find out whether you have IBD and, if so, which type.

Some tests used to diagnose IBD include:

- **Blood tests.** Your doctor will send a blood sample to a lab to test for inflammation, other signs of IBD, or anemia.

- **Stool (poop) sample**. Your doctor will send a sample of stool to test for blood and other signs of inflammation related to IBD.

- **Colonoscopy or sigmoidoscopy.** For both of these tests, doctors insert a long, thin tube with a lighted camera into the anus while you are under sedation (unconscious). The image appears on a screen. During a sigmoidoscopy, your doctor looks at the lining of the lower part of your large intestine. During a colonoscopy, your doctor looks at the lining of the entire large intestine and sometimes a small part of the small intestine. Your doctor looks for any inflammation, bleeding, or ulcers. During the exam, your doctor may do a biopsy to take a tissue sample from the lining of the digestive tract and view it under a microscope.

- **Upper endoscopy.** While you are under light sedation, your doctor puts an endoscope, a flexible tube with a camera, through the esophagus (food pipe) and stomach and into the small intestine to look at its lining. Your doctor may take a sample of tissue during this procedure.

- **Small bowel follow-through.** You will drink a liquid that contains a special dye that shows up on X-rays. As the dye moves from the stomach to the intestine, a radiologist will take X-rays to look for problems. This procedure is sometimes done after an upper endoscopy.

- **Computerized axial tomography (CT scan).** A CT scan takes X-rays from several different angles around your body. Your doctor studies the X-rays for signs of inflammation.

- **CT or magnetic resonance (MR) enterography.** CT enterography uses a special type of X-ray to look for problems in the digestive tract. An MR enterograph is another way to look at the digestive tract, but it does not use X-ray radiation. For both of these procedures, you drink a liquid with a dye or contrast solution. The solution colors your digestive tract and lets doctors see problem areas by using X-rays or magnetic fields.

- **Capsule endoscopy (CE).** A capsule endoscope is a small, pill-shaped camera that you swallow. The camera then travels through your digestive system. It records video of the small intestine and sends the video to a screen where your doctor can watch it.

How Is Inflammatory Bowel Disease Treated?

Treatments for IBD may include:

- **Medicines.** Most people with IBD take medicine to control their symptoms.

- **Surgery.** Surgery may be an option if medicine does not work to control your symptoms.

- **Steps you can take at home.** Your doctor can talk to you about steps you can take at home to help control your symptoms and prevent flare-ups.

- **Changes to your eating habits.** Avoiding certain foods, changing other eating habits, and limiting or avoiding alcohol may help control your symptoms during flare-ups.

Some forms of psychotherapy, sometimes called "talk therapy," may also help you cope with stress related to IBD symptoms and help make your pain less severe.

Some counselors specialize in working with people who have IBD. A counselor can help you talk about any distressing emotions you might have about IBD symptoms. A counselor can also treat anxiety, depression, or other mental-health concerns. Ask your doctor or nurse for a referral or recommendation for a counselor in your area.

What Medicines Treat Inflammatory Bowel Disease

Medicines used to treat IBD help reduce inflammation, relieve symptoms, and prevent future flare-ups. Your doctor may give you:

- Medicines to control inflammation, such as:

  - Aminosalicylates, which may also help prevent flare-ups. Most people with mild to moderate ulcerative colitis and some people with Crohn disease are treated with aminosalicylates.

  - Biologic therapies, which block substances in your body that cause inflammation

171

- Antibiotics, which may help if you have an infection or overgrowth of bacteria

- Medicines to calm your immune system, such as:

  - Corticosteroids, which are strong, fast-acting drugs to treat IBD flare-ups. You will take these for short periods of time only. If taken for too long, corticosteroids can cause serious side effects, including bone loss.

  - Immunosuppressants, which can take up to six months to work. But unlike corticosteroids, immunosuppressants can be taken long-term to prevent flare-ups.

You may need to try several different medicines before you find what works best for you.

Will I Need Surgery for Crohn Disease?

Maybe. More than half of people with Crohn disease need surgery within 20 years of being diagnosed. Surgery can relieve your symptoms, but it cannot cure the disease.

Surgeries for Crohn disease include:

- **Bowel resection.** In this surgery, your doctor removes the damaged part of your small or large intestine and sews the two healthy ends together.

- **Removal of your large intestine, including your rectum.** After this procedure, your body can no longer get rid of solid waste on its own. Your doctor will make a small opening in the front of your abdominal wall. Then your doctor will bring the end of your small intestine through the hole. This allows waste to drain out of your body. A pouch is worn over the opening to collect waste. You will need to empty the pouch several times a day.

- **Fistula surgery.** Some patients develop a collection of pus (an abscess) or drainage of pus from an opening (a fistula) around the anus. Surgery may be required to drain the pus and insert a small wire (a seton) to keep the pus from recollecting.

Will I Need Surgery for Ulcerative Colitis?

Maybe. Almost one in three people with ulcerative colitis may need surgery to treat the ulcerative colitis at some point.

Surgery to remove your entire large intestine and rectum may cure ulcerative colitis. After your large intestine and rectum are removed, your body can no longer get rid of solid waste on its own. Your doctor will do one of two types of procedures to allow your body to get rid of waste:

- Your doctor will make a small opening in the front of your abdominal wall. Then your doctor will bring the end of your small intestine through the hole. This allows waste to drain out of your body. A pouch is worn over the opening to collect waste. You will need to empty the pouch several times a day.

- Your doctor will attach the end of your small intestine to the inside of your anus, where the rectum used to create an internal pouch. This procedure is also called "ileoanal anastomosis." Waste is stored in the pouch and passes out of the anus in the usual way.

The type of procedure your doctor does depends on your symptoms and how severe they are, your age, and how the procedure will affect your quality of life (QOL), such as the types of activities you do.

What Can I Do at Home to Relieve My Inflammatory Bowel Disease Symptoms?

Your doctor will talk to you about steps you can take at home to relieve your IBD symptoms. Some steps may include:

- **Reducing stress.** Stress does not cause IBD, but it can make your IBD symptoms worse. Some studies show that mindfulness therapy, hypnotherapy, and psychotherapy may help. Get tips on relieving stress.

- **Changing your eating habits.** Some women report that limiting or avoiding certain foods helps relieve symptoms.

- **Taking vitamin supplements.** Your doctor may suggest vitamin supplements if your body does not get all of the nutrients you need from food because of IBD. You may need to take vitamin B_{12}, folic acid, vitamin D, calcium, or iron.

- **Taking probiotics.** Some research suggests that probiotics, which are live bacteria similar to what is found naturally in the body, may help some people with IBD. Probiotics are in foods such as yogurt that indicate there are "live and active cultures" on the label. Probiotics also come as a supplement you can buy in many stores. Vitamins and supplements are not regulated by the U.S. Food and Drug Administration (FDA) in the same way as medicines. Talk to your doctor or nurse about any supplements you take, including probiotics.

Can Changing My Eating Habits Help Treat Inflammatory Bowel Disease?

Maybe. Researchers don't have enough evidence yet to show which specific diets, foods, or ingredients may make IBD symptoms worse or better. Some women say that changing the foods they eat helps relieve their symptoms during flare-ups. Most doctors recommend avoiding processed foods and foods with a lot of additives, such as carrageenan and maltodextrin (thickeners).

Talk to your doctor about specific foods you may want to eat or avoid.

Can Inflammatory Bowel Disease Lead to Other Health Problems?

Yes. IBD can lead to other health problems. Some of the conditions include:

- **Weak bones.** Crohn disease can cause bone loss and osteoporosis. Medicines to treat ulcerative colitis may also lead to bone loss.

- **Iron-deficiency anemia.** Iron-deficiency anemia happens when your level of healthy red blood cells, which carry oxygen to all the parts of your body, is below normal. This can happen because of blood loss from your digestive system.

- **Dehydration or malnutrition.** Diarrhea and cramping pain can make it harder to eat or for your body to get the nutrients it needs. You may need an IV or feeding tube to replace lost fluids or nutrients.

- **Toxic megacolon.** Toxic megacolon happens when the large intestine swells quickly and stops working. Toxic megacolon is serious and can cause severe pain and even death.

- **Colon cancer.** Crohn disease can raise your risk of colon cancer. Talk to your doctor about your risk.

- **Inflammation inside your body.** IBD can cause liver problems, gallstones, and pancreatitis (inflammation of the pancreas).

- **Kidney stones.** Kidney stones are small, painful stones, sometimes formed from oxalate (a type of salt) in the kidneys. They are more common in people with Crohn disease.

Some of these other health problems get better when IBD is treated. Some other health problems must be treated separately from IBD.

Although these conditions are not necessarily caused by IBD, people with IBD are more likely to also have depression and anxiety, especially during flare-ups. Depression and anxiety are serious mental-health problems that can be treated.

Chapter 22

Multiple Myeloma

Multiple myeloma is a form of cancer that occurs due to abnormal and uncontrolled growth of plasma cells in the bone marrow. Some people with multiple myeloma, especially those with early stages of the condition, have no concerning signs or symptoms. When present, the most common symptom is anemia, which can be associated with fatigue and shortness of breath.

Other features of the condition may include multiple infections; abnormal bleeding; bone pain; weak and/or easily broken bones; and numbness and/or weakness of the arms and legs. The exact underlying cause of multiple myeloma is currently unknown. Factors that are associated with an increased risk of developing multiple myeloma include increasing age, male sex, African-American race, radiation exposure, a family history of the condition, obesity, and/or a personal history of monoclonal gammopathy of undetermined significance (MGUS).

Treatment varies based on many factors but may include one or more of the following interventions: chemotherapy, corticosteroid medications, targeted therapy, stem-cell transplant, biological therapy, radiation therapy, surgery, and/or watchful waiting.

Symptoms

In some cases, multiple myeloma is not associated with any signs and symptoms. When present, the most common symptom is anemia

This chapter includes text excerpted from "Multiple Myeloma," Genetic and Rare Diseases Information Center (GARD), National Center for Advancing Translational Sciences (NCATS), March 12, 2016.

(low red blood cell (RBC) count), which can be associated with fatigue, shortness of breath, and dizziness. Other features of the condition may include:

- Bone pain

- Nausea

- Constipation

- Loss of appetite

- Frequent infections

- Weight loss

- Excessive thirst

- Weakness and/or numbness in the arms and legs

- Confusion

- Abnormal bleeding

- Weak bones that may break easily

- Difficulty breathing

Cause

Although the exact underlying cause of multiple myeloma is poorly understood, the specific symptoms of the condition result from abnormal and excessive growth of plasma cells in the bone marrow. Plasma cells help the body fight infection by producing proteins called "antibodies." In people with multiple myeloma, excess plasma cells form tumors in the bone, causing bones to become weak and easily broken. The abnormal growth of plasma cells also makes it more difficult for the bone marrow to make healthy blood cells and platelets. The plasma cells produced in multiple myeloma produce abnormal antibodies that the immune system is unable to use. These abnormal antibodies build up in the body and cause a variety of problems.

Factors that are associated with an increased risk of developing multiple myeloma include increasing age, male sex, African American race, radiation exposure, a family history of the condition, obesity, and/or a personal history of monoclonal gammopathy of undetermined significance (MGUS).

Diagnosis

A diagnosis of multiple myeloma may be suspected based on the presence of characteristic signs and symptoms. Additional testing can then be ordered to confirm the diagnosis. This may include:

- Specialized blood tests including immunoglobulin studies, complete blood count with differential, and blood chemistry studies

- Urine tests such as immunoglobulin studies and a twenty-four-hour urine test

- Bone marrow aspiration and biopsy

- Imaging studies such as an X-ray of the bones (skeletal bone survey), magnetic resonance imaging (MRI), computerized tomography (CT) scan, and/or positron emission tomography (PET) scan

The American Cancer Society (ACS) offers more information regarding the diagnosis of multiple myeloma, including a summary of the many tests that may be recommended.

Some affected people may have no suspicious signs or symptoms of multiple myeloma, especially in the early stages of the condition. In these cases, multiple myeloma is sometimes diagnosed by chance when a blood test or urine test is ordered to investigate another condition.

Treatment

The treatment of multiple myeloma varies based on many factors, including the age and general health of the affected person; the associated signs and symptoms; and the severity of the condition. In general, one or more of the following interventions may be used to treat multiple myeloma:

- Chemotherapy

- Corticosteroid medications

- Targeted therapy

- Stem-cell transplant

- Biological therapy

- Radiation therapy

- Surgery

- Watchful waiting

Prognosis

The long-term outlook (prognosis) for people with multiple myeloma can be difficult to predict as some cases progress rapidly despite treatment, while others remain stable without therapy for a number of years. However, some general patterns have been observed. For example, prognosis appears to vary based on the affected person's age and the stage of the condition at the time of diagnosis. In general, survival is higher in younger people and lower in the elderly. Other factors that can be associated with a poor prognosis include a high tumor burden and kidney damage.

Infections are an important cause of early death among people with multiple myeloma. In fact, studies show that the risk of both bacterial infections and viral infections is approximately seven times higher in people affected by the condition.

Chapter 23

Oral Health and Bone Diseases

Osteoporosis and tooth loss are health concerns that affect many older men and women. Osteoporosis is a condition in which the bones become less dense and more likely to fracture. This disease can affect any bone in the body, although the bones in the hip, spine, and wrist are affected most often. In the United States, more than 53 million people either already have osteoporosis or are at high risk due to low bone mass.

Research suggests a link between osteoporosis and bone loss in the jaw. The bone in the jaw supports and anchors the teeth. When the jawbone becomes less dense, tooth loss can occur, a common occurrence in older adults.

Skeletal Bone Density and Dental Concerns

The portion of the jawbone that supports our teeth is known as the alveolar process. Several studies have found a link between the loss of alveolar bone and an increase in loose teeth (tooth mobility) and tooth loss. Women with osteoporosis are three times more likely to experience tooth loss than those who do not have the disease.

This chapter includes text excerpted from "Oral Health and Bone Disease," NIH Osteoporosis and Related Bone Diseases—National Resource Center (NIH ORBD—NRC), May 2016.

Low bone density in the jaw can result in other dental problems as well. For example, older women with osteoporosis may be more likely to have difficulty with loose or ill-fitting dentures and may have less optimal outcomes from oral surgical procedures.

Periodontal Disease and Bone Health

Periodontitis is a chronic infection that affects the gums and the bones that support the teeth. Bacteria and the body's own immune system break down the bone and connective tissue that hold teeth in place. Teeth may eventually become loose, fall out, or have to be removed. Although tooth loss is a well-documented consequence of periodontitis, the relationship between periodontitis and skeletal bone density is less clear. Some studies have found a strong and direct relationship among bone loss, periodontitis, and tooth loss. It is possible that the loss of alveolar bone mineral density leaves bone more susceptible to periodontal bacteria, increasing the risk for periodontitis and tooth loss.

Role of the Dentist and Dental X-Rays

Research supported by the National Institute of Arthritis and Musculoskeletal and Skin Diseases (NIAMS) suggests that dental X-rays may be used as a screening tool for osteoporosis. Researchers found that dental X-rays were highly effective in distinguishing people with osteoporosis from those with normal bone density.

Because many people see their dentist more regularly than their doctor, dentists are in a unique position to help identify people with low bone density and to encourage them to talk to their doctors about their bone health. Dental concerns that may indicate low bone density include loose teeth, gums detaching from the teeth or receding gums, and ill-fitting or loose dentures.

Effects of Osteoporosis Treatments on Oral Health

It is not known whether osteoporosis treatments have the same beneficial effect on oral health as they do on other bones in the skeleton. Additional research is needed to fully clarify the relationship between osteoporosis and oral bone loss; however, scientists are hopeful that efforts to optimize skeletal bone density will have a favorable impact on dental health.

Bisphosphonates, a group of medications available for the treatment of osteoporosis, have been linked to the development of osteonecrosis of the jaw (ONJ), which is cause for concern. The risk of ONJ has been greatest in patients receiving large doses of intravenous bisphosphonates, a therapy used to treat cancer. The occurrence of ONJ is rare in individuals taking oral forms of the medication for osteoporosis treatment.

Taking Steps for Healthy Bones

A healthy lifestyle can be critically important for keeping bones strong. You can take many important steps to optimize your bone health:

- Eat a well-balanced diet rich in calcium and vitamin D

- Engage in regular physical activity or exercise. Weight-bearing activities—such as walking, jogging, dancing, and weight training—are the best for keeping bones strong

- Don't smoke, and limit alcohol intake

- Report any problems with loose teeth, detached or receding gums, and loose or ill-fitting dentures to your dentist and your doctor

Chapter 24

Osteopetrosis

Osteopetrosis refers to a group of rare, inherited skeletal disorders characterized by increased bone density and abnormal bone growth. Symptoms and severity can vary greatly, ranging from neonatal onset with life-threatening complications (such as bone marrow failure) to the incidental finding of osteopetrosis on X-ray. Depending on severity and age of onset, features may include fractures, short stature, compressive neuropathies (pressure on the nerves), hypocalcemia with attendant tetanic seizures, and life-threatening pancytopenia. In rare cases, there may be neurological impairment or involvement of other body systems. Osteopetrosis may be caused by mutations in at least 10 genes. Inheritance can be autosomal recessive, autosomal dominant, or X-linked recessive with the most severe forms being autosomal recessive. Management depends on the specific symptoms and severity and may include vitamin D supplements, various medications, and/ or surgery. Adult osteopetrosis requires no treatment by itself, but complications may require intervention.

Symptoms

Table 24.1 lists symptoms that people with this disease may have. For most diseases, symptoms will vary from person to person. People with the same disease may not have all the symptoms listed.

This chapter includes text excerpted from "Osteopetrosis," Genetic and Rare Diseases Information Center (GARD), National Center for Advancing Translational Sciences (NCATS), July 20, 2016.

Table 24.1. Symptoms of Osteopetrosis

Medical Terms	Other Names
80 to 99% of people have these symptoms	
Abnormal cortical bone morphology	
Abnormal cranial nerve morphology	
Abnormal pelvis bone ossification	
Abnormality of the ribs	Rib abnormalities
Abnormality of vertebral epiphysis morphology	Abnormal shape of the end part of the vertebra bone
Abnormality of vision	Abnormality of sight; vision issue
Bone pain	
Cranial nerve paralysis	
Craniosynostosis	
Fever	
Growth delay	Delayed growth; growth deficiency; growth failure; growth retardation; poor growth; retarded growth
Hearing impairment	Deafness; hearing defect
Hypocalcemia	Low blood calcium levels
Hypophosphatemia	Low blood phosphate level
Lymphadenopathy	Swollen lymph nodes
Macrocephaly	Increased size of skull; large head; large head circumference
Osteomyelitis	Bone infection
Osteopetrosis	
Peripheral neuropathy	
Petechiae	
Recurrent fractures	Increased fracture rate; increased fractures; multiple fractures; multiple spontaneous fractures; varying degree of multiple fractures
Reduced bone mineral density	Low solidness and mass of the bones
Sandwich appearance of vertebral bodies	
Sclerotic vertebral endplates	
30 to 79% of people have these symptoms	
Bruising susceptibility	Bruise easily; easy bruisability; easy bruising

Table 24.1. Continued

Medical Terms	Other Names
30 to 79% of people have these symptoms	
Immunodeficiency	Decreased immune function
Leukocytosis	Elevated white blood count; high white blood count; increased blood leukocyte number
Persistence of primary teeth	Delayed loss of baby teeth; failure to lose baby teeth; retained baby teeth
5 to 29% of people have these symptoms	
Abnormal chorioretinal morphology	
Abnormal pulmonary valve morphology	
Bone marrow hypocellularity	Bone marrow failure
Carious teeth	Dental cavities; tooth cavities; tooth decay
Genu valgum	Knock knees
Intellectual disability	Mental deficiency; mental retardation; mental retardation, nonspecific; mental-retardation
Mandibular prognathism	Big lower jaw; increased projection of lower jaw; increased size of lower jaw; large lower jaw; prominent chin; prominent lower jaw
Nystagmus	Involuntary, rapid, rhythmic eye movements
Osteoarthritis	Degenerative joint disease
Renal tubular acidosis	
Sleep apnea	
Splenomegaly	Increased spleen size
Thrombocytopenia	Low platelet count

Cause

The various types of osteopetrosis are caused by genetic changes (mutations) in one of at least 10 genes. There is nothing a parent can do before, during, or after a pregnancy to cause osteopetrosis in a child.

The genes associated with osteopetrosis are involved in the development and/or function of osteoclasts, cells that break down bone tissue when old bone is being replaced by new bone (bone remodeling). This process is necessary to keep bones strong and healthy. Mutations in these genes can lead to abnormal osteoclasts, or having too few osteo-clasts. If this happens, old bone cannot be broken down as new bone is formed, so bones become too dense and prone to breaking.

- Mutations in the *CLCN7* gene cause most cases of autosomal dominant osteopetrosis, 10 to 15 percent of cases of autosomal recessive osteopetrosis (the most severe form), and all known cases of intermediate autosomal osteopetrosis

- Mutations in the *TCIRG1* gene cause about 50 percent of cases of autosomal recessive osteopetrosis

- Mutations in the *IKBKG* gene cause X-linked osteopetrosis

- Mutations in other genes are less common causes of osteopetrosis

- In about 30 percent of affected people, the cause is unknown

People with questions about the specific cause of osteopetrosis in themselves or a family member are encouraged to speak with a genetics professional.

Inheritance

Inheritance of the various subtypes of osteopetrosis can be auto-somal dominant (most commonly), autosomal recessive, or X-linked recessive. The most severe forms are autosomal recessive.

- In autosomal dominant inheritance, having a change (mutation) in only one copy of the responsible gene in each cell is enough to cause features of the condition. Most people with autosomal dominant osteopetrosis inherit the condition from an affected parent. Each child of a person with this form has a one in two (50%) chance of being affected.

- In autosomal recessive inheritance, in order to be affected a person must have a mutation in both copies of the responsible gene in each cell. Affected people inherit one mutated copy of the gene from each parent, who is referred to as a "carrier." Carriers of an autosomal recessive condition typically do not have any signs or symptoms (i.e., they are unaffected). When two carriers of an autosomal recessive condition have children, each child has a:

  - 25 percent (1 in 4) chance to be affected

- 50 percent (1 in 2) chance to be an unaffected carrier like each parent

- 25 percent chance to be unaffected and not be a carrier

- X-linked recessive conditions usually occur in males, who only have one X chromosome (and one Y chromosome). Females have two X chromosomes, so if they have a gene mutation on one of them, they still have a normal copy on their other X chromosome. For this reason, females are typically unaffected. While females can have an X-linked recessive condition, it is very rare.

If a mother is a carrier of an X-linked recessive condition and the father is not, the risk to children depends on each child's sex.

- Each male child has a 50 percent chance to be unaffected, and a 50 percent chance to be affected

- Each daughter has a 50 percent chance to be unaffected, and a 50 percent chance to be an unaffected carrier

If a father has the condition and the mother is not a carrier, all sons will be unaffected, and all daughters will be unaffected carriers.

Diagnosis

Genetic testing for the various subtypes of osteopetrosis is available. Genetic testing can be used to confirm the diagnosis and to differentiate between different subtypes of osteopetrosis. This may provide additional information regarding the long-term outlook (prognosis), likely response to treatment, and recurrence risks.

Treatment

Treatment for osteopetrosis depends on the specific symptoms present and the severity in each person. Therefore, treatment options must be evaluated on an individual basis. Nutritional support is important to improve growth and it also enhances responsiveness to other treatment options. A calcium-deficient diet has been beneficial for some affected people.

Treatment is necessary for the infantile form:

- Vitamin D (calcitriol) appears to stimulate dormant osteoclasts, which stimulates bone resorption. Large doses of calcitriol with restricted calcium intake sometimes improve osteopetrosis dramatically, but the improvement seen with calcitriol is not sustained when therapy is stopped.

- Gamma interferon can have long-term benefits. It improves white blood cell function (leading to fewer infections), decreases bone volume, and increases bone-marrow volume.

- Erythropoietin can be used for anemia, and corticosteroids can be used for anemia and to stimulate bone resorption.

Bone-marrow transplantation (BMT) markedly improves some cases of severe, infantile osteopetrosis associated with bone-marrow failure, and offers the best chance of longer-term survival for individuals with this type.

In pediatric (childhood) osteopetrosis, surgery is sometimes needed because of fractures.

Adult osteopetrosis typically does not require treatment, but complications of the condition may require intervention. Surgery may be needed for aesthetic or functional reasons (such as multiple fractures, deformity, and loss of function), or for severe degenerative joint disease.

Prognosis

The long-term outlook (prognosis) for people with osteopetrosis depends on the subtype and the severity of the condition in each person.

The severe infantile forms of osteopetrosis are associated with shortened life expectancy, with most untreated children not surviving past their first decade. Bone marrow transplantation seems to have cured some infants with early-onset disease.

However, the long-term prognosis after transplantation is unknown. For those with onset in childhood or adolescence, the effect of the condition depends on the specific symptoms (including how fragile the bones are and how much pain is present). Life expectancy in the adult-onset forms is normal.

Chapter 25

Osteogenesis Imperfecta

What Is Osteogenesis Imperfecta?

Osteogenesis imperfecta (OI) is a disease that affects your bones. OI is also called "brittle bone disease." If you have OI, you have bones that are weak and break easily.

Who Gets Osteogenesis Imperfecta

OI is a genetic disease, which means it runs in certain families. About 20,000 to 50,000 people in the United States have OI. OI is present at birth and is a lifelong disease.

What Are the Symptoms of Osteogenesis Imperfecta?

All people with OI have weak bones that break easily. People with OI often have other symptoms, such as:

- Malformed bones
- Short, small body

This chapter includes text excerpted from "Osteogenesis Imperfecta," National Institute of Arthritis and Musculoskeletal and Skin Diseases (NIAMS), November 30, 2014. Reviewed January 2019.

- Skin the bruises easily

- Loose joints

- Weak muscles

- Whites of the eyes that look blue, purple, or gray

- A face shaped like a triangle

- A rib cage shaped like a barrel

- A curved spine

- Brittle teeth

- Hearing loss, often starting in twenties or thirties

- Breathing problems

OI symptoms vary from person to person. They can range from mild to severe. For example, some people with OI may have a few broken bones over their lifetime. Others may have hundreds of broken bones in their lifetime, including broken bones that occur before birth.

What Causes Osteogenesis Imperfecta

OI is caused by an abnormal gene. Genes carry information that determine which features are passed to you from your parents.

People with OI have a defect in one of the genes that help make collagen. Collagen is a substance in the body that makes bones strong. People with OI do not have enough collagen. Or, the collagen does not work properly. This causes weak bones that break easily.

Most people with OI inherit this gene from one parent. Others inherit it from both parents. Parents do not have to have OI to pass on the gene that causes it. Sometimes, neither parent passes on the gene. Instead, the gene stops working properly on its own before the child is born.

Is There a Test for Osteogenesis Imperfecta?

There is no single test to detect OI. Doctors look at several factors to diagnose OI. These include:

- Family history

- Medical history

- Results from a physical exam

- X-rays

OI can be diagnosed through a skin biopsy. A skin biopsy is a surgical procedure in which a doctor removes a small piece of skin. Then, a doctor looks at it under a microscope to see whether there are any collagen abnormalities.

Doctors can also diagnose OI through a blood test that detects the abnormal genes that causes OI.

How Is Osteogenesis Imperfecta Treated?

The goal of treatment is to prevent or control symptoms of OI.

Medicines

- **Bone-strengthening medicines:** Your doctor may prescribe bone-strengthening medicines to slow bone loss and reduce the frequency and seriousness of broken bones.
- **Pain medicines:** Your doctor may prescribe pain medicines to treat pain caused by broken bones.

Broken Bone Care

Your doctor may cast, splint, or brace a broken bone to help it heal correctly.

Surgery

Your doctor may recommend surgery for many reasons:

- To fix a broken bone

- To support or correct bones that are curved or bowed

- To support the spine

Many children with OI have surgery in which a metal rod is placed into a bone. This is called "rodding surgery." Rodding surgery is performed to support the bone and prevent the bone from breaking.

Mobility Aids

Your doctor may recommend a walker, cane, crutches, or wheelchair to reduce injuries.

Physical or Occupational Therapy

You may benefit from physical or occupational therapy, which can help you:

- Build muscle strength, which may help prevent broken bones
- Learn how to avoid injuries
- Safely perform activities of daily living
- Recover from broken bones

Dental Care

Some people with OI have brittle teeth that chip or crack easily. You may require special dental care.

Chapter 26

Paget Disease of the Bone

What Is Paget Disease of Bone?

Paget disease (PD) is a chronic disorder that can result in enlarged and misshapen bones. The excessive breakdown and formation of bone tissue causes affected bone to weaken—resulting in bone pain, misshapen bones, fractures, and arthritis in the joints near the affected bones. Paget disease typically is localized, affecting just one or a few bones, as opposed to osteoporosis, for example, which affects all the bones in the body.

Scientists do not know for sure what causes Paget disease. In some cases, the disease runs in families, and so far two genes have been identified that predispose affected people to develop Paget disease. In most cases, however, scientists suspect that environmental factors play a role. For example, scientists are studying the possibility that a slow-acting virus may cause Paget disease.

Who Is Affected?

The disease is more common in older people and those of northern European heritage. Research suggests that a close relative of someone with Paget disease is seven times more likely to develop the disease than someone without an affected relative.

This chapter includes text excerpted from "Information for Patients about Paget Disease of Bone," NIH Osteoporosis and Related Bone Diseases—National Resource Center (NIH ORBD—NRC), May 2015. Reviewed January 2019.

What Are the Symptoms?

Many patients do not know they have Paget disease because they have no symptoms. Sometimes the symptoms may be confused with those of arthritis or other disorders. In other cases, the diagnosis is made only after the patient has developed complications.

Symptoms can include:

- Pain, which can occur in any bone affected by the disease or result from arthritis, a complication that develops in some patients

- Headaches and hearing loss, which may occur when Paget disease affects the skull

- Pressure on nerves, which may occur when Paget disease affects the skull or spine

- Increased head size, bowing of a limb, or curvature of the spine, which may occur in advanced cases

- Hip pain, which may occur when Paget disease affects the pelvis or thighbone

- Damage to cartilage of joints, which may lead to arthritis

Any bone or bones can be affected, but Paget disease occurs most frequently in the spine, pelvis, legs, or skull. Generally, symptoms progress slowly, and the disease does not spread to normal bones.

How Is It Diagnosed?

Paget disease is almost always diagnosed using X-rays but may be discovered initially by either of the following tests:

- **Alkaline phosphatase blood test.** An elevated level of alkaline phosphatase in the blood can be suggestive of Paget disease.

- **Bone scans.** Bone scans are useful in determining the extent and activity of the condition.

If a blood test or bone scan suggests Paget disease, the affected bone(s) should be X-rayed to confirm the diagnosis.

Early diagnosis and treatment are important to minimize complications. Siblings and children of people with Paget disease may wish to have an alkaline phosphatase blood test every two or three years starting around the age of 40. If the alkaline phosphatase level is higher than normal, a bone scan may be used to identify which bone or bones are affected and an X-ray of these bones is used to verify the diagnosis of Paget disease.

Who Treats It

The following types of medical specialists are generally knowledgeable about treating Paget disease:

- **Endocrinologists**. Doctors who specialize in hormonal and metabolic disorders.

- **Rheumatologists**. Doctors who specialize in joint and muscle disorders.

- **Others**. Orthopedic surgeons, neurologists, and otolaryngologists (doctors who specialize in ear, nose, and throat disorders) may be called on to evaluate specialized symptoms.

How Is It Treated?

Drug therapy: The U.S. Food and Drug Administration (FDA) has approved several medications to treat Paget disease. The medications work by controlling the excessive breakdown and formation of bone that occurs in the disease. The goal of treatment is to relieve bone pain and prevent progression of the disease. People with Paget disease should talk to their doctors about which medication is right for them. It is also important to get adequate calcium and vitamin D through diet and supplements as prescribed by your doctor, except for patients who have had kidney stones.

Bisphosphonates are a class of drugs used to treat a variety of bone diseases. Several bisphosphonates are currently available to treat Paget disease. Calcitonin is a naturally occurring hormone made by the thyroid gland. The medication may be appropriate for some patients.

Surgery: Medical therapy before surgery helps decrease bleeding and other complications. Patients who are having surgery should discuss pretreatment with their doctor. Surgery may be advised for three major complications of Paget disease:

- **Fractures.** Surgery may allow fractures to heal in better position.

- **Severe degenerative arthritis.** Hip or knee replacement may be considered if disability is severe and medication and physical therapy are no longer helpful.

- **Bone deformity.** Cutting and realigning pagetic bone (a procedure called an "osteotomy") may reduce the pain in weight-bearing joints, especially the knees.

Complications resulting from enlargement of the skull or spine may injure the nervous system. However, most neurological symptoms, even those that are moderately severe, can be treated with medication and do not require neurosurgery.

Diet and exercise: There is no special diet to prevent or help treat Paget disease. However, according to the Institute of Medicine (IOM) of the National Academy of Sciences (NAS), women age 50 and older and men age 70 and older should get 1,200 mg of calcium and at least 600 IU (International Units) of vitamin D every day to maintain a healthy skeleton. People age 70 and older need to increase their vitamin D intake to 800 IU. People with a history of kidney stones should discuss calcium and vitamin D intake with their doctor.

Exercise is important because it helps preserve skeletal health, prevent weight gain, and maintain joint mobility. Patients should discuss any new exercise program with their doctor before beginning, to avoid any undue stress on affected bones.

What Other Medical Conditions May It Lead To?

Paget disease may lead to other medical conditions, including:

- **Arthritis.** Long bones in the leg may bow, distorting alignment and increasing pressure on nearby joints. In addition, pagetic bone may enlarge, causing joint surfaces to undergo excessive wear and tear. In these cases, pain may be caused by a combination of Paget disease and osteoarthritis.

- **Hearing loss.** Loss of hearing in one or both ears may occur when Paget disease affects the skull and the bone that surrounds the inner ear. Treating Paget disease may slow or stop hearing loss. Hearing aids also may help.

- **Heart disease.** In severe Paget disease, the heart works harder to pump blood to affected bones. This usually does not result in heart failure except in some people who also have hardening of the arteries.

- **Kidney stones.** Kidney stones are more common in patients with Paget disease.

- **Nervous system problems.** Pagetic bone can cause pressure on the brain, spinal cord, or nerves and reduced blood flow to the brain and spinal cord.

- **Sarcoma.** Rarely, Paget disease is associated with the development of a malignant tumor of the bone. When there is a sudden onset or worsening of pain, sarcoma should be considered.

- **Loose teeth.** When Paget disease affects the facial bones, the teeth may loosen. This may make chewing more difficult.

- **Vision loss.** Rarely, when the skull is involved, the nerves to the eye may be affected, causing some loss of vision.

Paget disease is not associated with osteoporosis. Although Paget disease and osteoporosis can occur in the same patient, they are completely different disorders. Despite their marked differences, several medications for Paget disease also are used to treat osteoporosis.

What Is the Prognosis?

The outlook for people diagnosed with Paget disease is generally good, particularly if treatment is given before major changes have occurred in the affected bones. Treatment can reduce symptoms but is not a cure. Osteogenic sarcoma (osteosarcoma), a form of bone cancer, is an extremely rare complication that occurs in less than one percent of all patients with Paget disease.

Part Four

Risk Factors and Prevention of Osteoporosis

Chapter 27

Genes and Osteoporosis

Chapter Contents

Section 27.1

Genetics of Bone Density

This section includes text excerpted from "Genetics of
Bone Density," National Institutes of Health (NIH),
April 23, 2012. Reviewed January 2019.

A study linked 32 novel genetic regions to bone mineral density. The
findings may help researchers understand why some people are more
susceptible to bone fractures. The research also points to potential
drug targets for preventing or treating osteoporosis.

Bones are made of a mineral and protein scaffold filled with bone
cells. Bone is continually broken down and replaced. When the rate
of bone loss outpaces the rate of replacement, bones weaken, eventually leading to osteoporosis and increased risk of fracture. More
than 40 million people nationwide either have osteoporosis or are at
increased risk for broken bones because of low bone mineral density
(osteopenia).

Past studies suggest that genetic differences may account for more
than half the variance in bone mineral density between people. Previous genome-wide association studies identified 24 genetic regions
that influence bone mineral density. However, these genetic variants
explained a small fraction of the variation in bone density, and none
were shown to influence the risk of fracture in a definitive way.

A worldwide consortium with multiple research groups set out to do
the largest search to date for variants related to bone mineral density.
The effort was funded by many sources, including the European Com-
mission and several National Institutes of Health (NIH) components,
such as the National Institute on Aging (NIA) and National Institute for Arthritis, Musculoskeletal and Skin Diseases (NIAMS). The
extensive research team—led by a group at Erasmus Medical Center
in Rotterdam, the Netherlands—also included scientists at NIA. The
study appeared online in *Nature Genetics* on April 15, 2012.

The researchers first combined data from 17 different studies
involving more than 80,000 people across North America, Europe,
East Asia, and Australia. They looked across the genome for genetic
variants associated with bone mineral density (BMD) of the femoral
neck and lumbar spine. The researchers found 96 independent variations from 87 genomic regions.

The scientists next tested these associations in over 50,000 more
people from 34 other studies. They confirmed the association with bone

mineral density in 56 regions, 32 of which hadn't been previously been tied to bone density.

The team also examined whether the 96 variants were associated with bone fractures. They analyzed data from 50 studies with fracture information. Combined, the studies involved over 31,000 people with fractures and over 102,000 controls. Fourteen of the regions, the researchers found, were also associated with bone fracture risk.

These findings reinforce the relationship between genetic factors and the risk of osteoporosis and bone fracture. However, the researchers found that the ability to use these factors to predict risk was modest relative to clinical risk factors such as age and weight.

"In reality, there may be 500 or more gene variants regulating osteoporosis," says Dr. John Ioannidis of the Stanford University School of Medicine, one of the senior authors. "Each variant conveys a small quantum of risk or benefit. We can't predict exactly who will or won't get a fracture."

"The ultimate goal of genetic studies like this is to develop personal, gene-based treatments for osteoporosis as well as to better identify those at high risk for the disease," says another of the senior authors, Dr. Douglas P. Kiel of Harvard Medical School (HMS). "The findings could lead to new therapies to prevent or treat osteoporosis."

Section 27.2

Genes Linked to Abnormal Bone Density and Fracture

This section includes text excerpted from "Genes Linked to Abnormal Bone Density and Fracture," National Institutes of Health (NIH), January 15, 2019.

Abnormally low bone mineral density (BMD), known as osteoporosis, is a common health problem that runs in families. About one of every four women and one of every 20 men over 65 have osteoporosis.

As these people age, the composition of their bone tissue changes, and voids form to make their bone porous. This condition increases the risk of bone fractures, which is a significant health challenge for older adults.

Previous studies have identified certain genetic factors related to BMD. To further investigate genetic variations associated with BMD and fracture, an international research team led by Dr. Brent Richards at McGill University analyzed hundreds of thousands of people's genomes. The study was supported in part by National Institutes of Health's (NIH) National Institute of Arthritis and Musculoskeletal and Skin Diseases (NIAMS). Results were published on December 31, 2018, in Nature Genetics.

First, the research team analyzed the UK Biobank's collection of genomes from more than 400,000 white British participants. The researchers identified 518 BMD-related regions of the genome (loci), 301 of which were previously unknown.

Next, the researchers analyzed genomes from the UK Biobank for fracture risk. They found evidence of 20,122 fractures using medical history, and participants reported 48,818 fractures. The team was able to identify 14 genetic variations associated with fracture that mapped to 13 loci. They then confirmed these associations using personal genetics data from hundreds of thousands of people collected by 23andMe, Inc. Using the larger data set, they also showed that the genetic factors for lower BMD were linked to increased risk of bone fracture.

Next, the researchers developed a method to use their data to identify genes likely to influence bone density and strength. They identified 126 target genes. The analysis suggested that a gene called *DAAM2* was important, so they chose it for more detailed analysis.

In a series of lab tests with bone cells and genetically modified mice, the scientists showed that DAAM2 influences bone density, mineralization, porosity, and strength. The team also highlighted five other genes that preliminary work suggests are important for BMD and fracture: CBX1, WAC, DSCC1, RGCC, and YWHAE.

"Although it might seem overwhelming to sort through the many genes we found to be associated with bone density, we are able to focus on those with the greatest effect to potentially target for drug development," explains coauthor Dr. Douglas Kiel of Harvard Medical School.

"Our findings represent significant progress in highlighting drug development opportunities," Richards says. "This set of genetic changes that influence BMD provides drug targets that are likely to be helpful for osteoporotic fracture prevention."

This work may also lead to the eventual development of more accurate methods to estimate a person's risk for having weaker bones. That could potentially help guide lifestyle choices, such as physical activity and diet, and appropriate screening.

Chapter 28

Risk Factors in Women

Chapter Contents

Section 28.1

Menopause and the Long-Term Effects of Estrogen Deficiency

This section includes text excerpted from "Osteoporosis,"
Office on Women's Health (OWH), U.S. Department of
Health and Human Services (HHS), October 26, 2016.

Osteoporosis is a disease of the bones that causes bones to become weak and break easily. Osteoporosis affects mostly older women, but prevention starts when you are younger. No matter your age, you can take steps to build bone mass and prevent bone loss. Broken bones from osteoporosis cause serious health problems and disability in older women.

Who Gets Osteoporosis

Of the estimated 10 million Americans with osteoporosis, more than 8 million (or 80%) are women. Osteoporosis is most common in older women. In the United States, osteoporosis affects one in four women 65 or older.

What Causes Osteoporosis

Osteoporosis is caused by bone loss. Most often, the reason for bone loss is very low levels of the hormone estrogen. Estrogen plays an important role in building and maintaining your bones.

The most common cause of low estrogen levels is menopause. After menopause, your ovaries make very little estrogen. Some women lose up to 25 percent of bone mass in the first 10 years after menopause.

Also, your risk for developing osteoporosis is higher if you did not develop strong bones when you were young. Girls develop 90 percent of their bone mass by age 18. If an eating disorder, poor eating, lack of physical activity, or another health problem prevents you from building bone mass early in life, you will have less bone mass to draw on later in life.

What Are the Symptoms of Osteoporosis?

Osteoporosis is called a "silent" disease. You may not have any symptoms of osteoporosis until you break (fracture) a bone. Fractures are most common in the hip, wrist, and spine (vertebrae). Vertebrae support your body and help you to stand and sit up.

Fractures in the vertebrae can cause the spine to collapse and bend forward. If this happens, you may get any or all of these symptoms:

- Sloping shoulders
- Curvature in the back
- Height loss
- Back pain
- Hunched posture

How Is Osteoporosis Diagnosed?

Your doctor will do a bone density test to see how strong or weak your bones are. A common test is a central dual-energy X-ray absorptiometry (DXA). A DXA is a special type of X-ray of your bones. This test uses a very low amount of radiation.

Your doctor may also use other screening tools to predict your risk of having low bone density or breaking a bone.

Do I Need to Be Tested for Osteoporosis?

Your doctor may suggest a bone density test for osteoporosis if:

- You are 65 or older
- You are younger than 65 but have risk factors for osteoporosis. Bone density testing is recommended for older women whose risk of breaking a bone is the same as or greater than that of a 65-year-old white woman with no risk factors other than age. Ask your doctor or nurse whether you need a bone density test before age 65.

How Is Osteoporosis Treated?

If you have osteoporosis, your doctor may prescribe medicine to prevent more bone loss or build new bone mass. Your doctor may also suggest getting more calcium, vitamin D, and physical activity.

These steps may help prevent fractures, especially in the hip and spine, that can cause serious pain and disability.

How Can I Prevent Osteoporosis?

You can take steps to slow the natural bone loss with aging and to prevent your bones from becoming weak and brittle.

- Get enough calcium and vitamin D each day.

- Get active. Choose weight-bearing physical activities such as running or dancing to build and strengthen your bones.

- Don't smoke.

- If you drink alcohol, drink in moderation (for women, this is one drink a day at most). Too much alcohol can harm your bones.

- Talk to your doctor about whether you need medicine to prevent bone loss.

Should I Take a Calcium Supplement?

It's best to get the calcium your body needs from food. But if you don't get enough calcium from the foods you eat, you may want to consider taking a calcium supplement.

Talk with your doctor or nurse before taking calcium supplements to see which kind is best for you and how much you need to take.

Section 28.2

Pregnancy, Lactation, and Osteoporosis

This section includes text excerpted from "Pregnancy, Breastfeeding, and Bone Health," NIH Osteoporosis and Related Bone Diseases—National Resource Center (NIH ORBD—NRC), May 2015. Reviewed January 2019.

Both pregnancy and breastfeeding cause changes in, and place extra demands on, women's bodies. Some of these may affect their bones. The good news is that most women do not experience bone problems during pregnancy and breastfeeding. And if their bones are affected during these times, the problem often is corrected easily. Nevertheless, taking care of one's bone health is especially important during pregnancy and breastfeeding, for the good health of both the mother and her baby.

Pregnancy and Bone Health

During pregnancy, the baby growing in its mother's womb needs plenty of calcium to develop its skeleton. This need is especially great during the last three months of pregnancy. If the mother doesn't get enough calcium, her baby will draw what it needs from the mother's bones. So, it is disconcerting that most women of childbearing years are not in the habit of getting enough calcium. Fortunately, pregnancy appears to help protect most women's calcium reserves in several ways:

- Pregnant women absorb calcium from food and supplements better than women who are not pregnant. This is especially true during the last half of pregnancy, when the baby is growing quickly and has the greatest need for calcium.

- During pregnancy, women produce more estrogen, a hormone that protects bones.

- Any bone mass lost during pregnancy is typically restored within several months after the baby's delivery (or several months after breastfeeding is stopped).

Some studies suggest that pregnancy may be good for bone health overall. Some evidence suggests that the more times a woman has been pregnant (for at least 28 weeks), the greater her bone density and the lower her risk of fracture.

In some cases, women develop osteoporosis during pregnancy or breastfeeding, although this is rare. Osteoporosis is bone loss that is serious enough to result in fragile bones and an increased risk of fracture.

In many cases, women who develop osteoporosis during pregnancy or breastfeeding will recover lost bone after childbirth or after they stop breastfeeding. It is less clear whether teenage mothers can recover lost bone and go on to optimize their bone mass.

Teen pregnancy and bone health. Teenage mothers may be at especially high risk for bone loss during pregnancy and for osteoporosis later in life. Unlike older women, teenage mothers are still building much of their own total bone mass. The unborn baby's need to develop its skeleton may compete with the young mother's need for calcium to build her own bones, compromising her ability to achieve optimal bone mass that will help protect her from osteoporosis later in life. To minimize any bone loss, pregnant teens should be especially careful to get enough calcium during pregnancy and breastfeeding.

Breastfeeding and Bone Health

Breastfeeding also affects a mother's bones. Studies have shown that women often lose three to five percent of their bone mass during breastfeeding, although they recover it rapidly after weaning. This bone loss may be caused by the growing baby's increased need for calcium, which is drawn from the mother's bones. The amount of calcium the mother needs depends on the amount of breast milk produced and how long breastfeeding continues. Women also may lose bone mass during breastfeeding because they're producing less estrogen, which is the hormone that protects bones. The good news is that, like bone lost during pregnancy, bone lost during breastfeeding is usually recovered within six months after breastfeeding ends.

Tips to Keep Bones Healthy during Pregnancy, Breastfeeding, and Beyond

Taking care of your bones is important throughout life, including before, during, and after pregnancy and breastfeeding. A balanced diet with adequate calcium, regular exercise, and a healthy lifestyle are good for mothers and their babies.

Calcium. Although this important mineral is important throughout your lifetime, your body's demand for calcium is greater during pregnancy and breastfeeding because both you and your baby need it. The National Academy of Sciences (NAS) recommends that women who are pregnant or breastfeeding consume 1,000 mg (milligrams) of calcium each day. For pregnant teens, the recommended intake is even higher: 1,300 mg of calcium a day.

Good sources of calcium include:

- Low-fat dairy products, such as milk, yogurt, cheese, and ice cream

- Dark green, leafy vegetables, such as broccoli, collard greens, and bok choy

- Canned sardines and salmon with bones

- Tofu, almonds, and corn tortillas

- Foods fortified with calcium, such as orange juice, cereals, and breads

In addition, your doctor probably will prescribe a vitamin and mineral supplement to take during pregnancy and breastfeeding to ensure that you get enough of this important mineral.

Exercise. Like muscles, bones respond to exercise by becoming stronger. Regular exercise, especially weight-bearing exercise that forces you to work against gravity, helps build and maintain strong bones. Examples of weight-bearing exercise include walking, climbing stairs, dancing, and weight training. Exercising during pregnancy can benefit your health in other ways, too. According to the American College of Obstetricians and Gynecologists (ACOG), being active during pregnancy can:

- Help reduce backaches, constipation, bloating, and swelling

- Help prevent or treat gestational diabetes (a type of diabetes that starts during pregnancy)

- Increase energy

- Improve mood

- Improve posture

- Promote muscle tone, strength, and endurance

- Help you sleep better

- Help you get back in shape after your baby is born

Before you begin or resume an exercise program, talk to your doctor about your plans.

Healthy lifestyle. Smoking is bad for your baby, bad for your bones, and bad for your heart and lungs. If you smoke, talk to your doctor about quitting. She or he can suggest resources to help you. Alcohol also is bad for pregnant and breastfeeding women and their babies, and excess alcohol is bad for bones. Be sure to follow your doctor's orders to avoid alcohol during this important time.

Section 28.3

Secondary Amenorrhea Leading to Osteoporosis

This section contains text excerpted from the following sources: Text in this sections begins with excerpts from "About Amenorrhea," *Eunice Kennedy Shriver* National Institute of Child Health and Human Development (NICHD), January 31, 2017; Text under the heading "Irregular Periods in Young Women Could Be Warning Sign for Later Osteoporosis" is excerpted from "Irregular Periods in Young Women Could Be Warning Sign for Later Osteoporosis," *Eunice Kennedy Shriver* National Institute of Child Health and Human Development (NICHD), May 29, 2002. Reviewed January 2019; Text under the heading "How Does Amenorrhea Affect Bone Health?" is excerpted from "Other Amenorrhea FAQs," *Eunice Kennedy Shriver* National Institute of Child Health and Human Development (NICHD), January 31, 2017.

Amenorrhea is the absence of a menstrual period. Amenorrhea is sometimes categorized as:

- Primary amenorrhea. This describes a young woman who has not had a period by age 16.

- Secondary amenorrhea. This occurs when a woman who once had regular periods experiences an absence of more than three cycles. Causes of secondary amenorrhea include pregnancy.

Having regular periods is an important sign of overall health. Missing a period, when not caused by pregnancy, breastfeeding, or menopause, is generally a sign of another health problem. If you miss your period, talk to your healthcare provider about possible causes, including pregnancy.

Irregular Periods in Young Women Could Be Warning Sign for Later Osteoporosis

Irregular menstrual periods in young women may be a warning sign of a hormonal shortage that could lead to osteoporosis, according to a preliminary study by researchers at the *Eunice Kennedy Shriver* National Institute of Child Health and Human Development (NICHD). The study, of women with a condition known as premature ovarian failure, appears in the May issue of *Obstetrics & Gynecology*.

216

Premature ovarian failure occurs when the ovaries stop producing eggs and reproductive hormones well in advance of natural menopause. An estimated one percent of American women develop the condition by age 40.

Most of the women who took part in the study reported a history of amenorrhea-absence of a menstrual period for three months or more before they were later diagnosed with premature ovarian failure. Moreover, the majority of these young women had not considered amenorrhea as a significant health problem.

"These findings suggest that women and their physicians may want to err on the side of caution and evaluate menstrual irregularities early," said Duane Alexander, M.D., Director of the NICHD.

The NICHD researchers surveyed 48 women with premature ovarian failure, to try to gain an understanding of the early signs of the disorder, according to the study's first author, Nahrain H. Alzubaidi.

The 48 women surveyed visited the National Institutes of Health Clinical Center between September 2000 and June 2001. Most of the women interviewed did not view a change in menstrual pattern as an important health issue and this factor may have contributed to a delay in their receiving a diagnosis of premature ovarian failure.

"Because missed periods are common symptoms in young women, it's understandable that more than half of our patients weren't concerned at first," said the study's senior author, Lawrence Nelson, M.D., of NICHD's Unit on Gynecologic Endocrinology "But the delay in evaluating and treating ovarian insufficiency may place young women at increased risk of developing osteoporosis in later years."

The diagnosis of premature ovarian failure can be problematic, Dr. Nelson said. Although three percent of young women will experience amenorrhea in a given year, most of them do not go on to develop premature ovarian failure. Yet by the time they receive a diagnosis, many women with premature ovarian failure experience bone loss serious enough to possibly place them at risk for later bone fractures.

In an earlier study of 89 women with premature ovarian failure, Dr. Nelson and his colleagues had found that 67 percent of the women had already developed osteopenia-the low bone density that precedes osteoporosis. Dr. Nelson said he suspects that the high rate of bone loss in women with premature ovarian failure might be due to a delay in diagnosing and treating the hormonal shortfall that accompanies the disorder.

Osteoporosis results from a loss of bone density, which, in turn, leads to weaker bones that are more likely to break. Estrogen and other reproductive hormones produced by the ovary help to maintain bone density. Although osteoporosis is more common after menopause, younger women who are lacking sufficient ovarian hormone production—particularly those with premature ovarian failure may also develop the condition.

In a study, the researchers found that 92 percent of the women with premature ovarian failure (POF) reported a change in menstrual cycle as the first symptom they experienced. Moreover, more than half of the women with amenorrhea reported seeing three or more different providers before they received their diagnosis. One-fourth of the women did not receive a diagnosis for five or more years after the beginning of menstrual irregularity.

In almost all cases, at least some laboratory testing will need to be performed to determine the cause of the irregular periods, Dr. Nelson said. Typically, tests to detect premature ovarian failure measure the amount of a reproductive hormone in the blood known as follicle stimulating hormone (FSH). Treatment for premature ovarian failure usually consists of replacing the missing reproductive hormones estrogen and progesterone.

"It's relatively easy to measure a blood FSH level to detect ovarian failure early," Dr. Nelson said. "When dealing with osteoporosis an ounce of prevention is worth a pound of cure."

How Does Amenorrhea Affect Bone Health?

An important part of the menstrual cycle is the production of the hormone estrogen. Estrogen also plays a role in bone health. If amenorrhea is caused by low estrogen or problems with estrogen production, a woman may be at risk for loss of bone mass.

Some common causes of estrogen deficiency are excessive exercise and eating disorders. These can have a negative effect on bone density. Adolescent girls, in particular, need a combination of calcium, vitamin D, and physical activity to build strong bones during this critical time. Years ago, researchers found that girls with amenorrhea who diet are at risk for low bone density and that this condition increases their risk for osteoporosis later in life.

Amenorrhea that results from fragile X-associated primary ovarian insufficiency (FXPOI) also increases the risk for osteoporosis. It is important to see your healthcare provider as early as possible to begin investigating the cause of amenorrhea. According to one study, two-thirds of adolescent girls who reported FXPOI also had osteopenia, an early stage of osteoporosis, at their first visit.

Section 28.4

Peak Bone Mass and Overtraining

This section contains text excerpted from the following sources: Text in this section begins with excerpts from "Osteoporosis: Peak Bone Mass in Women," NIH Osteoporosis and Related Bone Diseases—National Resource Center (NIH ORBD—NRC), June 2015. Reviewed January 2019; Text beginning with the heading "Fitness: Overtraining Risks" is excerpted from "Exercise and Bone Health for Women: The Skeletal Risk of Overtraining," NIH Osteoporosis and Related Bone Diseases—National Resource Center (NIH ORBD—NRC), May 2016.

Bones are the framework for your body. Bone is living tissue that changes constantly, with bits of old bone being removed and replaced by new bone. You can think of bone as a bank account, where you make "deposits" and "withdrawals" of bone tissue.

During childhood and adolescence, much more bone is deposited than withdrawn, so the skeleton grows in both size and density. Up to 90 percent of peak bone mass is acquired by age 18 in girls and by age 20 in boys, which makes youth the best time to "invest" in one's bone health.

The amount of bone tissue in the skeleton, known as bone mass, can keep growing until around age 30. At that point, bones have reached their maximum strength and density, known as peak bone mass. Women tend to experience minimal change in total bone mass between age 30 and menopause. But in the first few years after menopause, most women go through rapid bone loss, a "withdrawal" from the bone bank account, which then slows but continues throughout the postmenopausal years. This loss of bone mass can lead to osteoporosis. Given the knowledge that high peak bone density reduces osteoporosis risk later in life, it makes sense to pay more attention to those factors that affect peak bone mass.

Factors Affecting Peak Bone Mass

A variety of genetic and environmental factors influence peak bone mass. It has been suggested that genetic factors (those you were born with and cannot change, such as gender and race) may account for up to 75 percent of bone mass, and environmental factors (such as diet and exercise habits) account for the remaining 25 percent.

219

Gender. Peak bone mass tends to be higher in men than in women. Before puberty, boys and girls acquire bone mass at similar rates. After puberty, however, men tend to acquire greater bone mass than women.

Race. For reasons still not known, African American females tend to achieve higher peak bone mass than white females. These differences in bone density are seen even during childhood and adolescence.

Hormonal factors. The hormone estrogen has an effect on peak bone mass. For example, women who had their first menstrual cycle at an early age and those who use oral contraceptives, which contain estrogen, often have high bone mineral density. In contrast, young women whose menstrual periods stop because of extremely low body weight or excessive exercise, for example, may lose significant amounts of bone density, which may not be recovered even after their periods return.

Nutrition. Calcium is an essential nutrient for bone health. Calcium deficiencies in young people can account for a significant difference in peak bone mass and can increase the risk for hip fracture later in life. Surveys indicate that teenage girls in the United States are less likely than teenage boys to get enough calcium.

Physical activity. Girls and boys and young adults who exercise regularly generally achieve greater peak bone mass than those who do not. Women and men age 30 and older can help prevent bone loss with regular exercise. The best activity for your bones is weight-bearing exercise. This is exercise that forces you to work against gravity, such as walking, hiking, jogging, climbing stairs, playing tennis, dancing, and weight training.

Lifestyle behaviors. Smoking has been linked to low bone density in adolescents and is associated with other unhealthy behaviors, such as alcohol use and a sedentary lifestyle. People who begin smoking at a younger age are more likely to be heavier smokers later in life. This fact worsens the negative impact of smoking on peak bone bass and puts older smokers at additional risk for bone loss and fracture.

The impact of alcohol intake on peak bone mass is not clear. The effects of alcohol on bone have been studied more extensively in adults, and the results indicate that high consumption of alcohol has been linked to low bone density. Experts assume that high consumption of alcohol in youth has a similar adverse effect on skeletal health.

Fitness: Overtraining Risks

Are you exercising too much? Eating too little? Have your menstrual periods stopped or become irregular? If so, you may be putting yourself at high risk for several serious problems that could affect your health, your ability to remain active, and your risk for injuries. You also may be putting yourself at risk for developing osteoporosis, a disease in which bone density is decreased, leaving your bones vulnerable to fracture (breaking).

Why Is Missing My Period Such a Big Deal?

Some athletes see amenorrhea (the absence of menstrual periods) as a sign of successful training. Others see it as a great answer to a monthly inconvenience. And some young women accept it blindly, not stopping to think of the consequences. But missing your periods is often a sign of decreased estrogen levels. And lower estrogen levels can lead to osteoporosis, a disease in which your bones become brittle and more likely to break.

Usually, bones don't become brittle and break until women are much older. But some young women, especially those who exercise so much that their periods stop, develop brittle bones, and may start to have fractures at a very early age. Some 20-year-old female athletes have been said to have the bones of an 80-year-old woman. Even if bones don't break when you're young, low estrogen levels during the peak years of bone-building, the preteen and teen years, can affect bone density for the rest of your life. And studies show that bone growth lost during these years may never be regained.

Broken bones don't just hurt—they can cause lasting physical malformations. Have you noticed that some older women and men have stooped postures? This is not a normal sign of aging. Fractures from osteoporosis have left their spines permanently altered.

Overtraining can cause other problems besides missed periods. If you don't take in enough calcium and vitamin D (among other nutrients), bone loss may result. This may lead to decreased athletic performance, decreased ability to exercise or train at desired levels of intensity or duration, and increased risk of injury.

Who Is at Risk for These Problems?

Girls and women who engage in rigorous exercise regimens or who try to lose weight by restricting their eating are at risk for these health problems. They may include serious athletes, "gym rats" (who spend considerable time and energy working out), and girls and women who believe "you can never be too thin."

How Can I Tell If Someone I Know, Train with, or Coach May Be at Risk for Bone Loss, Fracture, and Other Health Problems?

Here are some signs to look for:

- Missed or irregular menstrual periods

- Extreme or "unhealthy-looking" thinness

- Extreme or rapid weight loss

- Behaviors that reflect frequent dieting, such as eating very little, not eating in front of others, trips to the bathroom following meals, preoccupation with thinness or weight, focus on low-calorie and diet foods, possible increase in the consumption of water and other no- and low-calorie foods and beverages, possible increase in gum chewing, limiting diet to one food group, or eliminating a food group

- Frequent intense bouts of exercise (e.g., taking an aerobics class, then running 5 miles, then swimming for an hour, followed by weight-lifting)

- An "I can't miss a day of exercise/practice" attitude

- An overly anxious preoccupation with an injury

- Exercising despite illness, inclement weather, injury, and other conditions that might lead someone else to take the day off

- An unusual amount of self-criticism or self-dissatisfaction

- Indications of significant psychological or physical stress, including: depression, anxiety or nervousness, inability to concentrate, low levels of self-esteem, feeling cold all the time, problems sleeping, fatigue, injuries, and constantly talking about weight

How Can I Make Needed Changes to Improve My Bone Health?

If you recognize some of these signs in yourself, the best thing you can do is to make your diet more healthful. That includes consuming enough calories to support your activity level. If you've missed periods, it's best to check with a doctor to make sure it's not a sign of some other problem and to get his or her help as you work toward a more healthy balance of food and exercise. Also, a doctor can help you take steps to protect your bones from further damage.

What Can I Do If I Suspect a Friend May Have Some of These Signs?

First, be supportive. Approach your friend or teammate carefully, and be sensitive. She probably won't appreciate a lecture about how she should be taking better care of herself. But maybe you could suggest that she talk to a trainer, coach, or doctor about the symptoms she's experiencing.

My Friend Drinks a Lot of Diet Sodas. She Says This Helps Keep Her Thin

Girls and women who may be dieting often drink diet sodas rather than milk. Yet, milk and other dairy products are a good source of calcium, an essential ingredient for healthy bones. Drinking sodas instead of milk can be a problem, especially during the teen years when rapid bone growth occurs. If you (or your friend) find yourself drinking a lot of sodas, try drinking half as many sodas each day, and gradually add more milk and dairy products to your diet. A frozen yogurt shake can be an occasional low-fat, tasty treat. Or try a fruit smoothie made with frozen yogurt, fruit, or calcium-enriched orange juice.

My Coach and I Think I Should Lose Just a Little More Weight. I Want to Be Able to Excel at My Sport!

Years ago, it was not unusual for coaches to encourage athletes to be as thin as possible for many sports (e.g., dancing, gymnastics, figure skating, swimming, diving, and running). However, many coaches now realize that being too thin is unhealthy and can negatively affect performance. It's important to exercise and watch what you eat. However, it's also important to develop and maintain healthy bones and bodies. Without these, it will not matter how fast you can run, how thin you are, or how long you exercise each day. Balance is the key!

I'm Still Not Convinced. If My Bones Become Brittle, So What? What's the Worst That Could Happen to Me?

Brittle bones may not sound as scary as a fatal or rare disease. The fact is that osteoporosis can lead to fractures. It can cause disability.

Imagine having so many spine fractures that you've lost inches in height and walk bent over. Imagine looking down at the ground everywhere you go because you can't straighten your back. Imagine not being able to find clothes that fit you. Imagine having difficulty breathing and eating because your lungs and stomach are compressed into a smaller space. Imagine having difficulty walking, let alone exercising, because of pain and misshapen bones. Imagine constantly having to be aware of what you are doing and having to do things so slowly and carefully because of a very real fear and dread of a fracture—a fracture that could lead to a drastic change in your life, including pain, loss of independence, loss of mobility, loss of freedom, and more.

Osteoporosis isn't just an "older person's" disease. Young women also experience fractures. Imagine being sidelined because of a broken bone and not being able to get those good feelings you get from regular activity.

Eating for Healthy Bones
How Much Calcium Do I Need?

It's very important to your bone health that you receive adequate daily amounts of calcium, vitamin D, phosphorus, and magnesium. These vitamins and minerals are the most influential in building bones and teeth. This chart will help you decide how much calcium you need.

Table 28.1. Recommended Calcium Intakes

Recommended Calcium Intakes (Mg/Day)	
Age	Amount
9 to 13	1,300
14 to 18	1,300
19 to 30	1,000

(Source: Food and Nutrition Board (FNB), Institute of Medicine (IOM), National Academy of Sciences (NAS), 2010.)

Where Can I Get Calcium and Vitamin D?

Dairy products are the primary food sources of calcium. Choose low-fat milk, yogurt, cheeses, ice cream, or products made or served with these choices to fulfill your daily requirement. Three servings of dairy products per day should give you at least 900 mg (milligrams) of calcium. Green vegetables are another source. A cup of broccoli, for example, has about 136 mg of calcium.

Milk and Dairy Products

Many great snack and meal items contain calcium. With a little planning and "know-how," you can make meals and snacks calcium-rich!

- **Milk:** Wouldn't a tall, cold glass of this refreshing thirst quencher be great right now? If you're concerned about fat and calories, choose reduced-fat or fat-free milk. You can drink it plain or with a low- or no-fat syrup or flavoring, such as chocolate syrup, vanilla extract, hazelnut flavoring, or cinnamon.

- **Cheese:** Again, you can choose the low- or no-fat varieties. Use all different types of cheese for sandwiches, bagels, omelets, vegetable dishes, pasta creations, or as a snack by itself!

- **Pudding (prepared with milk):** You can now purchase (or make from a mix) pudding in a variety of flavors with little or no fat, such as chocolate fudge, lemon, butterscotch, vanilla, and pistachio. Try them all!

- **Yogurt:** Add fruit. Eat it plain. Add a low- or no-fat sauce or syrup. No matter how you choose to eat this calcium-rich food, yogurt remains a quick, easy, and convenient choice. It's also available in a variety of flavors. Try mocha-fudge-peppermint-swirl if you're more adventurous at heart and vanilla if you're a more traditional yogurt snacker!

- **Frozen yogurt (or fat-free ice cream):** Everybody loves ice cream. And now, without the unnecessary fat, you can enjoy it more often! Mix yogurt, milk, and fruit to create a breakfast shake. Have a cone at lunchtime or as a snack. A scoop or two after dinner can be cool and refreshing.

What Are Other Sources of Calcium?

Many foods you already buy and eat may be "calcium-fortified." Try calcium-fortified orange juice or calcium-fortified cereal. Check food labels to see if some of your other favorite foods may be good sources of calcium. You also can take calcium supplements if you think you may not be getting enough from your diet.

Chapter 29

Female Athlete Triad and Bone Health

Being active is great. In fact, girls should be active at least an hour each day. Sometimes, though, a girl will be very active (such as running every day or playing a competitive sport), but not eat enough to fuel her activity. This can lead to health problems.

Read about what can happen when girls don't eat enough to fuel their activity:

- A problem called "low energy availability"
- Period (menstrual) problems
- Bone problems

These three sometimes are called the female athlete triad. ("Triad" means a group of three). They sometimes also are called "Athletic Performance and Energy Deficit." (This means you have a "deficit," or lack, of the energy your body needs to stay healthy)

A Problem Called "Low Energy Availability"

Your body needs healthy food to fuel the things it does, like fight infections, heal wounds, and grow. If you exercise, your body

This chapter includes text excerpted from "Do You Exercise a Lot?" girlshealth.gov, Office on Women's Health (OWH), March 27, 2015. Reviewed January 2019.

needs extra food for your workout. You can learn how much food to eat based on your activity level using the MyPlate Checklist Calculator (www.choosemyplate.gov/MyPlatePlan).

"Energy availability" means the fuel from food that is not burned up by exercise and so is available for growing, healing, and more. If you exercise a lot and don't get enough nutrition, you may have low energy availability. That means your body won't be as healthy and strong as it should be.

Some female athletes diet to lose weight. They may do this to qualify for their sport or because they think losing weight will help them perform better. But eating enough healthy food is key to having the strength you need to succeed. Also, your body needs good nutrition to make hormones that help with things like healthy periods and strong bones.

Sometimes, girls may exercise too much and eat too little because they have an eating disorder. Eating disorders are serious and can even lead to death, but they are treatable.

Period (Menstrual) Problems

If you are very active, or if you just recently started getting your period (menstruating), you may skip a few periods. But if you work out really hard and do not eat enough, you may skip a lot of periods (or not get your period to begin with) because your body can't make enough of the hormone estrogen.

You may think you wouldn't mind missing your period, but not getting your period should be taken seriously. Not having your period can mean your body is not building enough bone, and the teenage years are the main time for building strong bones.

If you have been getting your period regularly and then miss three periods in a row, see your doctor. Not having your period could be a sign of a serious health problem or of being pregnant. Also see your doctor if you are 15 years old and still have not gotten your period.

Bone Problems

Being physically active helps build strong bones. But you can hurt your bones if you don't eat enough healthy food to fuel all your activity. That's because your body won't be able to make the hormones needed to build strong bones.

One sign that your bones are weak is getting stress fractures, which are tiny cracks in bones. Some places you could get these cracks are your feet, legs, ribs, and spine.

Even if you don't have problems with your bones when you're young, not taking good care of them now can be a problem later in life. Your skeleton is almost completely formed by age 18, so it's important to build strong bones early in life. If you don't, then later on you could wind up with osteoporosis, which is a disease that makes it easier for bones to break.

Signs of Not Eating Enough and Eating Disorders

Sometimes, girls exercise a lot and do not eat enough because they want to lose weight. Sometimes, exercising just lowers a person's appetite. And sometimes limiting food can be a sign that a girl may be developing an eating disorder. Here are some signs that you or a friend may have a problem:

- Worrying about gaining weight if you don't exercise enough

- Trying harder to find time to exercise than to eat

- Chewing gum or drinking water to cope with hunger

- Often wanting to exercise rather than be with friends

- Exercising instead of doing homework or other responsibilities

- Getting very upset if you miss a workout, but not if you miss a meal

- Having people tell you they are worried you are losing too much weight

If you think you or a friend has a problem, talk to a parent, guardian, or trusted adult.

Sometimes girls exercise a lot because they feel pressure to look a certain way. Soccer star Brandi Chastain knows how bad that can feel. It took a while, she says, for her to realize that only she was in charge of how she felt about her body. "Body image is tough, but it is something we have to take charge of," Brandi says. "Because inside, only we know who we are."

Chapter 30

Influence of Sex and Gender

Sex and gender can influence health in important ways. While sex and gender are distinct concepts, their influence is often inextricably linked. The scientific studies that generate the most complete data consider sex and/or gender influences in study design, data collection and analysis, and reporting of findings.

Sex is a biological classification, encoded in our deoxyribonucleic acid (DNA). Males have XY chromosomes, and females have XX chromosomes. Sex makes us male or female. Every cell in your body has a sex—making up tissues and organs, like your skin, brain, heart, and stomach. Each cell is either male or female depending on whether you are a man or a woman.

Gender refers to the socially constructed roles, behaviors, expressions, and identities of girls, women, boys, men, and gender diverse people. It influences how people perceive themselves and each other, and how they act and interact. Gender is usually conceptualized as binary (girl/woman and boy/man), yet there is considerable diversity in how individuals and groups understand, experience, and express it.

Few examples of sex and gender influences are as follows:

Osteoporosis

- Osteoporosis is more common in women because they have less bone tissue than men and experience a rapid phase of bone loss due to hormonal changes at menopause.

This chapter includes text excerpted from "How Sex and Gender Influence Health and Disease," Office of Research on Women's Health (ORWH), National Institutes of Health (NIH), February 12, 2015. Reviewed January 2019.

- Osteoporosis in men older than 50 can go undetected and is often undertreated because patients and providers think of osteoporosis as a "woman's disease."

Knee Arthritis

- Women and girls are more likely to injure their knees when playing sports, in part due to their knee and hip anatomy, imbalanced leg muscle strength, and looser tendons and ligaments. Knee injuries such as ACL tears dramatically increase a person's risk of developing osteoarthritis later in life.

- Walking in high-heeled shoes increases stress on the knee joint, placing women at increased risk of developing osteoarthritis.

Mental Health

- Women are twice as likely as men to experience depression, with some women experiencing mood symptoms related to hormone changes during puberty, pregnancy, and perimenopause.

- Women are more likely to admit to negative mood states and to seek treatment for mental-health issues, in contrast to men.

Smoking Cessation

- Women have a harder time quitting smoking than men do. Women metabolize nicotine, the addictive ingredient in tobacco, faster than men. Differences in metabolism may help explain why nicotine replacement therapies, like patches and gum, work better in men than in women. Men appear to be more sensitive to nicotine's pharmacologic effects related to addiction.

- Although men are more sensitive than women to nicotine's addiction-related effects, women maybe more susceptible than men to nonnicotine factors, such as the sensory and social stimuli associated with smoking.

Cardiovascular Risk

- The blood vessels in a woman's heart are smaller in diameter and much more intricately branched than those of a man. Those differences offer one explanation for why women's vessels may become blocked in a different pattern than those in men.

Women's heart attack symptoms and the patterns seen on a heart-screening test can differ, sometimes leading to a wrong diagnosis– or worse–missing the signs of an oncoming heart attack.

- Women are often the primary caretakers of children, household needs, and aging family members, and they are more likely to delay prevention and treatment for chronic conditions such as heart disease.

Chapter 31

Diseases and Disorders That Affect Bone Health

Chapter Contents

Section 31.1

Breast Cancer and Bone Health

This section includes text excerpted from "What Breast
Cancer Survivors Need to Know about Osteoporosis," NIH
Osteoporosis and Related Bone Diseases—National Resource
Center (NIH ORBD—NRC), April 2016.

The Impact of Breast Cancer

Other than skin cancer, breast cancer is the most common cancer
in women. It can occur in both men and women, but it is very rare
in men.

Although the exact cause is not known, the risk of developing breast
cancer increases with age. The risk is particularly high in women
age 60 and older. Because of their age, these women are already at
increased risk for osteoporosis. Given the rising incidence of breast
cancer and the improvement of long-term survival rates, bone health
and fracture prevention have become important health issues among
breast cancer survivors.

Facts about Osteoporosis

Osteoporosis is a condition in which the bones become less dense
and more likely to fracture. Fractures from osteoporosis can result
in significant pain and disability. In the United States, more than 53
million people either already have osteoporosis or are at high risk due
to low bone mass.

Risk factors for developing osteoporosis include:

- Thinness or small frame

- Family history of the disease

- Being postmenopausal and particularly having had early
  menopause

- Abnormal absence of menstrual periods (amenorrhea)

- Prolonged use of certain medications, such as those used to treat
  lupus, asthma, thyroid deficiencies, and seizures

- Low calcium intake

- Lack of physical activity

- Smoking

- Excessive alcohol intake

Osteoporosis often can be prevented. It is known as a "silent disease" because, if undetected, bone loss can progress for many years without symptoms until a fracture occurs. Osteoporosis has been called a "childhood disease with old age consequences" because building healthy bones in youth helps prevent osteoporosis and fractures later in life. However, it is never too late to adopt new habits for healthy bones.

The Link between Breast Cancer and Osteoporosis

Women who have had breast cancer treatment may be at increased risk for osteoporosis and fracture. Estrogen has a protective effect on bone, and reduced levels of the hormone trigger bone loss. Because of treatment medications or surgery, many breast-cancer survivors experience a loss of ovarian function and, consequently, a drop in estrogen levels. Women who were premenopausal before their cancer treatment may go through menopause earlier than those who have not had breast cancer.

Results from the National Institutes of Health (NIH)-supported Women's Health Initiative Observational Study (WHI-OS) found an increase in fracture risk among breast-cancer survivors.

Osteoporosis Management Strategies

Several strategies can reduce one's risk for osteoporosis or lessen the effects of the disease in women who have already been diagnosed.

Nutrition: Some studies have found a link between diet and breast cancer. However, it is not yet clear which foods or supplements may play a role in reducing breast cancer risk. As far as bone health is concerned, a well-balanced diet rich in calcium and vitamin D is important. Good sources of calcium include low-fat dairy products; dark green, leafy vegetables; and calcium-fortified foods and beverages. Supplements can help ensure that the calcium requirement is met each day, especially in people with a proven milk allergy. The Institute of Medicine recommends a daily calcium intake of 1,000 mg (milligrams) for men and women up to age 50. Women over age 50 and men over age 70 should increase their intake to 1,200 mg daily.

Vitamin D plays an important role in calcium absorption and bone health. Food sources of vitamin D include egg yolks, saltwater fish, and liver. Many people, especially those who are older or housebound, may need vitamin D supplements to achieve the recommended intake of 600 to 800 IU (International Units) each day.

Exercise: Like muscle, bone is living tissue that responds to exercise by becoming stronger. The best activity for your bones is weight-bearing exercise that forces you to work against gravity. Some examples include walking, climbing stairs, weight training, and dancing. Regular exercise, such as walking, may help prevent bone loss and will provide many other health benefits. A research suggests that exercise also may reduce breast cancer risk in younger women.

Healthy lifestyle: Smoking is bad for bones as well as the heart and lungs. Women who smoke tend to go through menopause earlier, resulting in earlier reduction in levels of the bone-preserving hormone estrogen and triggering earlier bone loss. In addition, smokers may absorb less calcium from their diets. Some studies have found a slightly higher risk of breast cancer in women who drink alcohol, and evidence suggests that alcohol can have a negative effect on bone health. Those who drink heavily are more prone to bone loss and fracture, because of both poor nutrition and an increased risk of falling.

Bone density test: A bone mineral density (BMD) test measures bone density in various parts of the body. This safe and painless test can detect osteoporosis before a fracture occurs and can predict one's chances of fracturing in the future. The BMD test can help determine whether medication should be considered. A woman recovering from breast cancer should ask her doctor whether she might be a candidate for a bone density test.

Medication: There is no cure for osteoporosis. However, several medications are available to prevent and treat this disease. Bisphosphonates, a class of osteoporosis treatment medications, have demonstrated some success in their ability to treat breast cancers that have spread to bone.

Another osteoporosis treatment medication, raloxifene, is a selective estrogen receptor modulator (SERM) that has been shown to reduce the risk of breast cancer in women with osteoporosis. The National Institutes of Health's (NIH) Study of Tamoxifen and Raloxifene (STAR) found that raloxifene was as effective as tamoxifen in reducing the risk of postmenopausal breast cancer in high-risk women.

Section 31.2

Anorexia Nervosa and Bone Health

This section includes text excerpted from "What People
with Anorexia Nervosa Need to Know about Osteoporosis,"
NIH Osteoporosis and Related Bone Diseases—National
Resource Center (NIH ORBD—NRC), April 2016.

What Is Anorexia Nervosa?

Anorexia nervosa is an eating disorder characterized by an irrational fear of weight gain. People with anorexia nervosa believe that they are overweight even when they are extremely thin.

Individuals with anorexia become obsessed with food and severely restrict their dietary intake. The disease is associated with several health problems and, in rare cases, even death. The disorder may begin as early as the onset of puberty. The first menstrual period is typically delayed in girls who have anorexia when they reach puberty. For girls who have already reached puberty when they develop anorexia, menstrual periods are often infrequent or absent.

What Is Osteoporosis?

Osteoporosis is a condition in which the bones become less dense and more likely to fracture. Fractures from osteoporosis can result in significant pain and disability. In the United States, more than 53 million people either already have osteoporosis or are at high risk due to low bone mass.

Risk factors for developing osteoporosis include:

- Thinness or small frame

- Family history of the disease

- Being postmenopausal and particularly having had early menopause

- Abnormal absence of menstrual periods (amenorrhea)

- Prolonged use of certain medications, such as those used to treat lupus, asthma, thyroid deficiencies, and seizures

- Low calcium intake

- Lack of physical activity

- Smoking

- Excessive alcohol intake

Osteoporosis often can be prevented. It is known as a "silent disease" because, if undetected, bone loss can progress for many years without symptoms until a fracture occurs. Osteoporosis has been called a childhood disease with old age consequences because building healthy bones in youth helps prevent osteoporosis and fractures later in life. However, it is never too late to adopt new habits for healthy bones.

The Link between Anorexia Nervosa and Osteoporosis

Anorexia nervosa has significant physical consequences. Affected individuals can experience nutritional and hormonal problems that negatively impact bone density. Low body weight in females can cause the body to stop producing estrogen, resulting in a condition known as amenorrhea, or absent menstrual periods. Low estrogen levels contribute to significant losses in bone density.

In addition, individuals with anorexia often produce excessive amounts of the adrenal hormone cortisol, which is known to trigger bone loss. Other problems, such as a decrease in the production of growth hormone and other growth factors, low body weight (apart from the estrogen loss it causes), calcium deficiency, and malnutrition, may contribute to bone loss in girls and women with anorexia. Weight loss, restricted dietary intake, and testosterone deficiency may be responsible for the low bone density found in males with the disorder.

Studies suggest that low bone mass is common in people with anorexia and that it occurs early in the course of the disease. Girls with anorexia may be less likely to reach their peak bone density, and therefore, may be at increased risk for osteoporosis and fracture throughout life.

Osteoporosis Management Strategies

Up to one-third of peak bone density is achieved during puberty. Anorexia is often identified during mid to late adolescence, a critical period for bone development. The longer the duration of the disorder, the greater the bone loss and the less likely it is that bone mineral density will ever return to normal. The primary goal of medical therapy for individuals with anorexia is weight gain and, in females, the return of normal menstrual periods. However, attention to other aspects of bone health is also important.

Nutrition: A well-balanced diet rich in calcium and vitamin D is important for healthy bones. Good sources of calcium include low-fat dairy products; dark green, leafy vegetables; and calcium-fortified foods and beverages. Supplements can help ensure that people get adequate amounts of calcium each day, especially in people with a proven milk allergy. The Institute of Medicine (IOM) recommends a daily calcium intake of 1,000 mg (milligrams) for men and women up to age 50. Women over age 50 and men over age 70 should increase their intake to 1,200 mg daily.

Vitamin D plays an important role in calcium absorption and bone health. Food sources of vitamin D include egg yolks, saltwater fish, and liver. Many people may need vitamin D supplements to achieve the recommended intake of 600 to 800 International Units (IU) each day.

Exercise: Like muscle, bone is living tissue that responds to exercise by becoming stronger. The best activity for your bones is weight-bearing exercise that forces you to work against gravity. Some examples include walking, climbing stairs, lifting weights, and dancing.

Although walking and other types of regular exercise can help prevent bone loss and provide many other health benefits, these potential benefits need to be weighed against the risk of fractures, delayed weight gain, and exercise-induced amenorrhea in people with anorexia and those recovering from the disorder.

Healthy lifestyle: Smoking is bad for bones as well as the heart and lungs. In addition, smokers may absorb less calcium from their diets. Alcohol also can have a negative effect on bone health. Those who drink heavily are more prone to bone loss and fracture, because of both poor nutrition and increased risk of falling.

Bone density test: A bone mineral density (BMD) test measures bone density in various parts of the body. This safe and painless test can detect osteoporosis before a fracture occurs and can predict one's chances of fracturing in the future. The BMD test can help determine whether medication should be considered.

Medication: There is no cure for osteoporosis. However, medications are available to prevent and treat the disease in postmenopausal women, men, and both women and men taking glucocorticoid medication.

Section 31.3

Diabetes and Bone Health

This section includes text excerpted from "What People with Diabetes Need to Know about Osteoporosis," NIH Osteoporosis and Related Bone Diseases—National Resource Center (NIH ORBD—NRC), April 2016.

What Is Diabetes?

Diabetes is a disorder of "metabolism," a term that describes the way our bodies chemically change the foods we eat into growth and energy. After we digest food, glucose (sugar) enters the bloodstream, where it is used by the cells for energy. For glucose to get into the cells, insulin must be present.

Insulin is a hormone produced by the pancreas, an organ located behind the stomach. It is responsible for moving glucose from the bloodstream into the cells to provide energy needed for daily life. In people with diabetes, the body produces too little or no insulin or it does not respond properly to the insulin that is produced. As a result, glucose builds up in the blood and may overflow into the urine where it is excreted from the body. Therefore, the cells lose their main source of energy.

According to the Center for Disease Control and Prevention (CDC), 29.1 million people have diabetes.

- In type 1 diabetes, the body produces little or no insulin. This form of the disease typically appears in children and young adults, but it can develop at any age.

- In type 2 diabetes, the body produces insulin but not enough, and the body does not respond properly to the insulin that is produced. This form of the disease is more common in people who are older, overweight, and inactive.

What Is Osteoporosis?

Osteoporosis is a condition in which the bones become less dense and more likely to fracture. Fractures from osteoporosis can result in pain and disability. In the United States, more than 53 million people either already have osteoporosis or are at high risk due to low bone mass.

Risk factors for developing osteoporosis include:

- Being thin or having a small frame
- Having a family history of the disease
- For women, being postmenopausal, having an early menopause, or not having menstrual periods (amenorrhea)
- Using certain medications, such as glucocorticoids
- Not getting enough calcium
- Not getting enough physical activity
- Smoking
- Drinking too much alcohol

Osteoporosis is a disease that often can be prevented. If undetected, it can progress for many years without symptoms until a fracture occurs.

The Link between Diabetes and Osteoporosis

Type 1 diabetes is linked to low bone density, although researchers don't know exactly why. Insulin, which is deficient in type 1 diabetes, may promote bone growth and strength. The onset of type 1 diabetes typically occurs at a young age when bone mass is still increasing. It is possible that people with type 1 diabetes achieve lower peak bone mass, the maximum strength and density that bones reach. People usually reach their peak bone mass by age 30. Low peak bone mass can increase one's risk of developing osteoporosis later in life. Some people with type 1 diabetes also have celiac disease, which is associated with reduced bone mass. It is also possible that cytokines, substances produced by various cells in the body, play a role in the development of both type 1 diabetes and osteoporosis.

Research also suggests that women with type 1 diabetes may have an increased fracture risk, since vision problems and nerve damage associated with the disease have been linked to an increased risk of falls and related fractures. Hypoglycemia, or low blood sugar reactions, may also contribute to falls.

Increased body weight can reduce one's risk of developing osteoporosis. Since excessive weight is common in people with type 2 diabetes, affected people were long believed to be protected against osteoporosis. However, although bone density is increased in people with type 2 diabetes, fractures are increased. As with type 1 diabetes, this may be due to increased falls because of vision problems and nerve damage. Moreover, the sedentary lifestyle common in many people with type 2 diabetes also interferes with bone health; and the disease disproportionately affects older individuals. As well, researchers suspect that the increased fracture risk in people with type 2 diabetes may be due to the negative impact of the disease on bone structure and quality.

Osteoporosis Management Strategies

Strategies to prevent and treat osteoporosis in people with diabetes are the same as for those without diabetes.

Nutrition. A diet rich in calcium and vitamin D is important for healthy bones. Good sources of calcium include low-fat dairy products; dark green, leafy vegetables; and calcium-fortified foods and beverages. Many low-fat and low-sugar sources of calcium are available. Also, supplements can help you meet the daily requirements of calcium and other important nutrients.

Vitamin D plays an important role in calcium absorption and bone health. It is synthesized in the skin through exposure to sunlight. Although many people are able to obtain enough vitamin D naturally, older individuals are often deficient in this vitamin due, in part, to limited time spent outdoors. They may require vitamin D supplements to ensure an adequate daily intake.

Exercise. Like muscle, bone is living tissue that responds to exercise by becoming stronger. The best exercise for your bones is weight-bearing exercise that forces you to work against gravity. Some examples include walking, stair climbing, and dancing. Regular exercise can help prevent bone loss and, by enhancing balance and flexibility, reduce the likelihood of falling and breaking a bone. Exercise is especially important for people with diabetes since exercise helps insulin lower blood glucose levels.

Healthy lifestyle. Smoking is bad for bones as well as for the heart and lungs. Women who smoke tend to go through menopause earlier, triggering earlier bone loss. In addition, smokers may absorb less calcium from their diets. Alcohol can also negatively affect bone health. Heavy drinkers are more prone to bone loss and fracture because of poor nutrition as well as an increased risk of falling. Avoiding smoking and alcohol can also help with managing diabetes.

Bone density test. Specialized tests are known as bone mineral density (BMD) tests measure bone density in various parts of the body. These tests can detect osteoporosis before a bone fracture occurs and predict one's chances of fracturing in the future. It can measure bone density at your hip and spine. People with diabetes should talk to their doctors about whether they might be candidates for a bone density test.

Medication. Like diabetes, there is no cure for osteoporosis. However, several medications are approved by the U.S. Food and Drug Administration (FDA) for the prevention and treatment of osteoporosis in postmenopausal women and men. Medications are also approved for use in both women and men with glucocorticoid-induced osteoporosis.

Section 31.4

Inflammatory Bowel Disease and Bone Health

This section includes text excerpted from "What People with Inflammatory Bowel Disease Need to Know about Osteoporosis," NIH Osteoporosis and Related Bone Diseases—National Resource Center (NIH ORBD—NRC), April 2016.

What Is Inflammatory Bowel Disease?

Crohn disease and ulcerative colitis are also known as inflammatory bowel diseases (IBD). Crohn disease tends to affect the small intestine, although any part of the digestive tract may be involved. Ulcerative colitis usually causes an inflammation in all or part of the large intestine. People with inflammatory bowel disease (IBD) often have diarrhea, abdominal pain, fever, and weight loss.

The causes of Crohn disease and ulcerative colitis are unknown. It is sometimes difficult to distinguish one disease from the other, and there is no cure for either condition. Medications are often prescribed to control the symptoms of IBD; in some cases, surgical removal of the involved intestine may be necessary.

What Is Osteoporosis?

Osteoporosis is a condition in which the bones become less dense and more likely to fracture. Fractures from osteoporosis can result in significant pain and disability. In the United States, more than 53 million people either already have osteoporosis or are at high risk due to low bone mass. Although postmenopausal white women have the highest risk for the disease, men and certain ethnic populations are also at risk.

Risk factors for developing osteoporosis include:

- Thinness or small frame

- Family history of the disease

- Being postmenopausal and particularly having had early menopause

- Abnormal absence of menstrual periods (amenorrhea)

- Prolonged use of certain medications, such as those used to treat lupus, asthma, thyroid deficiencies, and seizures

- Low calcium intake

- Lack of physical activity

- Smoking

- Excessive alcohol intake

Osteoporosis often can be prevented. It is known as a "silent disease" because if undetected, bone loss can progress for many years without symptoms until a fracture occurs. Osteoporosis has been called a childhood disease with old age consequences because building healthy bones in youth helps prevent osteoporosis and fractures later in life. However, it is never too late to adopt new habits for healthy bones.

The Link between Inflammatory Bowel Disease and Osteoporosis

People with IBD are often treated with medications known as glucocorticoids (such as prednisone or cortisone) to reduce the inflammation caused by their disease. Over time, these drugs interfere with the development and maintenance of healthy bones. Bone loss increases with the amount and length of glucocorticoid therapy.

In addition, people with severe inflammation of the small bowel or those who have parts of the small bowel surgically removed may have difficulty absorbing calcium and vitamin D. This is an additional concern for bone health.

Osteoporosis Management Strategies

To protect and promote bone health, people with IBD should eat a diet rich in calcium and vitamin D and participate in an appropriate exercise program. Not smoking and avoiding excessive use of alcohol are also important. In some cases, medication to prevent further bone loss may be recommended, especially for those on long-term glucocorticoid therapy.

Nutrition. A well-balanced diet rich in calcium and vitamin D is important for healthy bones. Good sources of calcium include low-fat dairy products; dark green, leafy vegetables; and calcium-fortified foods and beverages. Supplements can help ensure that you get adequate amounts of calcium each day, especially in people with a proven milk allergy. The Institute of Medicine (IOM) recommends a daily calcium intake of 1,000 mg (milligrams) for adults up to age 50. Women over age 50 and men over age 70 should increase their intake to 1,200 mg daily.

Vitamin D plays an important role in calcium absorption and bone health. Many people, especially those who are older, may need vitamin D supplements to achieve the recommended intake of 600 to 800 IU (International Units) each day.

Exercise. Like muscle, bone is living tissue that responds to exercise by becoming stronger. The best activity for your bones is weight-bearing exercise that forces one to work against gravity. Some examples include walking, climbing stairs, dancing, and weight training. These and other types of exercise also strengthen muscles that support bone, enhance balance and flexibility, and preserve joint mobility, all of which help reduce the likelihood of falling and breaking a bone, especially among older people.

Healthy lifestyle. Smoking is bad for bones as well as the heart and lungs. Women who smoke tend to go through menopause earlier, resulting in earlier reduction in levels of the bone-preserving hormone estrogen and triggering earlier bone loss. In addition, smokers may absorb less calcium from their diets. Alcohol also can have a negative effect on bone health. Those who drink heavily are more prone to bone loss and fracture, because of both poor nutrition and increased risk of falling.

Bone density test. A bone mineral density (BMD) test measures bone density in various parts of the body. This safe and painless test can detect osteoporosis before a fracture occurs and can predict one's chances of fracturing in the future. Adults with IBD should talk to their doctors about whether they might be candidates for a BMD test. This test can help determine whether medication should be considered and can be used to monitor the effects of an osteoporosis treatment program.

Medication. Like Crohn disease and ulcerative colitis, osteoporosis is a disease with no cure. However, several medications are available for the prevention and/or treatment of osteoporosis, including: bisphosphonates; estrogen agonists/antagonists (also called selective estrogen receptor modulators or SERMs); calcitonin; parathyroid hormone; estrogen therapy; hormone therapy; and a receptor activator of nuclear factor kappa-β ligand (RANKL) inhibitor.

Section 31.5

Lactose Intolerance and Bone Health

This section includes text excerpted from "What People with
Lactose Intolerance Need to Know about Osteoporosis," NIH
Osteoporosis and Related Bone Diseases—National
Resource Center (NIH ORBD—NRC), April 2016.

What Is Lactose Intolerance?

Lactose intolerance is a common problem. It happens when your
body does not have enough lactase, which is an enzyme produced in
the small intestine. Lactase is necessary to digest lactose—the natural sugar found in milk and other dairy products. In the intestines,
undigested lactose leads to the buildup of gas. Within 30 minutes to
2 hours after eating dairy products containing lactose, people with
lactose intolerance start to develop stomach cramps and diarrhea.
These two symptoms must be present for a person to be diagnosed
with lactose intolerance.

Lactose intolerance is a common condition that is more likely to
occur in adulthood, with a higher incidence in older adults. Some
ethnic and racial populations are more affected than others, including African Americans, Hispanic Americans, American Indians, and
Asian Americans. The condition is least common among Americans of
northern European descent.

What Is Osteoporosis?

Osteoporosis is a condition in which bones become less dense and
more likely to fracture. Fractures from osteoporosis can result in pain
and disability. In the United States, more than 53 million people either
already have osteoporosis or are at high risk due to low bone mass.

Risk factors for developing osteoporosis include:

- Thinness or small frame

- Family history of the disease

- Being postmenopausal and particularly having had early
  menopause

- Abnormal absence of menstrual periods (amenorrhea) prolonged
  use of certain medications, such as those used to treat lupus,
  asthma, thyroid deficiencies, and seizures

- Low calcium intake

- Lack of physical activity

- Smoking

- Excessive alcohol intake

Osteoporosis often can be prevented. It is known as a "silent disease" because if undetected, bone loss can progress for many years without symptoms until a fracture occurs. Osteoporosis has been called a childhood disease with old age consequences because building healthy bones in youth helps prevent osteoporosis and fractures later in life. However, it is never too late to adopt new habits for healthy bones.

The Link between Lactose Intolerance and Osteoporosis

One of the primary risk factors for developing osteoporosis is not getting enough calcium in your diet. Because dairy products are a major source of calcium, you might assume that people with lactose intolerance who avoid dairy products could be at increased risk for osteoporosis. However, research exploring the role of lactose intolerance in calcium intake and bone health has produced conflicting results. Some studies have found that people with lactose intolerance are at higher risk for low bone density, but other studies have not. Regardless, people with lactose intolerance should follow the same basic strategies to build and maintain healthy bones and should pay extra attention to getting enough calcium.

Bone Health Strategies

Calcium and vitamin D. A well-balanced diet rich in calcium and vitamin D is important for healthy bones. Besides low-fat dairy products, good sources of calcium include dark green, leafy vegetables and calcium-fortified foods and beverages. Many low-fat and low-sugar sources of calcium are available. Also, supplements can help people with lactose intolerance meet their daily requirements of calcium and other important nutrients. The Institute of Medicine (IOM) recommends a daily calcium intake of 1,000 mg for men and women up to age 50, increasing to 1,200 mg for women over age 50 and men over age 70.

Studies have shown that people who have at least some intestinal lactase can increase their tolerance to lactose by gradually introducing dairy products into the diet. These people can often eat small portions of dairy products without developing symptoms. The key for them is to consume small amounts of dairy products at a time so that there is enough lactase available in the intestine to digest the lactose. When the lactose is fully digested, symptoms do not develop.

Also, certain sources of dairy products may be easier for people with lactose intolerance to digest. For example, ripened cheese may contain up to 95 percent less lactose than whole milk. Yogurt containing active cultures also lessens gastrointestinal symptoms. A variety of lactose-reduced dairy products, including milk, cottage cheese, and processed cheese slices, are also available. Lactose replacement pills and liquid are also available to help with the digestion of dairy products.

Vitamin D plays an important role in calcium absorption and bone health. Food sources of vitamin D include egg yolks, fish oil, saltwater fish, liver, fortified margarine, and breakfast cereals. Many people may need vitamin D supplements to achieve the recommended intake of 600 IU (international units) each day. Men and women over age 70 should increase their uptake to 800 IU daily.

Exercise. Like muscle, bone is living tissue that responds to exercise by becoming stronger. The best activity for your bones is weight-bearing exercise that forces you to work against gravity. Some examples include walking, climbing stairs, weight training, and dancing. Regular exercise, such as walking, may help prevent bone loss and, by enhancing balance and flexibility, can reduce the likelihood of falling and breaking a bone.

Healthy lifestyle. Smoking is bad for bones as well as the heart and lungs. Women who smoke tend to go through menopause earlier, which triggers earlier bone loss. In addition, smokers may absorb less calcium from their diets. Alcohol also can have a negative effect on bone health. Those who drink heavily are more prone to bone loss and fracture because of both poor nutrition and increased risk of falling.

Bone density testing. A bone mineral density (BMD) test measures bone density in various parts of the body. This safe and painless test can detect osteoporosis before a bone fracture occurs and can predict one's chances of fracturing in the future. People with lactose intolerance should talk to their doctors about whether they might be candidates for a BMD test, which can help determine whether increased attention to bone health is warranted.

Medication. Like lactose intolerance, osteoporosis has no cure. However, several medications are available for the prevention and/or treatment of the disease, including: bisphosphonates; estrogen agonists/antagonists (also called selective estrogen receptor modulators or SERMs); calcitonin; parathyroid hormone; estrogen therapy; hormone therapy; and a receptor activator of nuclear factor kappa-β ligand (RANKL) inhibitor.

Section 31.6

Lupus and Bone Health

This section includes text excerpted from "What People with Lupus Need to Know about Osteoporosis," NIH Osteoporosis and Related Bone Diseases—National Resource Center (NIH ORBD—NRC), April 2016.

What Is Lupus?

Lupus is an autoimmune disease, a disorder in which the body attacks its own healthy cells and tissues. As a result, various parts of the body—such as the joints, skin, kidneys, heart, and lungs—can become inflamed and damaged. There are many different kinds of lupus. Systemic lupus erythematosus (SLE) is the form of the disease that is commonly referred to as lupus.

People with lupus can have a wide range of symptoms. Some of the most commonly reported symptoms are fatigue, painful or swollen joints, fever, skin rashes, and kidney problems. Typically, these symptoms come and go. When symptoms are present in a person with the disease, it is known as a flare. When symptoms are not present, the disease is said to be in remission.

We know that many more women than men have lupus. Lupus is more common in African American women than in white women and is also more common in women of Hispanic, Asian, and Native American descent. African American and Hispanic women are also more likely to have active disease and serious organ system involvement. In addition, lupus can run in families, but the risk that a child or a brother or sister of a patient will also have lupus is still quite low. It is difficult to estimate how many people in the United States have the disease because its symptoms vary widely and its onset is often hard to pinpoint. Unfortunately, there is no cure for the disease.

What Is Osteoporosis?

Osteoporosis is a condition in which the bones become less dense and more likely to fracture. Fractures from osteoporosis can result in significant pain and disability. In the United States, more than 53 million people either already have osteoporosis or are at high risk due to low bone mass.

Risk factors for developing osteoporosis include:

- Thinness or small frame
- Family history of the disease
- Being postmenopausal and particularly having had early menopause
- Abnormal absence of menstrual periods (amenorrhea)
- Prolonged use of certain medications, such as those used to treat lupus, asthma, thyroid deficiencies, and seizures
- Low calcium intake
- Lack of physical activity
- Smoking
- Excessive alcohol intake

Osteoporosis often can be prevented. It is known as a "silent disease" because, if undetected, bone loss can progress for many years without symptoms until a fracture occurs. Osteoporosis has been called a childhood disease with old age consequences because building healthy bones in youth helps prevent osteoporosis and fractures later in life. However, it is never too late to adopt new habits for healthy bones.

The Link between Lupus and Osteoporosis

Studies have found an increase in bone loss and fracture in individuals with SLE. Individuals with lupus are at increased risk for osteoporosis for many reasons. To begin with, the glucocorticoid medications often prescribed to treat SLE can trigger significant bone loss. In addition, pain and fatigue caused by the disease can result in inactivity, further increasing osteoporosis risk. Studies also show that bone loss in lupus may occur as a direct result of the disease. Of concern is the fact that 90 percent of the people affected with lupus are women, a group already at increased risk for osteoporosis.

Osteoporosis Management Strategies

Strategies for the prevention and treatment of osteoporosis in people with lupus are not significantly different from the strategies for those who do not have the disease.

Nutrition. A well-balanced diet rich in calcium and vitamin D is important for healthy bones. Good sources of calcium include low-fat dairy products; dark green, leafy vegetables; and calcium-fortified foods and beverages. Supplements can help ensure that you get adequate amounts of calcium each day, especially in people with a proven milk allergy. The Institute of Medicine recommends a daily calcium intake of 1,000 mg (milligrams) for men and women up to age 50. Women over age 50 and men over age 70 should increase their intake to 1,200 mg daily.

Vitamin D plays an important role in calcium absorption and bone health. Food sources of vitamin D include egg yolks, saltwater fish, and liver. Many people obtain enough vitamin D naturally, but some individuals may need vitamin D supplements to achieve the recommended intake of 600 to 800 IU (International Units) each day.

Exercise. Like muscle, bone is living tissue that responds to exercise by becoming stronger. The best activity for your bones is weight-bearing exercise that forces you to work against gravity. Some examples include walking, climbing stairs, weight training, and dancing.

Exercising can be challenging for people with lupus who are affected by joint pain and inflammation, muscle pain, and fatigue. However, regular exercise, such as walking, may help prevent bone loss and provide many other health benefits.

Healthy lifestyle. Smoking is bad for bones as well as the heart and lungs. Women who smoke tend to go through menopause earlier, resulting in earlier reduction in levels of the bone-preserving hormone estrogen and triggering earlier bone loss. In addition, smokers may absorb less calcium from their diets. Alcohol also can have a negative effect on bone health. Those who drink heavily are more prone to bone loss and fracture, both because of poor nutrition and an increased risk of falling.

Bone density test. A bone mineral density (BMD) test measures bone density at various parts of the body. This safe and painless test can detect osteoporosis before a fracture occurs and predict one's chances of fracturing in the future. Lupus patients, particularly those receiving glucocorticoid therapy for two months or more, should talk to their doctors about whether they might be candidates for a bone density test. The BMD test can help determine whether medication should be considered.

Medication. Like lupus, osteoporosis is a disease with no cure. However, several medications are available for the prevention and/or treatment of osteoporosis, including: bisphosphonates; estrogen agonists/antagonists (also called selective estrogen receptor modulators or SERMS); calcitonin; parathyroid hormone; estrogen therapy; hormone therapy; and a RANK ligand (RANKL) inhibitor.

Section 31.7

Depression Linked to Bone Loss

This section includes text excerpted from "Depression and Osteoporosis," National Institute of Mental Health (NIMH), January 30, 2017.

Depression not only affects your brain and behavior—it affects your entire body. Depression has been linked with other health problems, including osteoporosis. Dealing with more than one health problem at a time can be difficult, so proper treatment is important.

What Is Depression?

Major depressive disorder, or depression, is a serious mental illness. Depression interferes with your daily life and routine and reduces your quality of life (QOL). about 6.7 percent of U.S. adults ages 18 and older have depression.

Signs and Symptoms of Depression

- Ongoing sad, anxious, or empty feelings

- Feeling hopeless

- Feeling guilty, worthless, or helpless

- Feeling irritable or restless

- Loss of interest in activities or hobbies once enjoyable, including sex

- Feeling tired all the time

- Difficulty concentrating, remembering details, or making decisions

- Difficulty falling asleep or staying asleep, a condition called insomnia or sleeping all the time

- Overeating or loss of appetite

- Thoughts of death and suicide or suicide attempts

- Ongoing aches and pains, headaches, cramps, or digestive problems that do not ease with treatment

What Is Osteoporosis?

Osteoporosis is a disease that thins and weakens your bones to the point that they become fragile and break easily. About 10 million people in the United States have osteoporosis. About 50 percent of women and 25 percent of men age 50 or older will fracture a bone due to osteoporosis.

The Link between Depression and Osteoporosis

Studies show that older people with depression are more likely to have low bone mass than older people who aren't depressed. Bone mass refers to the number of minerals, such as calcium, in your bones. Low bone mass can lead to osteoporosis. Younger women with depression may also be at risk for osteoporosis. One study found that, among women who have not yet reached menopause, those with mild depression have less bone mass than those who aren't depressed.

Although osteoporosis affects more women than men, one study has recommended checking for osteoporosis in older men with depression. The same study suggested checking for depression in older men with osteoporosis, because osteoporosis increases the risk of depression.

If you have osteoporosis, you may need to make many lifestyle changes, and these changes may increase your risk of depression.

For example:

- To prevent falls that could cause already-fragile bones to fracture or break, you may not be able to take part in some activities you once enjoyed.

- Weakened bones may make it harder to perform everyday tasks, and you could lose some of your independence.

- You may feel nervous about going to crowded places, such as malls or movie theaters, for fear of falling and breaking a bone.

How Is Depression Treated in People Who Have Osteoporosis?

Depression is diagnosed and treated by a healthcare provider. Treating depression can help you manage your osteoporosis and improve your overall health. Recovery from depression takes time but treatments are effective.

At present, the most common treatments for depression include:

- Cognitive-behavioral therapy (CBT), a type of psychotherapy, or talk therapy, that helps people change negative thinking styles and behaviors that may contribute to their depression

- Selective serotonin reuptake inhibitor (SSRI), a type of antidepressant medication that includes citalopram (Celexa), sertraline (Zoloft), and fluoxetine (Prozac)

- Serotonin and norepinephrine reuptake inhibitor (SNRI), a type of antidepressant medication similar to SSRI that includes venlafaxine (Effexor) and duloxetine (Cymbalta)

While currently, available depression treatments are generally well tolerated and safe, some medications, including some antidepressants, anticonvulsants, and lithium, can increase your risk for osteoporosis. Certain medications can also increase your risk of falling, which is dangerous if you already have osteoporosis. Talk with your healthcare provider about side effects, possible drug interactions, and other treatment options that best suit your situation.

For the latest information on medications, visit the U.S. Food and Drug Administration (FDA) website at www.fda.gov. Not everyone responds to treatment the same way. Medications can take several weeks to work, may need to be combined with ongoing talk therapy, or may need to be changed or adjusted to minimize side effects and achieve the best results. But treatment can be effective.

Osteoporosis treatment may include medications that slow or stop bone loss or build new bone. exercise is an important part of osteoporosis treatment, particularly activities in which you support your weight on your feet. These activities help to strengthen bones and muscles that can prevent falls. These activities can also boost your mood and treat your depression. Your healthcare provider can recommend exercises that are right for you.

Section 31.8

Asthma and Bone Health

This section includes text excerpted from "What People with Asthma Need to Know about Osteoporosis," NIH Osteoporosis and Related Bone Diseases—National Resource Center (NIH ORBD—NRC), April 2015. Reviewed January 2019.

What Is Asthma?

According to the National Heart, Lung, and Blood Institute (NHLBI), asthma is a chronic lung disease that affects more than 25 million Americans, nearly 7 million of whom are children. For people with asthma, everyday things can trigger an attack. These triggers include air pollution, allergens, exercise, infections, emotional upset, or certain foods.

Typical asthma symptoms include coughing, wheezing, tightness in the chest, difficulty breathing, rapid heart rate, and sweating. Children with asthma often complain of an itchy upper chest or develop a dry cough. These may be the only signs of an asthma attack.

Asthma itself does not pose a threat to bone health. However, certain medications used to treat asthma and some behaviors triggered by concern over the disease can have a negative impact on the skeleton.

What Is Osteoporosis?

Osteoporosis is a condition in which the bones become less dense and more likely to fracture. Fractures from osteoporosis can result in pain and disability. In the United States, more than 53 million people either already have osteoporosis or are at high risk due to low bone mass.

Risk factors for developing osteoporosis include:

- Thinness or small frame
- Family history of the disease
- Being postmenopausal and particularly having had early menopause
- Abnormal absence of menstrual periods (amenorrhea)
- Prolonged use of certain medications, such as those used to treat lupus, asthma, thyroid deficiencies, and seizures
- Low calcium intake
- Lack of physical activity
- Smoking
- Excessive alcohol intake

Osteoporosis often can be prevented. It is known as a "silent disease" because, if undetected, it can progress for many years without symptoms until a fracture occurs. Osteoporosis has been called a childhood disease with consequences in old age because building healthy bones in youth can help prevent the disease and fractures later in life. However, it is never too late to adopt new habits for healthy bones.

The Link between Asthma and Osteoporosis

People with asthma tend to be at increased risk for osteoporosis, especially in the spine, for several reasons. First, anti-inflammatory medications, known as glucocorticoids, are commonly prescribed for asthma. When taken by mouth, these medications can decrease calcium absorbed from food, increase calcium loss from the kidneys, decrease bone formation, and increase bone loss. Corticosteroids also interfere with the production of sex hormones in both women and men, which can contribute to bone loss, and they can cause muscle weakness, which can increase the risk of falling and related fractures. Even inhaled forms of corticosteroids can negatively impact bone health.

People with asthma may think that milk and other dairy products trigger asthma attacks, although the evidence shows that this is only likely to be true if they also have a dairy allergy. This unnecessary avoidance of calcium-rich dairy products can be especially damaging for children with asthma who need calcium to build strong bones.

Because exercise often can trigger an asthma attack, many people with asthma avoid weight-bearing physical activities that are known to strengthen bone. Those people who remain physically active often choose swimming as their first exercise of choice because it is less likely than other activities to trigger an asthma attack. Unfortunately, swimming does not have the same beneficial impact on bone health as weight-bearing exercises, which work the body against gravity. Weight-bearing exercises include walking, jogging, racquet sports, basketball, volleyball, aerobics, dancing, and weight training.

Osteoporosis Management Strategies

Strategies to prevent and treat osteoporosis in people with asthma are not significantly different from those used to treat people who do not have asthma.

Nutrition. A well-balanced diet rich in calcium and vitamin D is important for healthy bones. Good sources of calcium include low-fat dairy products; dark green, leafy vegetables; and calcium-fortified foods and beverages. Supplements can help ensure that the calcium requirement is met each day, especially in those with a proven milk allergy. The Institute of Medicine recommends a daily calcium intake of 1,000 mg each day for men and women up to age 50. Women over age 50 and men over age 70 should increase their intake to 1,200 mg daily.

Vitamin D plays an important role in calcium absorption and bone health. Food sources of vitamin D include egg yolks, saltwater fish, and liver. Many people obtain enough vitamin D from eating fortified foods. Other individuals, especially those who are older, live in northern climates, or use sunscreen, may require vitamin D supplements to achieve the recommended intake of 600 to 800 International Units (IU) each day.

Exercise. Like muscle, bone is living tissue that responds to exercise by becoming stronger. The best kind of activity for your bones is weight-bearing exercise that forces you to work against gravity. Some examples include walking, climbing stairs, weight training, and dancing. Regular exercise, such as walking, may help prevent bone loss and provide many other health benefits.

People who experience exercise-induced asthma should exercise in an environmentally controlled facility and participate in activities that fall within their limitations. They may also use medication when necessary to enable them to exercise.

Healthy lifestyle. Smoking is bad for bones as well as the heart and lungs. Women who smoke tend to go through menopause earlier, triggering earlier bone loss. In addition, people who smoke may absorb less calcium from their diets. Alcohol also can affect bone health negatively. Those who drink heavily are more prone to bone loss and fracture because of both poor nutrition and an increased risk of falling.

Reducing exposure to asthma triggers, such as irritants and allergens, can help lessen a person's reliance on glucocorticoid medication. Avoiding people with colds and other respiratory infections and minimizing emotional stress can also be important.

Bone density test. A bone mineral density (BMD) test measures bone density at various sites of the body. This safe and painless test can detect osteoporosis before a fracture occurs and can predict one's chances of future fracture. People with asthma, particularly those receiving glucocorticoid therapy for two months or more, should talk to their doctors about whether they might be candidates for a BMD test.

Medication. Like asthma, osteoporosis is a disease with no cure. However, there are medications available to prevent and treat osteoporosis, including bisphosphonates; estrogen agonists/antagonists (also called selective estrogen receptor modulators or SERMs); calcitonin; parathyroid hormone; estrogen therapy; hormone therapy; and a receptor activator of nuclear factor kappa-β ligand (RANKL) inhibitor.

Because of their effectiveness in controlling asthma with fewer side effects, inhaled glucocorticoids are preferred to oral forms of the medication. Bone loss tends to increase with increased glucocorticoid doses and prolonged use; therefore, the lowest possible dose for the shortest period of time that controls asthma symptoms is recommended.

Section 31.9

Rheumatoid Arthritis and Bone Health

This section includes text excerpted from "What People with
Rheumatoid Arthritis Need to Know about Osteoporosis," NIH
Osteoporosis and Related Bone Diseases—National Resource
Center (NIH ORBD—NRC), April 2016.

What Is Rheumatoid Arthritis?

Rheumatoid arthritis is an autoimmune disease, a disorder in which the body attacks its own healthy cells and tissues. When someone has rheumatoid arthritis, the membranes around his or her joints become inflamed and release enzymes that cause the surrounding cartilage and bone to wear away. In severe cases, other tissues and body organs also can be affected.

Individuals with rheumatoid arthritis often experience pain, swelling, and stiffness in their joints, especially those in the hands and feet. Motion can be limited in the affected joints, curtailing one's ability to accomplish even the most basic everyday tasks. About one-quarter of those with rheumatoid arthritis develop nodules (bumps) that grow under the skin, usually close to the joints. Fatigue, anemia (low red blood cell count), neck pain, and dry eyes and dry mouth also can occur in individuals with the disease.

Scientists estimate that about 1.5 million people in the United States have rheumatoid arthritis. The disease occurs in all racial and ethnic groups, but affects two to three times as many women as men. Rheumatoid arthritis is more commonly found in older individuals, although the disease typically begins in middle age. Children and young adults can also be affected.

What Is Osteoporosis?

Osteoporosis is a condition in which the bones become less dense and more likely to fracture. Fractures from osteoporosis can result in significant pain and disability. In the United States, more than 53 million people either already have osteoporosis or are at high risk due to low bone mass.

Risk factors for developing osteoporosis include:

- Thinness or small frame

- Family history of the disease

- Being postmenopausal and particularly having had early menopause

- Abnormal absence of menstrual periods (amenorrhea)

- Prolonged use of certain medications, such as those used to treat lupus, asthma, thyroid deficiencies, and seizures

- Low calcium intake

- Lack of physical activity

- Smoking

- Excessive alcohol intake

Osteoporosis often can be prevented. It is known as a "silent disease" because, if undetected, bone loss can progress for many years without symptoms until a fracture occurs. Osteoporosis has been called a childhood disease with old age consequences because building healthy bones in youth helps prevent osteoporosis and fractures later in life. However, it is never too late to adopt new habits for healthy bones.

The Link between Rheumatoid Arthritis and Osteoporosis

Studies have found an increased risk of bone loss and fracture in individuals with rheumatoid arthritis. People with rheumatoid arthritis are at increased risk for osteoporosis for many reasons. To begin with, the glucocorticoid medications often prescribed for the treatment of rheumatoid arthritis can trigger significant bone loss. In addition, pain and loss of joint function caused by the disease can result in inactivity, further increasing osteoporosis risk. Studies also show that bone loss in rheumatoid arthritis may occur as a direct result of the disease. The bone loss is most pronounced in areas immediately surrounding the affected joints. Of concern is the fact that women, a group already at increased risk for osteoporosis, are two to three times more likely than men to have rheumatoid arthritis as well.

Osteoporosis Management Strategies

Strategies for preventing and treating osteoporosis in people with rheumatoid arthritis are not significantly different from the strategies for those who do not have the disease.

Nutrition. A well-balanced diet rich in calcium and vitamin D is important for healthy bones. Good sources of calcium include low-fat dairy products; dark green, leafy vegetables; and calcium-fortified foods and beverages. Supplements can help ensure that you get adequate amounts of calcium each day, especially in people with a proven milk allergy. The Institute of Medicine recommends a daily calcium intake of 1,000 mg (milligrams) for men and women up to age 50. Women over age 50 and men over age 70 should increase their intake to 1,200 mg daily.

Vitamin D plays an important role in calcium absorption and bone health. Food sources of vitamin D include egg yolks, saltwater fish, and liver. Many people, especially those who are older, may need vitamin D supplements to achieve the recommended intake of 600 to 800 IU (International Units) each day.

Exercise. Like muscle, bone is living tissue that responds to exercise by becoming stronger. The best activity for your bones is weight-bearing exercise that forces you to work against gravity. Some examples include walking, climbing stairs, weight training, and dancing.

Exercising can be challenging for people with rheumatoid arthritis, and it needs to be balanced with rest when the disease is active. However, regular exercise, such as walking, can help prevent bone loss and, by enhancing balance and flexibility, can reduce the likelihood of falling and breaking a bone. Exercise is also important for preserving joint mobility.

Healthy lifestyle. Smoking is bad for bones as well as the heart and lungs. Women who smoke tend to go through menopause earlier, resulting in earlier reduction in levels of the bone-preserving hormone estrogen and triggering earlier bone loss. In addition, smokers may absorb less calcium from their diets. Alcohol also can have a negative effect on bone health. Those who drink heavily are more prone to bone loss and fracture, because of both poor nutrition and increased risk of falling.

Bone density test. A bone mineral density (BMD) test measures bone density in various parts of the body. This safe and painless test can detect osteoporosis before a fracture occurs and can predict one's chances of fracturing in the future. The BMD test can help determine whether medication should be considered. People with rheumatoid arthritis, particularly those who have been receiving glucocorticoid therapy for two months or more, should talk to their doctor about whether a BMD test is appropriate.

Medication. Like rheumatoid arthritis, osteoporosis has no cure. However, medications are available to prevent and treat osteoporosis. Several medications are available for people with rheumatoid arthritis who have or are at risk for glucocorticoid-induced osteoporosis.

Section 31.10

Celiac Disease and Bone Health

This section includes text excerpted from "What People with Celiac Disease Need to Know about Osteoporosis," NIH Osteoporosis and Related Bone Diseases—National Resource Center (NIH ORBD—NRC), April 2016.

What Is Celiac Disease?

Celiac disease, sometimes called sprue or celiac sprue, is an inherited intestinal disorder in which the body cannot tolerate gluten. Gluten is a protein found in wheat, rye, barley, farina, and bulgur. When people with celiac disease eat foods containing gluten, their immune systems respond by attacking and damaging the lining of the small intestine. The small intestine is responsible for absorbing nutrients from food into the bloodstream for the body to use. When the lining is damaged, so is its ability to absorb these nutrients.

Celiac disease affects people differently. Some people develop symptoms as children and others as adults. Symptoms vary and may or may not occur in the digestive system. They may include diarrhea, abdominal pain, weight loss, irritability, and depression, among others. Irritability is one of the most common symptoms among children. In some cases, a diagnosis of celiac disease is missed because the symptoms are so varied and may only flare up occasionally.

Children and adults with untreated celiac disease may become malnourished, meaning they do not get enough nutrients, resulting in anemia, weight loss, and, in children, delayed growth and small stature. Among the possible complications of untreated celiac disease is the inability to develop optimal bone mass in children and the loss of bone in adults, both of which increase the risk of osteoporosis. The only treatment for celiac disease is to follow a gluten-free diet.

What Is Osteoporosis?

Osteoporosis is a condition in which the bones become less dense and more likely to fracture. Fractures from osteoporosis can result in pain and disability. In the United States, more than 53 million people either already have osteoporosis or are at high risk due to low bone mass. Although postmenopausal white women have the highest risk for the disease, men and certain ethnic populations are also at risk.

Risk factors for developing osteoporosis include:

- Thinness or small frame

- Family history of the disease

- Being postmenopausal and particularly having an early menopause

- Abnormal absence of menstrual periods (amenorrhea)

- Prolonged use of certain medications, such as those used to treat lupus, asthma, thyroid deficiencies, and seizures

- Low calcium intake

- Lack of physical activity

- Smoking

- Excessive alcohol intake

Osteoporosis often can be prevented. However, it is known as a "silent disease" because, if undetected, osteoporosis can progress for many years without symptoms until a fracture occurs. It has been called a childhood disease with old age consequences because building healthy bones in youth helps prevent osteoporosis and fractures later in life. However, it is never too late to adopt new habits for healthy bones.

The Link between Celiac Disease and Osteoporosis

Osteoporosis is a complication of untreated celiac disease. The small intestine is responsible for absorbing important nutrients, such as calcium. Calcium is essential for building and maintaining healthy bones. Even people with celiac disease who consume enough calcium are often deficient in this nutrient. And because calcium is needed to keep bones healthy, low bone density is common in both children and adults with untreated and newly diagnosed celiac disease.

Osteoporosis Management Strategies

When people with celiac disease eliminate foods containing gluten from their diet, normal absorption of nutrients from the intestines is usually restored within a few months, although it may take up to two years in older adults. Eventually, most children and adults have significant improvements in bone density.

People with celiac disease who have successfully adopted a gluten-free diet also need to follow the same basic strategies for bone health that apply to others who don't have the disease. These strategies include getting adequate calcium and vitamin D, performing weight-bearing exercise, not smoking, and avoiding excessive use of alcohol. In some cases, an osteoporosis treatment medication may be recommended.

Nutrition. A well-balanced diet rich in calcium and vitamin D is important for healthy bones. Good sources of calcium include low-fat dairy products; dark green, leafy vegetables; and calcium-fortified foods and beverages. Supplements can help ensure that the calcium requirement is met each day, especially in people with a proven milk allergy. The Institute of Medicine recommends a daily calcium intake of 1,000 mg (milligrams) for men and women up to age 50. Women over age 50 and men over age 70 should increase their intake to 1,200 mg daily.

Vitamin D plays an important role in calcium absorption and bone health. Food sources of vitamin D include egg yolks, saltwater fish, and liver. Older individuals—especially those who are housebound, live in northern climates, or use sunscreen—are often deficient in this vitamin and may need vitamin D supplements to achieve the recommended intake of 600 to 800 IU (International Units) each day.

Exercise. Like muscle, bone is living tissue that responds to exercise by becoming stronger. The best kind of activity for your bones is weight-bearing exercise that forces you to work against gravity. Some examples include walking, climbing stairs, weight training, and dancing. These and other types of exercise also strengthen muscles that support bone, enhance balance and flexibility, and preserve joint mobility, all of which help reduce the likelihood of falling and breaking a bone, especially among older people.

Healthy lifestyle. Smoking is bad for bones as well as the heart and lungs. Women who smoke tend to go through menopause earlier, resulting in earlier reduction in levels of the bone-preserving hormone estrogen and triggering earlier bone loss. In addition, smokers may absorb less calcium from their diets. Alcohol also can have a negative effect on bone health. Those who drink heavily are more prone to bone loss and fracture, because of both poor nutrition and increased risk of falling.

Bone density test. A bone mineral density (BMD) test measures bone density in various sites of the body. This safe and painless test usually can detect osteoporosis before a fracture occurs and predict one's chances of fracturing in the future. Adults with celiac disease should talk to their doctors about whether they might be candidates for a BMD test. The test can help determine whether medication should be considered.

Medication. Several medications are available to prevent and treat osteoporosis, including: bisphosphonates; estrogen agonists/antagonists (also called selective estrogen receptor modulators or SERMs); calcitonin; parathyroid hormone; estrogen therapy; hormone therapy; and a receptor activator of nuclear factor kappa-β ligand (RANKL) inhibitor.

Chapter 32

Fall and Fractures

Chapter Contents

Section 32.1

The Fall Itself

This section includes text excerpted from "Preventing
Falls and Related Fractures," NIH Osteoporosis and Related Bone
Diseases—National Resource Center (NIH ORBD—NRC),
April 2015. Reviewed January 2019.

Falls

Falls are serious at any age, and breaking a bone after a fall
becomes more likely as a person ages. Many of us know someone who
has fallen and broken a bone. While healing, the fracture limits the
person's activities and sometimes requires surgery. Often, the person wears a heavy cast to support the broken bone and needs physical therapy to resume normal activities. People are often unaware
of the frequent link between a broken bone and osteoporosis. It is
known as a silent disease because it progresses without symptoms,
osteoporosis involves the gradual loss of bone tissue or bone density and results in bones so fragile they break under the slightest
strain. Consequently, falls are especially dangerous for people who
are unaware that they have low bone density. If the patient and the
doctor fail to connect the broken bone to osteoporosis, the chance to
make a diagnosis with a bone density test and begin a prevention
or treatment program is lost. Bone loss continues, and other bones
may break.

Several factors can lead to a fall. Loss of footing or traction is a
common cause of falls. Loss of footing occurs when there is less than
total contact between one's foot and the ground or floor. Loss of traction
occurs when one's feet slip on wet or slippery ground or floor. Other
examples of loss of traction include tripping, especially over uneven
surfaces such as sidewalks, curbs, or floor elevations that result from
carpeting, risers, or scatter rugs. Loss of footing also happens from
using household items intended for other purposes—for example,
climbing on kitchen chairs or balancing on boxes or books to increase
height.

A fall may occur because a person's reflexes have changed. As people
age, reflexes slow down. Reflexes are automatic responses to stimuli
in the environment. Examples of reflexes include quickly slamming on
the car brakes when a child runs into the street or quickly moving out
of the way when something accidentally falls. Aging slows a person's

reaction time and makes it harder to regain one's balance following a sudden movement or shift of body weight.

Changes in muscle mass and body fat also can play a role in falls. As people get older, they lose muscle mass because they have become less active over time. Loss of muscle mass, especially in the legs, reduces one's strength to the point where she or he is often unable to get up from a chair without assistance. In addition, as people age, they lose body fat that has cushioned and protected bony areas, such as the hips. This loss of cushioning also affects the soles of the feet, which upsets the person's ability to balance. The gradual loss of muscle strength, which is common in older people but not inevitable, also plays a role in falling. Muscle-strengthening exercises can help people regain their balance, level of activity, and alertness no matter what their age.

Changes in vision also increase the risk of falling. Diminished vision can be corrected with glasses. However, often these glasses are bifocal or trifocal so that when the person looks down through the lower half of her or his glasses, depth perception is altered. This makes it easy to lose one's balance and fall. To prevent this from happening, people who wear bifocals or trifocals must practice looking straight ahead and lowering their head. For many other older people, vision changes cannot be corrected completely, making even the home environment hazardous.

Improving Balance

- Do muscle-strengthening exercises
- Obtain maximum vision correction
- Practice using bifocal or trifocal glasses
- Practice balance exercises daily

As people get older, they also are more likely to suffer from a variety of chronic medical conditions that often require taking several medications. People with chronic illnesses that affect their circulation, sensation, mobility, or mental alertness as well as those taking some types of medications are more likely to fall as a result of drug-related side effects such as dizziness, confusion, disorientation, or slowed reflexes.

Drinking alcoholic beverages also increases the risk of falling. Alcohol slows reflexes and response time; causes dizziness, sleepiness, or lightheadedness; alters balance; and encourages risky behaviors that can lead to falls.

Medications That May Increase the Risk of Falling

- Blood pressure pills
- Heart medicines
- Diuretics or water pills
- Muscle relaxers or tranquilizers

The Force and Direction of a Fall

The force of a fall (how hard a person lands) plays a major role in determining whether or not a person will break a bone. For example, the greater the distance between the hip bone and the floor, the greater the risk of fracturing a hip, so tall people appear to have an increased risk of fracture when they fall. The angle at which a person falls also is important. For example, falling sideways or straight down is more risky than falling backward.

Protective responses, such as reflexes and changes in posture that break the fall, can reduce the risk of fracturing a bone. Individuals who land on their hands or grab an object on their descent are less likely to fracture their hip, but they may fracture their wrist or arm. Although these fractures are painful and interfere with daily activities, they do not carry the high risks that a hip fracture does.

The type of surface on which one lands also can affect whether or not a bone breaks. Landing on a soft surface is less likely to cause a fracture than landing on a hard surface.

Preliminary research suggests that by wearing trochanteric (hip) padding, people can decrease the chances of fracturing a hip after a fall. The energy created by the fall is distributed throughout the pad, lessening the impact to the hip. Further research is needed to fully evaluate the role of these devices in decreasing the risk of a hip fracture following a fall.

Did You Know?

- Being tall appears to increase your risk of a hip fracture.
- How you land increases your fracture risk.
- Catching yourself so you land on your hands or grabbing onto an object as you fall can prevent a hip fracture.

Bone Fragility

Although most serious falls happen when people are older, steps to prevent and treat bone loss and falls can never begin too early. Many people begin adulthood with less than optimal bone mass, so the fact that bone mass or density is lost slowly over time puts them at increased risk for fractures.

Bones that once were strong become so fragile and thin that they break easily. Activities that once were done without a second thought are now avoided for fear that they will lead to another fracture.

Steps to Prevent Fragile Bones

• Consume adequate amounts of calcium and vitamin D.

• Exercise several times a week.

• Ask your doctor about a bone mineral density test.

• Ask about medications to slow bone loss and reduce fracture risk.

Section 32.2

Prevention of Falls and Fractures

This section includes text excerpted from "Preventing Falls and Related Fractures," NIH Osteoporosis and Related Bone Diseases—National Resource Center (NIH ORBD—NRC), April 2015. Reviewed January 2019.

Safety First to Prevent Falls

At any age, people can change their environments to reduce their risk of falling and breaking a bone.

Outdoor safety tips:

• In nasty weather, use a walker or cane for added stability.

• Wear warm boots with rubber soles for added traction.

- Look carefully at floor surfaces in public buildings. Many floors are made of highly polished marble or tile that can be very slippery. If floors have plastic or carpet runners in place, stay on them whenever possible.

- Identify community services that can provide assistance, such as 24-hour pharmacies and grocery stores that take orders over the phone and deliver. It is especially important to use these services in bad weather.

- Use a shoulder bag, fanny pack, or backpack to leave hands free.

- Stop at curbs and check their height before stepping up or down. Be cautious at curbs that have been cut away to allow access for bikes or wheelchairs. The incline up or down may lead to a fall.

Indoor safety tips:

- Keep all rooms free from clutter, especially the floors.

- Keep floor surfaces smooth but not slippery. When entering rooms, be aware of differences in floor levels and thresholds.

- Wear supportive, low-heeled shoes, even at home. Avoid walking around in socks, stockings, or floppy, backless slippers.

- Check that all carpets and area rugs have skid-proof backing or are tacked to the floor, including carpeting on stairs.

- Keep electrical and telephone cords and wires out of walkways.

- Be sure that all stairwells are adequately lit and that stairs have handrails on both sides. Consider placing fluorescent tape on the edges of the top and bottom steps.

- For optimal safety, install grab bars on bathroom walls beside tubs, showers, and toilets. If you are unstable on your feet, consider using a plastic chair with a back and nonskid leg tips in the shower.

- Use a rubber bath mat in the shower or tub.

- Keep a flashlight with fresh batteries beside your bed.

- Add ceiling fixtures to rooms lit by lamps only, or install lamps that can be turned on by a switch near the entry point into the room. Another option is to install voice- or sound-activated lamps.

- Use bright light bulbs in your home.

- If you must use a step-stool for hard-to-reach areas, use a sturdy one with a handrail and wide steps. A better option is to reorganize work and storage areas to minimize the need for stooping or excessive reaching.

- Consider purchasing a portable phone that you can take with you from room to room. It provides security because you can answer the phone without rushing for it and you can call for help should an accident occur.

- Don't let prescriptions run low. Always keep at least one weeks worth of medications on hand at home. Check prescriptions with your doctor and pharmacist to see if they may be increasing your risk of falling. If you take multiple medications, check with your doctor and pharmacist about possible interactions between the different medications.

- Arrange with a family member or friend for daily contact. Try to have at least one person who knows where you are.

- If you live alone, you may wish to contract with a monitoring company that will respond to your call 24 hours a day.

- Watch yourself in a mirror. Does your body lean or sway back and forth or side to side? People with decreased ability to balance often have a high degree of body sway and are more likely to fall.

Practice Balance Exercises Every Day

- While holding the back of a chair, sink, or countertop, practice standing on one leg at a time for a minute. Gradually increase the time. Try balancing with your eyes closed. Try balancing without holding on.

- While holding the back of a chair, sink, or countertop, practice standing on your toes, then rock back to balance on your heels. Hold each position for a count of 10.

- While holding the back of chair, sink, or countertop with both hands, make a big circle to the left with hips, then repeat to the right. Do not move your shoulders or feet. Repeat five times.

Reducing the Force of a Fall

Take steps to lessen your chances of breaking a bone in the event that you do fall:

- Remember that falling sideways or straight down is more likely to result in a hip fracture than falling in other directions. If possible, try to fall forward or to land on your buttocks.

- If possible, land on your hands or use objects around you to break a fall.

- Walk carefully, especially on hard surfaces.

- When possible, wear protective clothing for padding.

- Talk to your doctor about whether you may be a candidate for hip padding.

Decreasing Bone Fragility

Individuals can protect bone health by following osteoporosis prevention and treatment strategies:

- Consume a calcium-rich diet that provides between 1,000 mg (milligrams) daily for men and women up to age 50. Women over age 50 and men over age 70 should increase their intake to 1,200 mg daily from a combination of foods and supplements.

- Obtain 600 IU (International Units) of vitamin D daily up to age 70. Men and women over age 70 should increase their uptake to 800 IU daily.

- Participate in weight-bearing and resistance-training exercises most days, preferably daily.

- Talk with your doctor about having a bone mineral density (BMD) test. The most widely recognized BMD test is called a dual-energy X-ray absorptiometry, or DXA test. It is painless, a bit like having an X-ray, but with much less exposure to radiation. It can measure bone density at your hip and spine.

- Talk with your doctor about possibly beginning a medication approved by the U.S. Food and Drug Administration (FDA) for osteoporosis to stop bone loss, improve bone density, and reduce fracture risk.

People need to know whether they are at risk for developing osteoporosis or whether they have lost so much bone that they already have osteoporosis. Although risk factors can alert a person to the possibility of low bone density, only a BMD test can measure current bone density, diagnose osteoporosis, and determine fracture risk. Many different techniques measure bone mineral density painlessly and safely. Most of them involve machines that use extremely low levels of radiation to complete their readings. Sometimes, ultrasound machines, which rely on sound waves, are used instead.

Individuals may wish to have a BMD test to determine current bone health. Today, Medicare and many private insurance carriers cover bone density tests to detect osteoporosis for individuals who meet certain criteria. Talk with your doctor about whether or not this test would be appropriate for you. Falls are serious, but simple, inexpensive steps can be taken to reduce your risk of falling and of breaking a bone if you do fall.

Table 32.1. Recommended Calcium and Vitamin D Intakes

Life-Stage Group	Calcium (mg/day)	Vitamin D (IU/day)
Infants 0 to 6 months	200	400
Infants 6 to 12 months	260	400
1 to 3 years old	700	600
4 to 8 years old	1,000	600
9 to 13 years old	1,300	600
14 to 18 years old	1,300	600
19 to 30 years old	1,000	600
31 to 50 years old	1,000	600
51- to 70-year-old males	1,000	600
51- to 70-year-old females	1,200	600
>70 years old	1,200	800
14 to 18 years old, pregnant/lactating	1,300	600
19 to 50 years old, pregnant/lactating	1,000	600

Definitions: mg = milligrams; IU = International Units
(Source: Food and Nutrition Board (FNB), Institute of Medicine (IOM), National Academy of Sciences (NAS), 2010.)

Chapter 33

Alcohol and Osteoporosis

Chapter Contents

Section 33.1

Alcohol's Harmful Effects on Bone

This section includes text excerpted from "Alcohol's Harmful
Effects on Bone," National Institute on Alcohol Abuse and
Alcoholism (NIAAA), February 1, 2002. Reviewed January 2019.

Adolescent Bone Development and Alcohol

Achieving an optimal peak bone mass during adolescence may
reduce a person's risk for developing osteoporosis (i.e., bone loss with
fracture) later in life. A high peak bone mass should withstand a
longer duration and greater level of bone loss before reaching the
fracture threshold. Although peak bone mass appears to be largely
under genetic control, it can be influenced by hormonal, nutritional,
environmental, and lifestyle factors, including tobacco and alcohol
consumption.

A significant proportion of the adolescent population may be at
risk for alcohol's harmful effects on bone. A nationwide survey of more
than 50,000 high school students found that 63 percent of seniors had
been drunk at least once and 51 percent had consumed alcohol in the
month before the survey. Most respondents had consumed alcohol for
the first time before age 13.

Results of experiments using laboratory animals suggest potential consequences of alcohol consumption during adolescent bone
growth. Long-term alcohol administration to young, rapidly growing rats significantly reduced bone growth, volume, density, and
strength. The longitudinal growth rate and the rate of proliferation of cells in the growing region near the ends of long bones (i.e.,
growth plates) stop during long-term alcohol administration. If those
effects occur in humans, they could significantly decrease bone mass.
The decreased bone mass that occurs from early, long-term alcohol
consumption could result in increased fracture and early onset of
osteoporosis.

Alcohol's Effects on Hormones That Regulate Bone

In addition to providing structural support, bone is a major storage
depot for calcium and other minerals. The small intestine absorbs
calcium from ingested food, and the kidneys excrete excess calcium.
An adequate concentration of calcium in the bloodstream is required
for the proper functioning of nerves and muscle. The body monitors

calcium concentration and responds through the action of hormones, vitamins, and local growth factors to regulate the distribution of calcium between blood and bone. Alcohol may disrupt this balance by affecting the hormones that regulate calcium metabolism as well as the hormones that influence calcium metabolism indirectly (e.g., steroid reproductive hormones and growth hormone [GH]) (Sampson 1997).

Calcium-Regulating Hormones

Parathyroid hormone. Parathyroid hormone (PTH) is secreted into the bloodstream by four small glands located behind the thyroid gland in the neck. The hormone, which is produced in response to decreasing levels of calcium in the blood, stimulates the activity of specialized bone cells called osteoclasts. Osteoclasts dissolve small areas of bone, releasing calcium into the blood. (The role of osteoclasts in bone remodeling is discussed in the section "Alcohol's Effects on Bone Remodeling,") In addition, PTH inhibits the excretion of calcium by the kidney and activates vitamin D, which promotes the absorption of calcium from the intestine. The resulting increase in calcium levels eventually inhibits further PTH production.

Short-term alcohol consumption increases PTH secretion, possibly by causing calcium to leave body fluids (e.g., blood) and flow into cells. Laitinen and colleagues administered intoxicating doses of alcohol over a 3-hour period to men and women who were moderate drinkers, with each person receiving approximately 5 to 11 standard drinks. Levels of PTH declined sharply until the end of the drinking period and rose over the next nine hours, eventually exceeding levels measured before alcohol consumption. Urinary calcium excretion increased during the first three hours and subsequently decreased. Long-term heavy drinking was associated with low blood calcium (i.e., hypocalcemia) but normal PTH levels. Those findings indicate that the hypocalcemia did not result from reduced PTH secretion and also suggest that alcohol administration impaired the ability of the parathyroid glands to increase PTH production in response to the presence of hypocalcemia.

Calcitonin. Specialized cells in the thyroid gland produce calcitonin, a hormone that protects the skeleton from calcium loss by inhibiting osteoclast activity. In contrast to the action of PTH, calcitonin increases the deposition of calcium in bone and lowers the level

281

of calcium in the blood. Calcitonin levels increase only briefly during acute and short-term alcohol consumption. The significance of this effect is uncertain.

Vitamin D. Vitamin D increases intestinal absorption of dietary calcium and has a function in normal bone metabolism. Vitamin D is formed in the skin through the action of sunlight and occurs in foods such as liver, eggs, and milk. The vitamin becomes physiologically active only after chemical modification in the liver and kidneys. Alcoholics normally have low levels of activated vitamin D, along with low levels of the proteins that bind with vitamin D to protect it during transport within the blood. Vitamin D levels are especially low in the presence of alcoholic liver disease (e.g., alcoholic cirrhosis). The alcohol-induced decrease in activated vitamin D results in decreased absorption of calcium, although calcium levels quickly return to normal following abstinence.

Reproductive Hormones

Osteoporosis can develop in postmenopausal women as well as in men with inadequate gonadal function. Alcoholic men frequently have decreased levels of the male steroid hormone testosterone (produced mainly in the testes), and female alcoholics experience increased metabolic conversion of testosterone (produced in the ovaries and adrenal glands) to the female steroid hormone estradiol. Because estrogen deficiency is a major contributing factor for the development of osteoporosis, alcohol might indirectly affect bone through estrogen. Estrogen replacement reduces a woman's risk of developing postmenopausal osteoporosis. In addition, moderate alcohol consumption has been reported to increase estrogen levels in the blood. A review of published research on alcohol and estrogen, however, concluded that moderate alcohol consumption (i.e., no more than one drink per day for women) does not appear to have a significant effect on levels of estradiol, the most potent of the estrogens.

Effects of Moderate Alcohol Consumption

Studies show a relationship between the consumption of large quantities of alcohol and bone loss. However, a few studies indicate that moderate alcohol consumption may help reduce osteoporosis and decrease fracture risk in postmenopausal women. For example, in a study of more than 14,000 subjects, Naves Diaz and colleagues reported that women age 65 and older who consume alcohol on more than five days per week had a reduced risk of vertebral deformity compared with those who consumed alcohol less than once per week.

Two recent studies investigated the influence of moderate alcohol consumption on rats following surgical removal of their ovaries (i.e., ovariectomy) to mimic menopause. In one study, rats were administered doses of alcohol equivalent to 18 percent of their total dietary caloric intake for three weeks. Sampson and Shipley administered the equivalent of two standard drinks, as previously defined, per day for six weeks. In both studies, ovariectomized rats exhibited decreased bone density and bone volume compared with nonovariectomized rats. However, these changes were not significantly affected by alcohol administration. Although Fanti and colleagues found fewer osteoclasts in ovariectomized alcohol-fed animals, this finding was not reflected in decreased bone volume. Therefore, neither study identified a beneficial effect of moderate alcohol consumption on bone quality.

Growth Hormone

Growth hormone, secreted by the pituitary gland, is important in bone growth and remodeling. Growth hormone exerts its effects largely through a hormone called insulin-like growth factor 1 (IGF-1), which is produced in the liver and other organs. Levels of IGF-1 are significantly reduced in alcohol-fed animals until seven months of age. The aforementioned findings might explain the greatly reduced rates of longitudinal growth and the proliferation of certain cell types in the growth plates of young, rapidly growing animals. The levels of IGF-1 in alcohol-fed animals become normal after six months of alcohol feeding, but bone deficiencies resulting from alcohol consumption continue, possibly through a mechanism independent of growth factors.

Alcohol's Effects on Bone Remodeling

Remodeling occurs in small, circumscribed areas scattered on the surface of the bone. Osteoclasts erode a cavity on the bone surface in a process known as resorption. When the resorption cavity is complete, the osteoclasts disappear, the floor of the cavity is smoothed off, and a thin layer of matrix or cement is deposited. Bone-forming cells (i.e., osteoblasts) fill the newly formed cavity with new bone.

Local imbalance of bone remodeling can occur when osteoclasts erode cavities that are too deep or when osteoblasts lay down layers of new bone which are too shallow. It is unclear whether alcohol's effects on bone remodeling result from improper bone formation or overactive osteoclast resorption.

Schnitzler and Solomon found that alcohol administration reduced bone formation and increased bone resorption. In a study of men who were daily drinkers and who had osteoporosis of unknown origin, De Vernejoul and colleagues found a markedly reduced mean wall thickness (i.e., the thickness of the newly formed structural unit formed during remodeling), which they took into account when measuring the quantity of resorbed bone. Based on their calculations, De Vernejoul and colleagues theorized that alcoholic osteoporosis is characterized by decreased bone formation but normal levels of resorption. A microscopic analysis of bone tissue from men with osteoporosis confirmed that alcohol consumption leads to delayed and impaired osteoblast activity associated with normal osteoclast function.

To determine whether alcohol has a direct effect on osteoblasts, researchers measured levels of osteocalcin, a protein secreted by osteoblasts and thought to be a measure of osteoblast function. Using in vitro preparations of osteoblasts from rats, most investigators reported a decrease in osteocalcin levels in response to alcohol administration, suggesting that alcohol decreases osteoblastic activity. Microscopic studies of bone tissue from rats demonstrated decreased trabecular bone volume, decreased numbers of osteoblasts, and decreased rates of bone formation, indicating impaired bone formation and mineralization, along with other characteristics indicative of osteoporosis. In addition, the amount of trabecular surface covered by active osteoblasts was significantly reduced in alcohol-fed rats, suggesting an inhibition of osteoblast proliferation. Wall thickness, another measure of osteoblast activity, was reduced by 52 percent in alcohol-fed animals compared with animals not administered alcohol. These findings agree with in vitro studies that demonstrate diminished osteoblast numbers and osteoblast function in humans. Overall, alcohol appears to suppress osteoblast function in adults, resulting in decreased bone formation.

Section 33.2

Managing Alcoholism and Osteoporosis

This section includes text excerpted from "What People Recovering from Alcoholism Need to Know about Osteoporosis," NIH Osteoporosis and Related Bone Diseases—National Resource Center (NIH ORBD—NRC), April 2016.

Alcoholism and Recovery

According to the National Institute on Alcohol Abuse and Alcoholism (NIAAA), approximately 17 million adults ages 18 and older have an alcohol-use disorder (AUD). Alcoholism is a disease characterized by a dependency on alcohol. Because alcohol affects almost every organ in the body, chronic heavy drinking is associated with many serious health problems, including pancreatitis, liver disease, heart disease, cancer, and osteoporosis.

Maintaining sobriety is undoubtedly the most important health goal for individuals recovering from alcoholism. However, attention to other aspects of health, including bone health, can help increase the likelihood of a healthy future, free from the devastating consequences of osteoporosis and fracture.

What Is Osteoporosis?

Osteoporosis is a condition in which bones become less dense and more likely to fracture. Fractures from osteoporosis can result in significant pain and disability. In the United States, more than 53 million people either already have osteoporosis or are at high risk due to low bone mass.

Risk factors for developing osteoporosis include:

- Thinness or small frame

- Being postmenopausal and particularly having had early menopause

- Abnormal absence of menstrual periods (amenorrhea)

- Prolonged use of certain medications, such as those used to treat lupus, asthma, thyroid deficiencies, and seizures

- Low calcium intake

- Lack of physical activity

- Smoking

- Excessive alcohol intake

Osteoporosis often can be prevented. It is known as a "silent disease" because, if undetected, bone loss can progress for many years without symptoms until a fracture occurs. Osteoporosis has been called a childhood disease with old age consequences because building healthy bones in one's youth helps prevent osteoporosis and fractures later in life. However, it is never too late to adopt new habits for healthy bones.

The Link between Alcohol and Osteoporosis

Alcohol negatively affects bone health for several reasons. To begin with, excessive alcohol interferes with the balance of calcium, an essential nutrient for healthy bones. Calcium balance may be further disrupted by alcohol's ability to interfere with the production of vitamin D, a vitamin essential for calcium absorption.

In addition, chronic heavy drinking can cause hormone deficiencies in men and women. Men with alcoholism may produce less testosterone, a hormone linked to the production of osteoblasts (the cells that stimulate bone formation). In women, chronic alcohol exposure can trigger irregular menstrual cycles, a factor that reduces estrogen levels, increasing the risk for osteoporosis. Also, cortisol levels may be elevated in people with alcoholism. Cortisol is known to decrease bone formation and increase bone breakdown.

Because of the effects of alcohol on balance and gait, people with alcoholism tend to fall more frequently than those without the disorder. Heavy alcohol consumption has been linked to an increase in the risk of fracture, including the most serious kind—hip fracture. Vertebral fractures are also more common in those who abuse alcohol.

Osteoporosis Management Strategies

The most effective strategy for alcohol-induced bone loss is abstinence. People with alcoholism who abstain from drinking tend to have a rapid recovery of osteoblastic (bone-building) activity. Some studies have even found that lost bone can be partially restored when alcohol abuse ends.

Nutrition. Because of the negative nutritional effects of chronic alcohol use, people recovering from alcoholism should make healthy nutritional habits a top priority. As far as bone health is concerned, a well-balanced diet rich in calcium and vitamin D is critical. Good sources of calcium include low-fat dairy products; dark green, leafy vegetables; and calcium-fortified foods and beverages. Supplements can help ensure that you get adequate amounts of calcium each day, especially in people with a proven milk allergy. The Institute of Medicine (IOM) recommends a daily calcium intake of 1,000 mg (milligrams) for men and women up to age 50. Women over age 50 and men over age 70 should increase their intake to 1,200 mg daily.

Vitamin D plays an important role in calcium absorption and bone health. Food sources of vitamin D include egg yolks, saltwater fish, and liver. Many people, especially those who are older or housebound, may need vitamin D supplements to achieve the recommended intake of 600 to 800 IU (International Units) each day.

Exercise. Like muscle, bone is living tissue that responds to exercise by becoming stronger. The best exercise for your bones is weight-bearing exercise that forces you to work against gravity. Some examples include walking, climbing stairs, weight training, and dancing. Regular exercise, such as walking, may help prevent bone loss and will provide many other health benefits.

Healthy lifestyle. Smoking is bad for bones as well as the heart and lungs. Women who smoke tend to go through menopause earlier, resulting in earlier reduction in levels of the bone-preserving hormone estrogen and triggering earlier bone loss. In addition, smokers may absorb less calcium from their diets.

Bone density test. A bone mineral density (BMD) test measures bone density in various parts of the body. This safe and painless test can detect osteoporosis before a fracture occurs and can predict one's chances of fracturing in the future. The BMD test can help determine whether medication should be considered. Individuals in recovery are encouraged to talk to their healthcare providers about whether they might be candidates for a BMD test.

Medication. Several medications are available for the prevention and/or treatment of osteoporosis, including: bisphosphonates; estrogen agonists/antagonists (also called selective estrogen receptor modulators or SERMs); calcitonin; parathyroid hormone; estrogen therapy; hormone therapy; and a receptor activator of nuclear factor kappa-β ligand (RANKL) inhibitor.

Chapter 34

Smoking and Bone Health

Many of the health problems caused by tobacco use are well known. Cigarette smoking causes heart disease, lung and esophageal cancer, and chronic lung disease. Additionally, several research studies have identified smoking as a risk factor for osteoporosis and bone fracture. According to the Centers for Disease Control and Prevention (CDC), more than 16 million Americans are living with a disease caused by smoking.

Facts about Osteoporosis

Osteoporosis is a condition in which bones weaken and are more likely to fracture. Fractures from osteoporosis can result in pain and disability. In the United States, more than 53 million people either already have osteoporosis or are at high risk due to low bone mass.

In addition to smoking, risk factors for developing osteoporosis include:

- Thinness or small frame

- Family history of the disease

- Being postmenopausal and particularly having had early menopause

---

This chapter includes text excerpted from "Smoking and Bone Health," NIH Osteoporosis and Related Bone Diseases—National Resource Center (NIH ORBD—NRC), May 2016.

- Abnormal absence of menstrual periods (amenorrhea)
- Prolonged use of certain medications, such as those used to treat lupus, asthma, thyroid deficiencies, and seizures
- Low calcium intake
- Lack of physical activity
- Excessive alcohol intake

Osteoporosis can often be prevented. It is known as a "silent disease" because, if undetected, bone loss can progress for many years without symptoms until a fracture occurs. It has been called a childhood disease with old age consequences because building healthy bones in youth helps prevent osteoporosis and fractures later in life. However, it is never too late to adopt new habits for healthy bones.

Smoking and Osteoporosis

Cigarette smoking was first identified as a risk factor for osteoporosis decades ago. Studies have shown a direct relationship between tobacco use and decreased bone density. Analyzing the impact of cigarette smoking on bone health is complicated. It is hard to determine whether a decrease in bone density is due to smoking itself or to other risk factors common among smokers. For example, in many cases, smokers are thinner than nonsmokers, tend to drink more alcohol, may be less physically active, and have poor diets. Women who smoke also tend to have an earlier menopause than nonsmokers. These factors place many smokers at an increased risk for osteoporosis apart from their tobacco use.

In addition, studies on the effects of smoking suggest that smoking increases the risk of having a fracture. As well, smoking has been shown to have a negative impact on bone healing after fracture.

Osteoporosis Management Strategies

Start by quitting: The best thing smokers can do to protect their bones is to quit smoking. Smoking cessation, even later in life, may help limit smoking-related bone loss.

Eat a well-balanced diet rich in calcium and vitamin D: Good sources of calcium include low-fat dairy products; dark green, leafy vegetables; and calcium-fortified foods and beverages. Supplements can help ensure that you get adequate amounts of calcium each day, especially in people with a proven milk allergy. The Institute of Medicine (IOM) recommends a daily calcium intake of 1,000 mg (milligrams) for men and women up to age 50. Women over age 50 and men over age 70 should increase their intake to 1,200 mg daily.

Vitamin D plays an important role in calcium absorption and bone health. Food sources of vitamin D include egg yolks, saltwater fish, and liver. Many people, especially those who are older, may need vitamin D supplements to achieve the recommended intake of 600 to 800 IU (International Units) each day.

Exercise for your bone health: Like muscle, bone is living tissue that responds to exercise by becoming stronger. Weight-bearing exercise that forces you to work against gravity is the best exercise for bone.

Some examples include walking, climbing stairs, weight training, and dancing. Regular exercise, such as walking, may help prevent bone loss and will provide many other health benefits.

Avoid excessive use of alcohol: Chronic alcohol use has been linked to an increase in fractures of the hip, spine, and wrist. Drinking too much alcohol interferes with the balance of calcium in the body. It also affects the production of hormones, which have a protective effect on bone, and of vitamins, which we need to absorb calcium. Excessive alcohol consumption also can lead to more falls and related fractures.

Talk to your doctor about a bone density test: A bone mineral density (BMD) test measures bone density at various sites of the body. This safe and painless test can detect osteoporosis before a fracture occurs and can predict one's chances of fracturing in the future. If you are a current or former smoker, you may want to ask your healthcare provider whether you are a candidate for a BMD test, which can help determine whether medication should be considered.

See if medication is an option for you: There is no cure for osteoporosis. However, several medications are available to prevent and treat the disease in postmenopausal women and in men. Your doctor can help you decide whether medication might be right for you.

Chapter 35

Drugs and Fracture Risk

Chapter Contents

Section 35.1

Fracture Risk with Osteoporosis Drugs

This section includes text excerpted from "Possible
Fracture Risk with Osteoporosis Drugs," U.S. Food and
Drug Administration (FDA), January 23, 2018.

The U.S. Food and Drug Administration (FDA) is warning there is
a possible risk of a rare type of thigh bone (femoral) fracture in people
who take drugs known as bisphosphonates to treat osteoporosis.

The agency warned patients and healthcare professionals of this
risk because the rare type of femoral fracture has been predominantly
reported in patients taking these prescription medications.

The FDA says the possible risk of thigh fracture will be reflected
in a labeling change for bisphosphonate medications that treat osteoporosis and in a medication guide that will be required to be given to
patients when they pick up their prescription.

Bisphosphonates are a class of drugs that slow or inhibit the loss
of bone mass. They have been used successfully since 1995 to prevent
and treat osteoporosis and similar diseases. Osteoporosis is a disease
in which the bones become weak and are more likely to break.

The FDA says it is not clear whether bisphosphonates are the cause
of the unusual bone breaks known as subtrochanteric femur fractures,
which occur just below the hip joint, and diaphyseal femur fractures,
which occur in the long part of the thigh.

Medication Guide, Labeling Change

The changes to labeling and the medication guide will affect only
bisphosphonates approved for osteoporosis. These include:

- Oral bisphosphonates such as Actonel, Actonel with Calcium,
  Atelvia, Boniva, Fosamax, Fosamax Plus D, and their generic
  products

- Injectable bisphosphonates such as Boniva and Reclast and their
  generic products

Labeling and the medication guides for bisphosphonates that are
used for other conditions will not change. The FDA says the optimal
duration of bisphosphonates treatment for osteoporosis is unknown—
an uncertainty the agency is highlighting because these fractures may
be related to use of bisphosphonates for longer than five years.

FDA medical officer Theresa Kehoe, M.D., says the agency continues to evaluate data about the safety and effectiveness of bisphosphonates when used long-term for osteoporosis treatment.

"In the interim, it's important for patients and healthcare professionals to have all the safety information available when determining the best course of treatment for osteoporosis," she says.

Advice for Consumers

If you are currently taking bisphosphonates for osteoporosis, the FDA advises that you:

- Keep taking your medication unless you are told to stop by your healthcare professional

- Read the medication guide. It will describe the symptoms of an atypical femur fracture. The guide also advises you to notify your healthcare professional if you develop symptoms

- Tell your healthcare professional if you develop new hip or thigh pain (commonly described as dull or aching pain), or have any concerns with your medications

- Report any side effects with your bisphosphonate medication to the FDA's MedWatch program:

  - Online: www.accessdata.fda.gov/scripts/medwatch/medwatch-online.htm

  - By Fax: 800-FDA-0178 (800-332-0178)

  - By phone: 800-FDA-1088 (800-332-1088)

The FDA also recommends that healthcare professionals be aware of the possible risk in patients taking bisphosphonates and consider periodic re-evaluation of the need for continued bisphosphonate therapy, particularly for patients who have been on bisphosphonates for longer than five years.

Section 35.2

Optimal Duration of Osteoporosis Drugs Intake

This section includes text excerpted from "How Long Should You Take Certain Osteoporosis Drugs?" U.S. Food and Drug Administration (FDA), December 30, 2017.

Researchers at the U.S. Food and Drug Administration (FDA) have taken a close look at the long-term benefit of bisphosphonates, a class of medications widely prescribed to treat osteoporosis.

An FDA review of clinical studies measuring the effectiveness of long-term bisphosphonates use shows that some patients may be able to stop using bisphosphonates after three to five years and still continue to benefit from their use, says Marcea Whitaker, M.D., a medical officer at the FDA's Center for Drug Evaluation and Research (CDER). Whitaker is one of the co-authors of the FDA review, which was published in the May 31, 2012 issue of *The New England Journal of Medicine*.

If you're one of the 44 million Americans at risk for osteoporosis—a disease in which bones become weak and are more likely to break—you may be taking bisphosphonates. This class of drugs has been successfully used since 1995 to slow or inhibit the loss of bone mass. Doctors commonly prescribe such brand name drugs as Actonel, Atelvia, Boniva, and Fosamax (as well as a number of generic products) for osteoporosis. In fact, more than 150 million prescriptions were dispensed to patients between 2005 and 2009.

According to the review, further investigation is needed on the long-term risks and benefits of these drugs.

"These drugs clearly work," Whitaker says. "We just don't know yet the optimum period of time individual patients should be on the drug to both maximize its effectiveness and minimize potential risks." More research is needed on patients' risk of fracture after they stop taking bisphosphonates, and whether taking them again later on could prove beneficial, she adds. As always, patients should talk to their healthcare provider about their continued need for therapy.

The studies suggest that patients at low risk of fracture (for example, younger patients without a fracture history and with a bone mineral density approaching normal) may be good candidates for discontinuation of bisphosphonate therapy after three to five years.

In contrast, patients at increased risk for fractures (for example, older patients with a history of fracture and a bone mineral density remaining in the osteoporotic range) may benefit further from continued bisphosphonate therapy.

How the Medication Works

Bones go through a continual process of remodeling, in the form of bone resorption (disintegration) and bone formation. Bone loss related to osteoporosis occurs when resorption is greater than formation. Bisphosphonates decrease bone resorption, thereby slowing bone loss.

During treatment, bisphosphonates become part of the newly formed bone and can stay there for years, through many cycles of resorption and formation. Patients continue to be exposed to the effects of the drug even long after they've stopped taking it.

According to Whitaker, the studies that the FDA considered focused on patients who had been using bisphosphonates for at least three years and as many as ten. They looked at outcomes related both to bone mineral density and bone fractures.

"Bisphosphonates have been proven very effective in protecting against bone fractures in clinical trials lasting three to four years," says Whitaker. But it's still unknown whether the benefit lasts longer than that in decreasing the risk of fractures.

Bisphosphonate labels have carried a safety warning about severe jaw bone decay (osteonecrosis of the jaw) since 2002. In October 2010, the FDA warned patients and healthcare professionals about the increased risk of unusual thigh bone fractures and directed manufacturers to include the warning in the safety labels and medication guides that come with prescription medications. The FDA continues to evaluate the possible association of bisphosphonates with esophageal cancer. These associations would suggest that healthcare professionals may want to reconsider how long patients should continue taking the drugs.

What Should a Patient Do?

Decisions to continue treatment must be based on individual assessments of risks and benefits and on patient preference, Whitaker says

If you are taking bisphosphonates:

- Talk to your physician about whether or not you should continue this therapy. Re-evaluate the decision on a periodic basis.

- Don't stop taking these (or any) prescribed drugs without talking to your physician first. If you do make the decision to discontinue use, talk to your physician before stopping therapy.

- Tell your healthcare professional if you develop new hip or thigh pain (commonly described as dull or aching pain), or have any concerns with your medications.

- Report unusual side effects of your bisphosphonate medication to the FDA's MedWatch program.

Section 35.3

HIV Drugs and Low Bone Mass

This section contains text excerpted from the following sources: Text in this section begins with excerpts from "Drug Used to Treat HIV Linked to Lower Bone Mass in Newborns," *Eunice Kennedy Shriver* National Institute of Child Health and Human Development (NICHD), September 30, 2015. Reviewed January 2019; Text under the heading "Researchers Recommend Monitoring, Exercise, Vitamin D to Prevent Future Fracture Risk" is excerpted from "NIH Study Finds HIV-Positive Young Men at Risk of Low Bone Mass," *Eunice Kennedy Shriver* National Institute of Child Health and Human Development (NICHD), June 19, 2012. Reviewed January 2019.

Infants exposed in the womb to a drug used to treat human immunodeficiency virus (HIV) and reduce the transmission of HIV from mother to child, may have lower bone mineral content than those exposed to other anti-HIV drugs, according to a National Institutes of Health (NIH) study.

Researchers found that pregnant women who received the drug tenofovir disoproxil fumarate in their third trimester gave birth to babies whose bone mineral content was 12 percent lower than that of infants who were not exposed to the drug in the uterus. Proper mineral content helps strengthen normal bones. The study appears in Clinical Infectious Diseases.

"At this point, we can say that those who care for pregnant women with HIV and their children should be aware that prescribing tenofovir to pregnant women could be a concern for their infants' bones," said George K. Siberry, M.D., the first author of the study and medical officer with the National Institutes of Health's (NIH) *Eunice Kennedy Shriver* National Institute of Child Health and Human Development (NICHD).

Although the study authors described the results as concerning, they cautioned against any changes in the use of tenofovir in pregnant women. The drug has proved successful as part of drug regimens that treat HIV in pregnant women, and often is used to prevent HIV transmission to infants. The researchers called for additional studies to understand bone health and development among children born to women who took tenofovir during their pregnancies.

"Families should keep in close touch with their physicians to monitor their child's bone development," Dr. Siberry added.

In the study, researchers enrolled a total of 143 infants at 14 sites across the United States from 2011 to 2013. Of these participants, 74 were exposed to tenofovir in the uterus, while 69 were given other anti-HIV drugs. Researchers used special, low-radiation X-ray scans, called Dual-energy X-ray absorptiometry (DXA) scans to measure bone mineral content within the first four weeks of birth.

The researchers then compared the bone mineral content of the two groups and found that the group of infants whose mothers took tenofovir, on average, had lower bone mineral content than the group of infants whose mothers were given other kinds of anti-HIV drugs. However, the researchers do not know whether the lower bone mineral content of the children in the tenofovir group is abnormal and will increase the risk of fractures. Dr. Siberry added that it is also unknown whether children can regain bone mineral content as they get older.

The study authors point out that tenofovir use has been associated with bone loss in adults and older children. A few NIH-funded studies have found that adults who used tenofovir were at increased risk for bone fracture.

The study was supported by several NIH institutes, including the National Institute of Drug Abuse (NIDA), the National Institute of Allergy and Infectious Diseases, the Office of AIDS Research, the National Institute of Mental Health (NIMH), the National Institute of Neurological Disorders and Stroke (NINDS), the National Institute of Deafness and Other Communication Disorders (NIDCD), the National Heart, Lung and Blood Institute (NHLBI), the National Institute of Dental and Craniofacial Research (NIDCR), and the National Institute of Alcohol Abuse and Alcoholism (NIAAA).

Researchers Recommend Monitoring, Exercise, Vitamin D to Prevent Future Fracture Risk

Young men being treated for HIV are more likely to experience low bone mass than are other men their age, according to results from a research network supported by the NIH. The findings indicate that physicians who care for these patients should monitor them regularly for signs of bone thinning, which could foretell a risk for fractures. The young men in the study did not have HIV at birth and had been diagnosed with HIV an average of two years earlier.

Earlier studies have shown that adults with HIV also have bone loss and increased risk for bone fractures, associated in part with the use of certain anti-HIV medications.

"The young men in the study had been taking anti-HIV medications for a comparatively short time, yet they still had lower bone mineral density than other men their age," said co-author Bill G. Kapogiannis, M.D., of the Pediatric, Adolescent, and Maternal AIDS Branch of the NICHD. "These findings suggest a short-term impact of HIV therapy on bone at ages when people are still growing and building bone mass. This raises concern about the risk of fracture as they age."

For the HIV-infected young men, on average, bone density in the hip was five to eight percent lower, and in the spine two to four percent lower, than for study participants without HIV.

The study was not designed to determine the cause of the bone loss and cannot rule out the possibility that low bone mass preceded the young men's HIV infection. The researchers noted that all the young men had several risk factors for bone loss, such as tobacco and alcohol use, and low intake of calcium and vitamin D (needed to absorb calcium.)

The study was conducted by lead authors Kathleen Mulligan, Ph.D., of the University of California (USC), San Francisco; Grace Aldrovandi, M.D., of Children's Hospital Los Angeles and the University of Southern California; Dr. Kapogiannis, and seven other researchers affiliated with the NICHD-supported Adolescent Medicine Trials Network for HIV/AIDS Interventions (ATN).

Their findings appear in *Clinical Infectious* Diseases.

Additional funding was provided by the NIH's NIDA, the NIMH, and the National Center for Research Resources (NCRR) and the National Center for Advancing Translational Sciences (NCATS).

Some 250 teens and young men (14 to 25 years old) participated in the study. About 88 percent of the study participants identified themselves as African American or Hispanic and all lived in urban areas. The participants underwent whole body scans to measure their bone density as well as the distribution of fat and lean muscle mass in certain regions of their bodies. Participants also answered questions about their medical history, diet, exercise and other lifestyle habits.

The researchers calculated the density of bones in the body as a whole, as well as the spine and hip bones. These bones are more susceptible than other bones to bone loss, Dr. Mulligan explained. The researchers also assessed total body fat and amounts of fat in the arms, legs, and trunk.

The researchers found that the HIV-positive participants who had not yet begun treatment tended to have less body fat than either their counterparts on medication or the study's HIV-negative participants.

Both bone density and the calcium and other mineral content of bones tended to be lowest in participants taking medication for HIV. Youth with HIV who had not begun treatment had higher bone mass levels than HIV positive youth who were on anti-HIV regimens, but lower bone mass levels than youth who did not have HIV. Participants' responses to questions about diet indicated that at least half of them did not consume sufficient calcium or vitamin D. The researchers also found that more than 30 percent of all the participants smoked. Half said they did not get regular exercise. Smoking and lack of exercise can contribute to weaker bones. The study authors noted that additional studies are needed to follow HIV-positive young men long term to determine whether bone loss during adolescence increases the risk of fractures later in life.

"None of the young men we saw is in immediate risk of fracture," said Dr. Mulligan. "However, our results indicated that it would be a good idea for young men newly diagnosed with HIV to make sure they exercise, get enough calcium and vitamin D, quit smoking, and limit alcohol consumption."

Chapter 36

Bed Rest and Immobilization

Like muscle, bone is living tissue that responds to exercise by becoming stronger. Young women and men who exercise regularly generally have greater bone mass (bone density and strength) than those who do not. For most people, bone mass peaks by the late twenties. After the age of 30, women and men can help prevent bone loss with regular exercise. The best exercise for bones is weight-bearing exercise. This is exercise that forces you to work against gravity, such as walking, hiking, jogging, climbing stairs, playing tennis, dancing, and lifting weights. Swimming and bicycling are examples of non-weight-bearing exercises.

Although weight-bearing activities contribute to the development and maintenance of bone mass, weightlessness and immobility can result in bone loss. Space travel has provided significant research data on the subject of weightlessness and bone loss. Astronauts exposed to the microgravity of space experience significant bone loss, leaving their bones weak and less able to support the body's weight and movement upon return to Earth.

The Impact of Bed Rest and Inactivity

Some people can't perform weight-bearing activity. They include, for example, people who are on prolonged bed rest because of surgery,

This chapter includes text excerpted from "Bed Rest and Immobilization: Risk Factors for Bone Loss," NIH Osteoporosis and Related Bone Diseases—National Resource Center (NIH ORBD—NRC), May 2016.

serious illness, or complications of pregnancy; and those who are experiencing immobilization of some part of the body because of stroke, fracture, spinal cord injury, or other chronic conditions. These people often experience a significant bone loss and are at high risk for developing osteoporosis and having a fracture.

Bone loss typically occurs over several months and then gradually levels off as the bones adjust to the state of weightlessness.

Maintaining Bone Health

In general, healthy people who undergo prolonged periods of bed rest or immobilization can regain bone mass when they resume weight-bearing activities. Studies suggest that there is a good chance to fully recover the lost bone if the immobilization period is limited to one to two months. Additionally, even brief intervals of weight-bearing activity during periods of limited mobility or bed rest can help lessen bone loss.

The greatest concern is for people who cannot resume weight-bearing activities, and therefore, typically do not regain lost bone density. Studies suggest that taking an osteoporosis treatment medication and reducing or eliminating other risk factors for osteoporosis can help slow the rate of bone loss.

The Bottom Line

- A lifetime of weight-bearing exercise is important for building and maintaining bone mass, improving balance and coordination, and promoting overall good health.

- Weight-bearing exercise should be resumed and maintained after a prolonged period of bed rest or immobilization to help recover bone lost during disuse.

- Those who cannot resume weight-bearing exercise are at significant risk for osteoporosis. In this case, it is important to reduce or eliminate other risk factors for osteoporosis, such as smoking and excessive alcohol consumption, and to eat a diet rich in calcium and vitamin D. Taking an osteoporosis medication may also be an option to minimize bone loss.

Chapter 37

Preventing Osteoporosis

Chapter Contents

Section 37.1

Bone Health throughout Life

This section includes text excerpted from "Osteoporosis—Prevention of Osteoporosis," National Institute of Arthritis and Musculoskeletal and Skin Diseases (NIAMS), February 28, 2016.

Preventing osteoporosis is a lifelong endeavor. To reach optimal peak bone mass and minimize loss of bone as you get older, there are several factors you should consider. Addressing all of these factors is the best way to optimize bone health throughout life.

Screening for Osteoporosis

Prevention also includes screening for osteoporosis. The United States Preventive Services Task Force (USPSTF), an independent panel of experts in primary care and prevention, recommends screening for osteoporosis for:

- All women age 65 and older be screened for osteoporosis
- Women under the age of 65 who are at high risk for fractures

You should also ask your doctor about osteoporosis if you:

- Are over 50 and have broken a bone
- Have lost height or your posture has become stooped or hunched
- Experience sudden back pain
- Have a chronic disease or eating disorder known to increase the risk of osteoporosis
- Are taking one or more medications known to cause bone loss
- Have multiple risk factors for osteoporosis and osteoporosis-related fractures

Consider talking to your doctor about being evaluated for osteoporosis if:

- You are a man or woman over age 50 or a postmenopausal woman and you break a bone
- You are a woman age 65 or older
- You are a woman younger than 65 and at high risk for fractures

- You have lost height, developed a stooped or hunched posture, or experienced sudden back pain with no apparent cause

- You have a chronic illness or are taking a medication that is known to cause bone loss

- You have anorexia nervosa or a history of this eating disorder

- You are a premenopausal woman, not pregnant, and your menstrual periods have stopped, are irregular, or never started when you reached puberty

Overall Nutrition

A healthy, balanced diet that includes lots of fruits and vegetables and enough calories is also important for lifelong bone health. If you take in adequate amounts of calcium and vitamin D throughout your life, you are more likely to have optimal skeletal mass early in life and are less likely to lose bone later in life.

Calcium

Taking the recommended amount of calcium over a lifetime is thought to play an important role in the development of osteoporosis. Many published studies show that low calcium intakes are associated with:

- Low bone mass

- Rapid bone loss

- High fracture rates

National surveys suggest that the average calcium intake of individuals is far below the levels recommended for optimal bone health. The body's demand for calcium is greater in:

- Childhood and adolescence, when the skeleton is growing rapidly

- Women during pregnancy and breastfeeding

- Postmenopausal women and older men. Increased calcium requirements in older people may be related to vitamin D deficiencies that reduce intestinal absorption of calcium.

Also, as you age, your body becomes less efficient at absorbing calcium and other nutrients. Older adults are also more likely to have chronic medical problems and to use medications that may impair calcium absorption.

Adolescence is the most critical period for building bone mass that helps protect against osteoporosis later in life. Yet studies show that among children age 9 to 19 in the United States, few meet the recommended levels. Therefore, it is especially important for parents, other caregivers, and pediatricians to talk to children and young teens about developing bone-healthy habits, including eating calcium-rich foods and getting enough exercise.

Vitamin D

Vitamin D plays an important role in calcium absorption and bone health. It is made in the skin after exposure to sunlight and can also be obtained through the diet. Although many people are able to obtain enough vitamin D naturally, vitamin D production decreases if you:

- Are older

- Are housebound

- Do not get enough sun

- Have a chronic neurological or gastrointestinal diseases

If you are at for vitamin D deficiency your doctor may recommend vitamin D supplements.

Calcium and vitamin D supplements may help slow bone loss and prevent hip fracture.

Table 37.1. Recommended Calcium and Vitamin D Intakes

Life-Stage Group	Calcium mg/day	Vitamin D (IU/day)
Infants 0 to 6 months	200	400
Infants 6 to 12 months	260	400
1 to 3 years old	700	600
4 to 8 years old	1,000	600
9 to 13 years old	1,300	600
14 to 18 years old	1,300	600
19 to 30 years old	1,000	600
31 to 50 years old	1,000	600
51 to 70 years old males	1,000	600
51 to 70 years old females	1,200	600

Table 37.1. Continued

Life-Stage Group	Calcium mg/day	Vitamin D (IU/day)
>70 years old	1,200	800
14 to 18 years old, pregnant/lactating	1,300	600
19 to 50 years old, pregnant/lactating	1,000	600

Definitions: mg = milligrams; IU = International Units
(Source: Food and Nutrition Board (FNB), Institute of Medicine (IOM), National Academy of Sciences (NAS), 2010.)

Exercise

Like a muscle, bone is a living tissue that responds to exercise by becoming stronger. There is good evidence that physical activity early in life contributes to higher peak bone mass. The best exercise for building and maintaining bone mass is weight-bearing exercise: exercise that you do on your feet and that forces you to work against gravity. Weight-bearing exercises include:

- Jogging
- Aerobics
- Hiking
- Walking
- Stair climbing
- Gardening
- Weight training
- Tennis
- Dancing

High-impact exercises may provide the most benefit. Bicycling and swimming are not weight-bearing exercises, but they have other health benefits. Exercise machines that provide some degree of weight-bearing exercise include:

- Treadmills
- Stair-climbing machines
- Ski machines
- Exercise bicycles

Strength training to build and maintain muscle mass and exercises that help with coordination and balance are also important. Later in life, the benefits of exercise for building and maintaining bone mass are not nearly as great, but staying active and doing weight-bearing exercise is still important.

A properly designed exercise program that builds muscles and improves balance and coordination provides other benefits for older people, including helping to prevent falls and maintaining overall health and independence. Experts recommend 30 minutes or more of moderate physical activity on most (preferably all) days of the week, including a mix of weight-bearing exercises, strength training (two or three times a week), and balance training.

Smoking

Smoking is bad for your bones and for your heart and lungs. Women who smoke have lower levels of estrogen compared to nonsmokers and frequently go through menopause earlier.

Alcohol

People who drink heavily are more prone to bone loss and fractures because of poor nutrition and harmful effects on calcium balance and hormonal factors. Drinking too much also increases the risk of falling, which is likely to increase fracture risk.

Medications

The long-term use of glucocorticoids can lead to a loss of bone density and fractures. Other forms of drug therapy that can cause bone loss include:

- Long-term treatment with certain antiseizure drugs and barbiturates
- Some drugs used to treat endometriosis
- Excessive use of aluminum-containing antacids
- Certain cancer treatments; and excessive thyroid hormone

It is important to discuss the use of these drugs with your doctor, and not to stop or alter your medication dose on your own.

Section 37.2

Protecting Your Bone

This section includes text excerpted from "The Surgeon General's Report on Bone Health and Osteoporosis: What It Means to You," NIH Osteoporosis and Related Bone Diseases—National Resource Center (NIH ORBD—NRC), February 2017.

The average American eats too little calcium. And nearly half of us do not get enough physical activity to strengthen our bones.

The same healthy lifestyle that strengthens your bones strengthens your whole body. You might not hear as much about bone health as other health concerns. But healthy habits are good for all your organs, including your bones.

- Be physically active every day—at least 60 minutes for children, 30 minutes for adults. Do strength-building and weight-bearing activities to build strong bones.

- Eat a healthy diet. Educate yourself on proper nutrition. Be aware that certain foods are naturally rich in calcium and vitamin D. Get the recommended amounts of calcium and vitamin D daily.

- Reduce your risks of falling. Check your home for loose rugs, poor lighting, etc. Take classes that increase balance and strength—like tai chi or yoga. Make stretching a part of your workout.

Even people who know better don't always do what's good for their bones. Make yourself an exception. Be aware of your risks and work to reduce them. Get help from your family and friends and your doctor, nurse, pharmacist, or other healthcare professional. Building healthy bones begins at birth and lasts your whole life.

Your Doctor Can Help Protect Your Bones

Talk to your doctor about bone health. Together you can evaluate your risks. Some things to discuss include your current health, your diet and physical activity levels, and your family background.

Your doctor can look at your age, weight, height, and medical history. From that she or he can determine if you need a bone density test. Broken bones are a "red flag" for your doctor. If you break a bone after the age of 50, talk to your doctor about measuring your bone density. Even if you broke a bone in an accident, you might have weak bones. It is worth checking.

Your doctor might recommend a medical test called a bone mineral density test. Bone density tests use X-rays or sound waves to measure how strong your bones are. These tests are quick (5 to 10 minutes), safe, and painless. They will give you and your doctor an idea of how healthy your bones are. All women over age 65 should have a bone density test. Women who are younger than age 65 and at high risk for fractures should also have a bone density test.

Your doctor might also want to do a blood test to check for a vitamin D deficiency or abnormal calcium levels.

If your doctor finds that your bones are becoming weaker, there are things you can do to make them stronger. You can be more physically active, change your diet, and take calcium and vitamin D supplements. If your bones are already weak, there are medicines that stop bone loss. They can even build new bone and make it less likely that you will suffer a broken bone.

Your doctor might suggest medications to help you build stronger bones. To reduce the chance that you might fall, have your vision checked. When you speak to your doctor, be prepared with a list of questions and concerns. The list on the next page should help get you started.

See Your Doctor

Although osteoporosis is the most common disease that harms bones, certain other conditions can also be harmful. Your doctor can help you learn if you are at risk and can help you treat these conditions.

- **Rickets and osteomalacia**—Too little vitamin D causes these diseases in children and adults. They can lead to bone deformities and fractures

- **Kidney disease**—Renal osteodystrophy can cause fractures

- **Paget disease of bone**—Bones become deformed and weak, which can be caused by genetic and environmental factors

- **Genetic abnormalities**—Disorders like osteogenesis imperfecta cause bones to grow abnormally and break easily

- **Endocrine disorders**—Overactive glands can cause bone disease

Chapter 38

Calcium, Vitamins, and Bone Health

Chapter Contents

Section 38.1

Calcium and Vitamin D: Important at Every Age

This section includes text excerpted from "Calcium and Vitamin D: Important at Every Age," NIH Osteoporosis and Related Bone Diseases—National Resource Center (NIH ORBD—NRC), May 2015. Reviewed January 2019.

The foods we eat contain a variety of vitamins, minerals, and other important nutrients that help keep our bodies healthy. Two nutrients in particular, calcium and vitamin D, are needed for strong bones.

The Role of Calcium

Calcium is needed for our heart, muscles, and nerves to function properly and for blood to clot. Inadequate calcium significantly contributes to the development of osteoporosis. Many published studies show that low calcium intake throughout life is associated with low bone mass and high fracture rates. National nutrition surveys have shown that most people are not getting the calcium they need to grow and maintain healthy bones. To find out how much calcium you need, see the Recommended Calcium Intakes (in milligrams) chart below.

To learn how easily you can include more calcium in your diet without adding much fat, see the Selected Calcium-Rich Foods list below.

Table 38.1. Recommended Calcium Intakes

Life-Stage Group	Mg/Day
Infants 0 to 6 months	200
Infants 6 to 12 months	260
1 to 3 years old	700
4 to 8 years old	1,000
9 to 13 years old	1,300
14 to 18 years old	1,300
19 to 30 years old	1,000
31 to 50 years old	1,000
51- to 70-year-old males	1,000

Table 38.1. Continued

Life-Stage Group	Mg/Day
51- to 70-year-old females	1,200
70 years old	1,200
14 to 18 years old, pregnant/lactating	1,300
19 to 50 years old, pregnant/lactating	1,000

(Source: Food and Nutrition Board (FNB), Institute of Medicine (IOM), National Academy of Sciences (NAS), 2010.)

Table 38.2. Selected Calcium-Rich Foods

Food	Calcium (mg)
Fortified oatmeal, 1 packet	350
Sardines, canned in oil, with edible bones, 3 oz.	324
Cheddar cheese, 1½ oz. shredded	306
Milk, nonfat, 1 cup	302
Milkshake, 1 cup	300
Yogurt, plain, low-fat, 1 cup	300
Soybeans, cooked, 1 cup	261
Tofu, firm, with calcium, ½ cup	204
Orange juice, fortified with calcium, 6 oz.	200 to 260 (varies)
Salmon, canned, with edible bones, 3 oz.	181
Pudding, instant (chocolate, banana, etc.) made with 2% milk, ½ cup	153
Baked beans, 1 cup	142
Cottage cheese, 1% milk fat, 1 cup	138
Spaghetti, lasagna, 1 cup	125
Frozen yogurt, vanilla, soft serve, ½ cup	103
Ready-to-eat cereal, fortified with calcium, 1 cup	100 to 1,000 (varies)
Cheese pizza, 1 slice	100
Fortified waffles, 2	100
Turnip greens, boiled, ½ cup	99
Broccoli, raw, 1 cup	90
Ice cream, vanilla, ½ cup	85
Soy or rice milk, fortified with calcium, 1 cup	80 to 500 (varies)

(Source: The 2004 Surgeon General's Report on Bone Health and Osteoporosis: What It Means to You. U.S. Department of Health and Human Services (HHS), Office of the Surgeon General (OSG), 2004, pages 12–13.)

Calcium Culprits

Although a balanced diet aids calcium absorption, high levels of protein and sodium (salt) in the diet are thought to increase calcium excretion through the kidneys. Excessive amounts of these substances should be avoided, especially in those with low calcium intake.

Lactose intolerance also can lead to inadequate calcium intake. Those who are lactose intolerant have insufficient amounts of the enzyme lactase, which is needed to break down the lactose found in dairy products. To include dairy products in the diet, dairy foods can be taken in small quantities or treated with lactase drops, or lactase can be taken as a pill. Some milk products on the market already have been treated with lactase.

Calcium Supplements

If you have trouble getting enough calcium in your diet, you may need to take a calcium supplement. The amount of calcium you will need from a supplement depends on how much calcium you obtain from food sources. There are several different calcium compounds from which to choose, such as calcium carbonate and calcium citrate, among others. Except in people with gastrointestinal disease, all major forms of calcium supplements are absorbed equally well when taken with food.

Calcium supplements are better absorbed when taken in small doses (500 mg or less) several times throughout the day. In many individuals, calcium supplements are better absorbed when taken with food. It is important to check supplement labels to ensure that the product meets United States Pharmacopeia (USP) standards.

Vitamin D

The body needs vitamin D to absorb calcium. Without enough vitamin D, one can't form enough of the hormone calcitriol (known as the "active vitamin D"). This in turn leads to insufficient calcium absorption from the diet. In this situation, the body must take calcium from its stores in the skeleton, which weakens existing bone and prevents the formation of strong, new bone.

You can get vitamin D in three ways: through the skin, from the diet, and from supplements. Experts recommend a daily intake of 600 IU (International Units) of vitamin D up to age 70. Men and women over age 70 should increase their uptake to 800 IU daily, which also can be obtained from supplements or vitamin D-rich foods such as egg yolks, saltwater fish, liver, and fortified milk. The Institute of Medicine (IOM) recommends no more than 4,000 IU per day for adults. However, sometimes doctors prescribe higher doses for people who are deficient in vitamin D.

A Complete Osteoporosis Program

Remember, a balanced diet rich in calcium and vitamin D is only one part of an osteoporosis prevention or treatment program. Like exercise, getting enough calcium is a strategy that helps strengthen bones at any age. But these strategies may not be enough to stop bone loss caused by lifestyle, medications, or menopause. Your doctor can determine the need for an osteoporosis medication in addition to diet and exercise.

Section 38.2

Calcium and Children's Bone Health

This section includes text excerpted from "Children's Bone Health and Calcium: Condition Information," *Eunice Kennedy Shriver* National Institute of Child Health and Human Development (NICHD), December 1, 2016.

Overall Bone Health

Healthy bones enable children to stand up straight, walk, run, and lead an active life. Calcium is one of the key dietary building blocks to develop strong bones. Because bone growth is rapid during the adolescent years, this is when excellent nutrition, including adequate amounts of calcium is especially important.

Developing strong and healthy bones during childhood may help prevent fractures and avoid osteoporosis later in life. Osteoporosis is a disease in which the bones become thin and weak and break easily. This condition usually appears later in life, but it develops slowly, and early signs of this bone disorder may start in childhood. The best defenses against osteoporosis are eating a well-balanced diet that contains plenty of calcium and taking part in regular physical activity.

Bone Health and Childhood

About one in ten girls and fewer than one in four boys ages 9 to 13 are at or above their adequate intake of calcium. This lack of calcium has a big impact on bones and teeth. Your body continually removes and replaces small amounts of calcium from your bones. If your body removes more calcium than it replaces, your bones will become weaker and have a greater chance of breaking. Children and adolescents establish bone health, which serves as an important foundation to last a lifetime.

The adolescent years are a time of rapid bone growth. For example, teenagers can build more than 25 percent of their adult bone mass during the adolescent years of peak skeletal growth. By the time teens finish their growth spurts at around age 17 years, more than 90 percent of their adult bone mass is established.

Section 38.3

Calcium: Shopping List

This section includes text excerpted from "Calcium: Shopping List," Office of Disease Prevention and Health Promotion (ODPHP), U.S. Department of Health and Human Services (HHS), September 18, 2018.

Many Americans don't get enough calcium. Your body needs calcium to build strong bones and help prevent osteoporosis (bone loss).

The best way to get enough calcium is to eat more dairy products. Foods with added calcium and vitamin D can also help, and so can certain vegetables.

These tips can help you get enough calcium:

- Use the Nutrition Facts label to find foods and drinks with at least 20%DV (Daily Value) of calcium.

- Also, include foods and drinks with less than 20% DV of calcium throughout the day. This will help you meet your daily goal.
- Don't forget vitamin D. Vitamin D helps your body absorb (take in) calcium.

Dairy Products

Look for fat-free or low-fat dairy products.

- Fat-free or low-fat (1%) milk
- Fat-free or low-fat yogurt (choose options with no added sugars)
- Low-fat cheese (3 grams of fat or less per serving)
- Soymilk with added calcium, vitamin A, and vitamin D

Vegetables

You can also get calcium from vegetables like:

- Soybeans (edamame)
- Kale
- Turnip greens
- Chinese cabbage (bok choy)
- Collard greens
- Broccoli

If you buy canned vegetables, watch out for sodium. Read the Nutrition Facts label and choose the option with the least sodium.

If you buy frozen vegetables, check the Nutrition Facts label and choose ones without butter or cream sauces.

Foods with Added Calcium

Check the Nutrition Facts label to look for foods that have 10 percent or more DV of calcium added:

- Breakfast cereal
- Tofu
- 100 percent orange juice
- Soymilk, almond milk, or rice milk

Foods with Vitamin D

- Vitamin D is added to some foods, like milk, breakfast cereals, and juice. Check the Nutrition Facts label.

- You can also get some vitamin D from many types of fish like salmon, tuna, and trout.

Section 38.4

Vitamin A and Bone Health

This section includes text excerpted from "Vitamin A and Bone Health," NIH Osteoporosis and Related Bone Diseases—National Resource Center (NIH ORBD—NRC), May 2015. Reviewed January 2019.

Vitamin A is essential for good health. It promotes growth, the immune system, reproduction, and vision. However, recent research suggests that too much vitamin A, particularly in the form of retinol, may be bad for your bones. This section explains where we get vitamin A, how much of this important vitamin we need, how it can build up in the body to excessive levels, and how you can assess your own vitamin A intake.

What Is Vitamin A?

Vitamin A is a family of compounds that play an important role in vision, bone growth, reproduction, cell division, and cell differentiation. We get vitamin A from a variety of sources. Two of the most common sources are retinol and beta-carotene.

Retinol is sometimes called "true" vitamin A because it is nearly ready for the body to use. Retinol is found in such animal foods as liver, eggs, and fatty fish. It also can be found in many fortified foods, such as breakfast cereals, and in dietary supplements.

Beta-carotene is a precursor for vitamin A. The body needs to convert it to retinol or vitamin A for use. Beta-carotene is found naturally in mostly orange and dark green plant foods, such as carrots, sweet potatoes, mangos, and kale.

The body stores both retinol and beta-carotene in the liver, drawing on this store whenever more vitamin A is needed.

How Much Vitamin A Do I Need?

The Institute of Medicine (IOM) developed the Recommended Dietary Allowance (RDA) for vitamin A (retinol). The recommended intakes are listed in International Units (IU) in the table, below:

Table 38.3. Recommended Dietary Allowance (RDA) for Vitamin A (Retinol) in International Units (IU)

Age (yrs)	Children	Men	Women	Pregnancy	Lactation
1 to 3	1,000				
4 to 8	1,320				
9 to 13	2,000				
14 to 18		3,000	2,310	2,500	4,000
19+		3,000	2,310	2,565	4,300

(Source: Institute of Medicine (IOM), 2001.)

The body can convert beta-carotene into vitamin A to help meet these requirements. Although there is no RDA for beta-carotene, the National Institutes of Health (NIH) Office of Dietary Supplements recommends eating five or more servings of fruits and vegetables per day, including dark green and leafy vegetables and deep yellow or orange fruits to get appropriate amounts of beta-carotene.

How Does Vitamin A Affect My Bones?

Vitamin A is a family of fat-soluble compounds that play an important role in vision, bone growth, reproduction, cell division, and cell differentiation. Vitamin A is important for healthy bones. However, too much vitamin A has been linked to bone loss and an increase in the risk of hip fracture. Scientists believe that excessive amounts of vitamin A trigger an increase in osteoclasts, the cells that break down bone. They also believe that too much vitamin A may interfere with vitamin D, which plays an important role in preserving bone.

Retinol is the form of vitamin A that causes concern. In addition to getting retinol from their diets, some people may be using synthetic retinoid preparations that are chemically similar to vitamin A to treat acne, psoriasis, and other skin conditions. These preparations have been shown to have the same negative impact on bone health as dietary retinol. Use of these medications in children and teens also has been linked to delays in growth.

Beta-carotene, on the other hand, is largely considered to be safe and has not been linked to adverse effects in bone or elsewhere in the body.

How Can I Make Sure I Get the Right Amount of Vitamin A?

Surveys suggest that most Americans are getting adequate amounts of vitamin A. The Institute of Medicine cautions against daily intakes of retinol above 10,000 IU.

The chart below identifies some common food sources of retinol. Most of the reported cases of vitamin A toxicity have been blamed on the use of supplements. Healthy individuals who eat a balanced diet generally do not need a vitamin A supplement.

Table 38.4. Common Food Sources of Retinol

Food Sources of Retinol	Vitamin A (IU)
Liver, beef, cooked 3 oz.	30,325
Liver, chicken, cooked, 3 oz.	13,920
Egg substitute, fortified, ¼ cup	1,355
Fat-free milk, fortified with vitamin A, 1 cup	500
Cheese pizza, ⅛ of a 12-inch pie	380
Milk, whole, 3.25% fat, 1 cup	305
Cheddar cheese, 1 oz	300
Whole egg, 1 medium	280

(Source: National Institutes of Health (NIH), Office of Dietary Supplements (ODS).)

Plant sources of beta-carotene are not as well absorbed as the animal sources of vitamin A listed in the chart, but they are still an important source of this vitamin. Dark orange and green vegetables and fruit, including carrots, sweet potatoes, spinach, cantaloupe, and kale are excellent sources of beta-carotene. Because of concerns about the negative effects of too much retinol, some people prefer to eat more foods rich in beta-carotene to satisfy their need for vitamin A.

Are Some People at Special Risk of Getting Too Much Vitamin A?

The 1988 to 1994 National Health and Nutrition Examination Survey (NHANES III) found high levels of retinol in 5 to 10 percent of the survey participants. Increased levels were more common in men age 30 and older and in women age 50 and older.

Older people who regularly take dietary supplements containing vitamin A may be at higher risk of getting too much vitamin A.

Studies suggest that taking dietary supplements is a common practice among many older adults. However, the routine use of vitamin A supplements, as well as fortified foods, in older men and women is increasingly being questioned. Older adults are at significant risk for osteoporosis and related fractures, and their serum (blood) levels of retinol increase with age. As a result, fortified foods and supplements containing vitamin A in the form of beta-carotene may be a better choice for bone health in this population.

The supplement label provides information about how much vitamin A is provided, in both International Units (IU) and as a percentage of the RDA. The list of ingredients will contain information about which forms of vitamin A are included. Other names for retinol include retinyl, palmitate, and retinyl acetate.

Section 38.5

Magnesium and Bone Health

This section includes text excerpted from "Magnesium Fact Sheet for Consumers," Office of Dietary Supplements (ODS), National Institutes of Health (NIH), February 17, 2016.

What Is Magnesium and What Does It Do?

Magnesium is a nutrient that the body needs to stay healthy. Magnesium is important for many processes in the body, including regulating muscle and nerve function, blood sugar levels, and blood pressure and making protein, bone, and deoxyribonucleic acid (DNA).

How Much Magnesium Do I Need?

The amount of magnesium you need depends on your age and sex. Average daily recommended amounts are listed below in milligrams (mg):

Table 38.5. Average Daily Recommended Amounts of Magnesium

Life Stage	Recommended Amount
Birth to 6 months	30 mg
Infants 7 to 12 months	75 mg
Children 1 to 3 years	80 mg
Children 4 to 8 years	130 mg
Children 9 to 13 years	240 mg
Teen boys 14 to 18 years	410 mg
Teen girls 14 to 18 years	360 mg
Men	400 to 420 mg
Women	310 to 320 mg
Pregnant teens	400 mg
Pregnant women	350 to 360 mg
Breastfeeding teens	360 mg
Breastfeeding women	310 to 320 mg

What Foods Provide Magnesium?

Magnesium is found naturally in many foods and is added to some fortified foods. You can get recommended amounts of magnesium by eating a variety of foods, including the following:

- Legumes, nuts, seeds, whole grains, and green leafy vegetables (such as spinach)

- Fortified breakfast cereals and other fortified foods

- Milk, yogurt, and some other milk products

What Kinds of Magnesium Dietary Supplements Are Available?

Magnesium is available in multivitamin-mineral supplements and other dietary supplements. Forms of magnesium in dietary supplements that are more easily absorbed by the body are magnesium aspartate, magnesium citrate, magnesium lactate, and magnesium chloride.

Magnesium is also included in some laxatives and some products for treating heartburn and indigestion.

Am I Getting Enough Magnesium?

The diets of most people in the United States provide less than the recommended amounts of magnesium. Men older than 70 and teenage girls are most likely to have low intakes of magnesium. When the amount of magnesium people get from food and dietary supplements are combined, however, total intakes of magnesium are generally above recommended amounts.

What Happens If I Don't Get Enough Magnesium?

In the short term, getting too little magnesium does not produce obvious symptoms. When healthy people have low intakes, the kidneys help retain magnesium by limiting the amount lost in urine. Low magnesium intakes for a long period of time, however, can lead to magnesium deficiency. In addition, some medical conditions and medications interfere with the body's ability to absorb magnesium or increase the amount of magnesium that the body excretes, which can also lead to magnesium deficiency. Symptoms of magnesium deficiency include loss of appetite, nausea, vomiting, fatigue, and weakness. Extreme magnesium deficiency can cause numbness, tingling, muscle cramps, seizures, personality changes, and an abnormal heart rhythm.

The following groups of people are more likely than others to get too little magnesium:

- People with gastrointestinal diseases (such as Crohn disease and celiac disease)

- People with type 2 diabetes

- People with long-term alcoholism

- Older people

What Are Some Effects of Magnesium on Health?

Scientists are studying magnesium to understand how it affects health. Here are some examples of what this research has shown.

Osteoporosis

Magnesium is important for healthy bones. People with higher intakes of magnesium have a higher bone mineral density, which is important in reducing the risk of bone fractures and osteoporosis. Getting more magnesium from foods or dietary supplements might help older women improve their bone mineral density. More research is needed to better understand whether magnesium supplements can help reduce the risk of osteoporosis or treat this condition.

High Blood Pressure and Heart Disease

High blood pressure is a major risk factor for heart disease and stroke. Magnesium supplements might decrease blood pressure, but only by a small amount. Some studies show that people who have more magnesium in their diets have a lower risk of some types of heart disease and stroke. But in many of these studies, it's hard to know how much of the effect was due to magnesium as opposed to other nutrients.

Type 2 Diabetes

People with higher amounts of magnesium in their diets tend to have a lower risk of developing type 2 diabetes. Magnesium helps the body break down sugars and might help reduce the risk of insulin resistance (a condition that leads to diabetes). Scientists are studying whether magnesium supplements might help people who already have type 2 diabetes control their disease. More research is needed to better understand whether magnesium can help treat diabetes.

Can Magnesium Be Harmful?

Magnesium that is naturally present in food is not harmful and does not need to be limited. In healthy people, the kidneys can get rid of any excess in the urine. But magnesium in dietary supplements and medications should not be consumed in amounts above the upper limit unless recommended by a healthcare provider.

The upper limits for magnesium from dietary supplements and/or medications are listed below. For many age groups, the upper limit appears to be lower than the recommended amount. This occurs because the recommended amounts include magnesium from all sources—food, dietary supplements, and medications. The upper limits include magnesium from only dietary supplements and medications; they do not include magnesium found naturally in food.

Table 38.6. Upper Limit for Magnesium in Dietary Supplements and Medications

Ages	Upper Limit for Magnesium in Dietary Supplements and Medications
Birth to 12 months	Not established
Children 1 to 3 years	65 mg
Children 4 to 8 years	110 mg
Children 9 to 18 years	350 mg
Adults	350 mg

High intakes of magnesium from dietary supplements and medications can cause diarrhea, nausea, and abdominal cramping. Extremely high intakes of magnesium can lead to irregular heartbeat and cardiac arrest.

Are There Any Interactions with Magnesium That I Should Know About?

Yes. Magnesium supplements can interact or interfere with some medicines. Here are several examples:

- Bisphosphonates, used to treat osteoporosis, are not well absorbed when taken too soon before or after taking dietary supplements or medications with high amounts of magnesium.

- Antibiotics might not be absorbed if taken too soon before or after taking a dietary supplement that contains magnesium.

- Diuretics can either increase or decrease the loss of magnesium through urine, depending on the type of diuretic.

- Prescription drugs used to ease symptoms of acid reflux or treat peptic ulcers can cause low blood levels of magnesium when taken over a long period of time.

- Very high doses of zinc supplements can interfere with the body's ability to absorb and regulate magnesium.

Tell your doctor, pharmacist, and other healthcare providers about any dietary supplements and prescription or over-the-counter (OTC) medicines you take. They can tell you if the dietary supplements might interact with your medicines or if the medicines might interfere with how your body absorbs, uses, or breaks down nutrients.

Magnesium and Healthful Eating

People should get most of their nutrients from food, advises the federal government's *Dietary Guidelines for Americans*. Foods contain vitamins, minerals, dietary fiber, and other substances that benefit health. In some cases, fortified foods and dietary supplements may provide nutrients that otherwise may be consumed in less-than-recommended amounts.

Chapter 39

Bone Builders: Support Your Bones with Healthy Habits

Chapter Contents

Section 39.1

Building Strong Bones

This section includes text excerpted from "Building Strong Bones:
Calcium Information for Healthcare Providers," *Eunice Kennedy
Shriver* National Institute of Child Health and Human
Development (NICHD), January 2006. Reviewed January 2019.

You can play a critical role in making sure tweens and teens get
1,300 mg of calcium every day at least 3 cups of low-fat or fat-free milk,
plus other calcium-rich foods—to build strong bones for life. Calcium
is essential to overall health and bone development, but most children
and teenagers are not getting enough. In fact, fewer than one in 10
girls and just more than one in four boys ages 9 to 13 are at or above
their adequate intake of calcium.

You can help children achieve lifelong bone health by talking to
parents and young people about the importance of calcium consumption, especially during ages 11 to 15, a time of critical bone growth.
Children and teenagers can get most of their daily calcium from 3
cups of low-fat or fat-free milk (900 mg), but they also need additional
servings of calcium-rich foods to get the 1,300 mg of calcium necessary
for optimal bone development. Research suggests many parents don't
know that children and teenagers need almost twice as much calcium
as children younger than age 9.

How Does Pediatric Bone Development Influence
Osteoporosis Later in Life?

The tween and teen years are critical for bone development because
most bone mass accumulates during this time. In the years of peak
skeletal growth, teenagers accumulate more than 25 percent of adult
bone, and by the time teens finish their growth spurts around age 17,
90 percent of their adult bone mass is established.

Calcium is critical to building bone mass for supporting physical
activity throughout life, and for reducing the risk of bone fractures,
especially those due to osteoporosis. The onset of osteoporosis later in
life is influenced by two important factors:

- Peak bone mass attained in the first two to three decades of
  life

- The rate at which bone is lost in the later years

Although the consequences of low calcium consumption may not be visible in childhood, the *Eunice Kennedy Shriver* National Institute of Child Health and Human Development (NICHD) recognizes lack of calcium intake as a serious and growing threat to the health of young people later in life. At a time when they require more nutrients to feed their rapidly growing and developing bodies, tweens and teens who don't get enough calcium are at increased risk for osteoporosis later in life.

Why Are Milk and Dairy Products Especially Good Sources of Calcium?

- Although calcium is found in a variety of foods, the 1994 National Institutes of Health (NIH) *Consensus Statement on Optimal Calcium Intake* designated dairy products as the preferred source of calcium because of their high calcium content.

- The 2005 *Dietary Guidelines for Americans* also recommends milk and milk products as sources of dietary calcium based on studies that show a positive relationship between intake of milk and milk products and bone mineral content or bone mineral density in one or more skeletal sites.

- The NICHD has described low-fat or fat-free milk as the best source of calcium because it has high calcium content without added fat, and because the calcium is easily absorbed by the body.

- Other foods, including dark green, leafy vegetables such as kale and spinach, are also healthy dietary sources of calcium, but it takes many servings of these vegetables to get the same amount of calcium in 3 to 4 cups of milk.

In addition to calcium, milk provides other essential nutrients that are important for optimal bone health and development, including:

- Vitamins D, A, and B_{12}
- Phosphorous
- Potassium
- Riboflavin
- Magnesium
- Protein

What Kind of Milk Is Best for Children?

Children 1 to 2 years old should drink whole milk. After age 2, low-fat or fat-free milk should become the regular drink. Regardless of fat content, an 8-ounce glass of milk contains about 300 mg of calcium.

What If Children Don't Like Milk?

If it is a question of taste, there are plenty of ways to get calcium into the diet:

- Try flavored low-fat or fat-free milk, such as chocolate, vanilla, or strawberry. Flavored milk has the same amount of calcium as plain milk.

- Serve low-fat or fat-free milk or yogurt smoothies. These can be made at home or there are ready-made versions available at many grocery stores.

- In moderation, low-fat or fat-free ice cream and frozen yogurt are calcium-rich treats.

- Serve nonmilk sources of calcium, such as broccoli, spinach, or orange juice with added calcium.

How Does Bioavailability Affect Calcium Absorption?

Bioavailability, the degree to which the intestinal system absorbs calcium, depends on the overall level of calcium in a food and the type of food being consumed. Calcium in foods such as milk and milk products is highly bioavailable, meaning that it is easily absorbed. Absorption is similarly high in grain foods.

However, calcium in foods high in oxalic acid (such as spinach, sweet potatoes, and beans) or phytic acid (such as unleavened bread, raw beans, seeds, and nuts) may be poorly absorbed. Oxalates in particular are strong inhibitors of calcium absorption. As a result, additional servings of certain calcium-rich foods are needed to compensate for their low calcium bioavailability.

According to the National Academy of Sciences' 1997 *Report on Dietary Reference Intakes*, the body absorbs about one-tenth as much calcium from spinach as it does from milk. High bioavailability is one of the reasons that the NICHD describes low-fat and fat-free milk and milk products as the best dietary sources of calcium.

What about People Who Have Trouble Digesting Milk or Milk Products

Individuals with lactose intolerance are unable to digest significant amounts of lactose due to an inadequate amount of the enzyme lactase.

Research shows that lactase is high at birth in all infants regardless of race or ethnicity, but wanes in non-Caucasians and other populations that don't traditionally include dairy products in their diets by age 5 to 7.

There are three main types of lactose intolerance:

- Primary lactose intolerance, in which individuals who were able to digest lactose previously begin experiencing symptoms of digestive discomfort with no history or signs of underlying intestinal disease, is the most common form of lactase deficiency.

- Secondary lactose intolerance is the result of a gastrointestinal disease, such as severe gastroenteritis.

- Congenital lactose intolerance, such as galactosemia, is a lifelong complete absence of lactase, and it is relatively rare. However, it is not uncommon for secondary lactose intolerance to be misdiagnosed during the newborn period as congenital lactose intolerance.

Clinical symptoms of lactose intolerance can include abdominal pain, diarrhea, flatulence, and bloating. The severity of symptoms differs, often depending on the amount of lactase remaining in the body and how much lactose has been consumed.

Individuals vary in their degree of lactose intolerance, but even children and teenagers with primary lactose intolerance can usually consume 8 to 12 ounces (1 to 1½ cups) of milk without experiencing symptoms.

What Is the Role of Physical Activity in Bone Development?

Weight-bearing activity determines the strength, shape, and mass of bone. Activities such as running, dancing, and climbing stairs, as well as those that increase strength, such as weight lifting, can help bone development. For children and teenagers, some of the best weight-bearing activities include team sports, such as basketball, volleyball, soccer, and softball.

Studies show that absence of physical activity results in a loss of bone mass, especially during long periods of immobilization or inactivity.

Are There Any Special Calcium Recommendations for Lactating or Pregnant Teens?

Increasing dietary calcium does not prevent the loss of calcium that occurs during lactation, and the calcium lost seems to be regained after weaning. Therefore, the Dietary Reference Intakes do not recommend increasing calcium intake for lactating adolescents above normal levels for that age group. However, the 1994 NIH Consensus Statement on Optimal Calcium Intake recommends that lactating teenagers and young adults increase their calcium intake to up to 1,500 mg per day.

What about Calcium Supplements

Experts suggest that the preferred source of calcium is through calcium-rich foods. However, if calcium cannot be obtained through the diet, calcium supplements can be given to children.

Section 39.2

Exercises and Bone Health

This section contains text excerpted from the following sources: Text beginning with the heading "Why Exercise" is excerpted from "Exercise for Your Bone Health," NIH Osteoporosis and Related Bone Diseases—National Resource Center (NIH ORBD—NRC), April 2015. Reviewed January 2019; Text under the heading "How Does Physical Activity Help Build Healthy Bones?" is excerpted from "How Does Physical Activity Help Build Healthy Bones?" *Eunice Kennedy Shriver* National Institute of Child Health and Human Development (NICHD), January 12, 2016.

Why Exercise

Like muscle, bone is living tissue that responds to exercise by becoming stronger. Young women and men who exercise regularly generally achieve greater peak bone mass (maximum bone density and strength) than those who do not. For most people, bone mass peaks during the third decade of life. After that time, we can begin to lose bone. Women and men older than age 20 can help prevent bone loss with regular exercise. Exercising allows us to maintain muscle strength, coordination, and balance, which in turn helps to prevent falls and related fractures. This is especially important for older adults and people who have been diagnosed with osteoporosis.

The Best Bone Building Exercise

The best exercise for your bones is the weight-bearing kind, which forces you to work against gravity. Some examples of weight-bearing exercises include weight training, walking, hiking, jogging, climbing stairs, tennis, and dancing. Examples of exercises that are not weight-bearing include swimming and bicycling. Although these activities help build and maintain strong muscles and have excellent cardiovascular benefits, they are not the best way to exercise your bones.

Exercise Tips

If you have health problems—such as heart trouble, high blood pressure, diabetes, or obesity—or if you are age 40 or older, check with your doctor before you begin a regular exercise program.

According to the Surgeon General, the optimal goal is at least 30 minutes of physical activity on most days, preferably daily.

Listen to your body. When starting an exercise routine, you may have some muscle soreness and discomfort at the beginning, but this should not be painful or last more than 48 hours. If it does, you may be working too hard and need to ease up. Stop exercising if you have any chest pain or discomfort, and see your doctor before your next exercise session.

If you have osteoporosis, ask your doctor which activities are safe for you. If you have low bone mass, experts recommend that you protect your spine by avoiding exercises or activities that flex, bend, or twist it. Furthermore, you should avoid high-impact exercise to lower the risk of breaking a bone. You also might want to consult with an exercise specialist to learn the proper progression of activity, how to stretch and strengthen muscles safely, and how to correct poor posture habits. An exercise specialist should have a degree in exercise physiology, physical education, physical therapy, or a similar specialty. Be sure to ask if she or he is familiar with the special needs of people with osteoporosis.

A Complete Osteoporosis Program

Remember, exercise is only one part of an osteoporosis prevention or treatment program. Like a diet rich in calcium and vitamin D, exercise helps strengthen bones at any age. But proper exercise and diet may not be enough to stop bone loss caused by medical conditions, menopause, or lifestyle choices such as tobacco use and excessive alcohol consumption. It is important to speak with your doctor about your bone health. Discuss whether you might be a candidate for a bone mineral density test. If you are diagnosed with low bone mass, ask what medications might help keep your bones strong.

How Does Physical Activity Help Build Healthy Bones?

Bones are living tissue. Weight-bearing physical activity causes new bone tissue to form, and this makes bones stronger. This kind of physical activity also makes muscles stronger. Bones and muscles both become stronger when muscles push and tug against bones during physical activity.

Weight-bearing physical activity keeps you on your feet so that your legs carry your body weight. Some examples of weight-bearing physical activities include:

- Walking, jogging, or running

- Playing tennis or racquetball

- Playing field hockey

- Climbing stairs

- Jumping rope and other types of jumping

- Playing basketball

- Dancing

- Hiking

- Playing soccer

- Lifting weights

Swimming and bicycling are not weight-bearing activities, so they do not directly help build bones. But swimming and bicycling do help build strong muscles, and having strong muscles helps build strong bones. These activities are also good for the heart and for overall health.

Bone-strengthening activities are especially important for children and teens because the greatest gains in bone mass occur just before and during puberty. They obtain their lifetime peak bone mass in their teens.

- Children and teens aged 6 to 17 years should get a total of 60 minutes of physical activity every day. Short bursts of activity throughout the day can add up to the recommended total.

- Children and teens should participate in bone-strengthening activities at least 3 days each week.

- Younger children, aged 2 to 5 years, should play actively several times every day.

Best Bones Forever External Web Site Policy is a bone health campaign for girls and their friends to "grow strong together and stay strong forever!" Created by the U.S. Office on Women's Health (OWH), it includes an interactive and educational website to engage girls in learning about and participating in bone-strengthening activities.

Section 39.3

Physical Activity Brings Lasting Bone Benefits

This section includes text excerpted from "Physical Activity Brings Lasting Bone Benefits," National Institutes of Health (NIH), March 31, 2014. Reviewed January 2019.

A study of professional baseball players showed that some benefits of building bone during youth can last a lifetime. The research also confirmed that continued physical activity can help maintain bone strength as we age.

Bone is a living tissue that responds to physical activity by becoming heavier, bigger, and stronger. It does this best during youth. Bone mass usually peaks during the third decade of life. After that, we often begin to lose bone.

A team led by Dr. Stuart J. Warden of Indiana University explored whether any bone benefits of physical activity during youth persist with aging. Previous work found that mechanical loading during a period of rapid growth conferred lifelong benefits in bone size and strength in rodent models.

To test whether the same holds true for humans, the researchers recruited more than 100 professional baseball players at different stages of their careers. Baseball players have a unique internal control for such a study. Their throwing arms are exposed to repeated mechanical loads, while their nonthrowing arms aren't. Baseball players also often retire from stressful throwing activities once they stop professional play. This allowed the scientists to explore the effects of physical activity long after players return to more typical activity. Almost 100 age-matched controls were also studied for comparison.

The researchers focused on the humerus, the upper arm bone running from shoulder to elbow. They used quantitative CT scans and dual-energy X-ray absorptiometry (DXA) to measure bone size and bone mineral density. The study, which was funded by NIH's National Institute of Arthritis and Musculoskeletal and Skin Diseases (NIAMS), appeared online in Proceedings of the National Academy of Sciences on March 24, 2014.

The loads on humerus bones from repeated pitches, the researchers found, led the bones in throwing arms to nearly double in strength. The throwing arms of baseball players had more bone on the outer surface of the humerus (cortical bone), creating a bone with a bigger diameter. Compared to humeral bones in nonthrowing arms, those in throwing arms had about 50 percent greater mass, size (total cross-sectional area), and thickness.

The bone mass benefits from throwing were gradually lost after throwing activities ended. Bone loss during aging occurred mostly on the inside of bones rather than the outside. Because of this pattern of bone loss, about half the bone size benefits of physical activity during youth and one-third of the bone strength benefits were maintained lifelong. Players who continued throwing during aging experienced less bone loss on the inside of the bone and maintained even more of the strength benefits.

"Exercise during youth adds extra layers to the outer surface of a bone to essentially make the bone bigger," Warden says. "As bone loss during aging predominantly occurs on the inside rather than outside of a bone, the bigger bone generated by physical activity when young has a means of sticking around long-term to keep the skeleton stronger."

This study demonstrates the importance of building bone during youth. It also highlights the fact that physical activity during aging can continue to help fend off bone decay.

Section 39.4

Nutrition Fact Label

This section includes text excerpted from "Using the Nutrition Facts Label: A How-to Guide for Older Adults," U.S. Food and Drug Administration (FDA), July 31, 2018.

Why Nutrition Matters For You

Good nutrition is important throughout your life!

It can help you feel your best and stay strong. It can help reduce the risk of some diseases that are common among older adults. And, if you already have certain health issues, good nutrition can help you manage the symptoms.

Nutrition can sometimes seem complicated. But the good news is that the U.S. Food and Drug Administration (FDA) has a simple tool to help you know exactly what you're eating.

It's called the Nutrition Facts Label. You will find it on all packaged foods and beverages. It serves as your guide for making choices that can affect your long-term health.

Good nutrition can help you avoid or manage these common diseases:

• Certain cancers

• High blood pressure

• Type 2 diabetes

• Obesity

• Heart disease

• Osteoporosis

At-a-Glance: The Nutrition Facts Label

Understanding what the Nutrition Facts Label includes can help you make food choices that are best for your health.

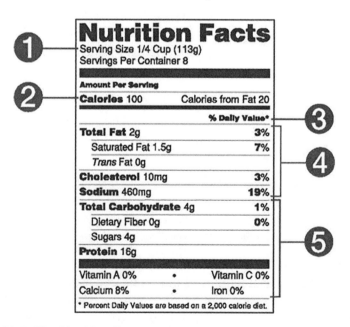

Figure 39.1. *The Nutrition Facts Label*

1. Serving Size

This section shows how many servings are in the package, and how big the serving is. Serving sizes are given in familiar measurements, such as "cups" or "pieces."

Remember: All of the nutrition information on the label is based upon one serving of the food. A package of food often contains more than one serving!

2. Amount of Calories

The calories listed are for one serving of the food. "Calories from fat" shows how many fat calories there are in one serving.

Remember—a product that's fat-free isn't necessarily calorie-free. Read the label!

3. Percent (%) Daily Value

This section tells you how the nutrients in one serving of the food contribute to your total daily diet. Use it to choose foods that are high in the nutrients you should get more of, and low in the nutrients you should get less of.

Daily Values are based on a 2,000-calorie diet. However, your nutritional needs will likely depend on how physically active you are. Talk to your healthcare provider to see what calorie level is right for you.

4. Limit these Nutrients

Eating too much total fat (especially saturated fat and trans fat), cholesterol, or sodium may increase your risk of certain chronic diseases, such as heart disease, some cancers, or high blood pressure.

Try to keep these nutrients as low as possible each day.

5. Get Enough of these Nutrients

Americans often don't get enough dietary fiber, vitamin A, vitamin C, calcium, and potassium in their diets. These nutrients are essential for keeping you feeling strong and healthy.

Eating enough of these nutrients may improve your health and help reduce the risk of some diseases.

Three Key Areas of Importance

As you use the Nutrition Facts Label, pay particular attention to serving size, percent daily value, and nutrients.

Serving Size

The top of the Nutrition Facts Label shows the serving size and the servings per container. Serving size is the key to the rest of the information on the Nutrition Facts Label.

- The nutrition information about the food—like the calories, sodium, and fiber—is based upon one serving.

- If you eat two servings of the food, you are eating double the calories and getting twice the amount of nutrients, both good and bad.

- If you eat three servings, that means three times the calories and nutrients—and so on.

That is why knowing the serving size is important. It's how you know for sure how many calories and nutrients you are getting.

Check Serving Size!

It is very common for a food package to contain more than one serving. One bottled soft drink or a small bag of chips can actually contain two or more serving.

Percent Daily Value (%DV)

The %DV is a general guide to help you link nutrients in one serving of food to their contribution to your total daily diet. It can help you determine if a food is high or low in a nutrient: five percent or less is low, 20 percent or more is high.

You can also use the %DV to make dietary trade-offs with other foods throughout the day.

%DV: Quick Tips

You can tell if a food is high or low in a particular nutrient by taking a quick look at the %DV.

- If it has five percent of the daily value or less, it is low in that nutrient.

This can be good or bad, depending on if it is a nutrient you want more of or less of.

- If it has 20 percent or more, it is high in that nutrient.

This can be good for nutrients like fiber (a nutrient to get more of) . . . but not so good for something like saturated fat (a nutrient to get less of).

Using %DV

- Once you are familiar with %DV, you can use it to compare foods and decide which is the better choice for you. Be sure to check for the particular nutrients you want more of or less of.

- Using %DV information can also help you "balance things out" for the day.

- For example: If you ate a favorite food at lunch that was high in sodium, a "nutrient to get less of," you would then try to choose foods for dinner that are lower in sodium.

Nutrients

A nutrient is an ingredient in a food that provides nourishment. Nutrients are essential for life and to keep your body functioning properly.

Nutrients to Get More Of

There are some nutrients that are especially important for your health. You should try to get adequate amounts of these each day. They are:

- Calcium

- Dietary fiber

- Potassium*

- Vitamin A

- Vitamin C

Note: The listing of potassium is optional on the Nutrition Facts Label.

Nutrients to Get Less Of

There are other nutrients that are important, but that you should eat in moderate amounts. They can increase your risk of certain diseases.

They are:

- Total fat (especially saturated fat)

- Cholesterol

- Sodium

Your Guide to a Healthy Diet

The Nutrition Facts Label can help you make choices for overall health. But some nutrients can also affect certain health conditions and diseases.

Use this section as a guide for those nutrients that could impact your own health. Each nutrient section discusses:

- What the nutrient is

- What it can mean for your health

- Label-reading tips

Watch for "nutrients to get less of" (the ones that you should try to limit), and "nutrients to get more of" (the ones that are very important to be sure to get enough of). You also might want to talk to your healthcare provider about which nutrients you should track closely for your continued health. And remember—the Nutrition Facts Label is a tool that is available to you on every packaged food and beverage!

Nutrients and Your Needs

On the following pages, you'll find specific information about certain nutrients.

Some are nutrients to get less of; others are nutrients to get more of. All of them can have an impact on your long-term health.

In addition, here is an example of how the Nutrition Facts Label can guide you in making good decisions for long-term health and nutrition.

Example

Heart disease is the number one cause of death in the United States. You can use the Nutrition Facts Label to compare foods and decide which ones fit with a diet that may help reduce the risk of heart disease. Choose foods that have fewer calories per serving and a lower percent DV of these "nutrients to get less of"

- Total fat

- Saturated fat

- Cholesterol

- Sodium

To lower your risk of heart disease, it is also recommended that you eat more fiber.

Dietary Salt/Sodium: Get Less Of
What It Is

Salt is a crystal-like compound that is used to flavor and preserve food. The words "salt" and "sodium" are often used interchangeably. Salt is listed as "sodium" on the Nutrition Facts Label.

What You Should Know

A small amount of sodium is needed to help certain organs and fluids work properly. But most people eat too much of it—and they may not even know it! That's because many packaged foods have a high amount of sodium, even when they don't taste "salty." Plus, when you add salt to food, you're adding more sodium.

Sodium has been linked to high blood pressure. In fact, eating less sodium can often help lower blood pressure, which in turn can help reduce the risk of heart disease.

And since blood pressure normally rises with age, limiting your sodium intake becomes even more important each year.

Label Reading Tips: Salt / Sodium

- Read the label to see how much sodium is in the food you are choosing.

  - 5 percent DV or less is low in sodium

  - 20 percent DV or more is high in sodium

- When you are deciding between two foods, compare the amount of sodium. Look for cereals, crackers, pasta sauces, canned vegetables, and other packaged foods that are lower in sodium.

Fiber: Get More Of
What It Is

Fiber, or "dietary fiber," is sometimes called "roughage." It's the part of food that can't be broken down during digestion. So because it moves through your digestive system "undigested," it plays an important role in keeping your system moving and "in working order."

What You Should Know

Fiber is a "nutrient to get more of." In addition to aiding in digestion, fiber has a number of other health-related benefits. These benefits are especially effective when you have a high fiber diet that is also low in saturated fat, cholesterol, trans fat, added sugars, salt, and alcohol.

- Eating a diet that is low in saturated fat and cholesterol and high in fruits, vegetables, and grain products that contain some types of dietary fiber, particularly soluble fiber, may help lower your cholesterol and reduce your chances of getting heart disease, a disease associated with many factors.

- Healthful diets that are low in fat and rich in fruits and vegetables that contain fiber may reduce the risk of some types of cancer, including colon cancer, a disease associated with many factors. In addition, such healthful diets are also associated with a reduced risk of type 2 diabetes.

- Fiber also aids in the regularity of bowel movements and preventing constipation. It may help reduce the risk of diverticulosis, a common condition in which small pouches form in the colon wall. This condition often has few or no symptoms; people who already have diverticulosis and do have symptoms often find that increased fiber consumption can reduce these symptoms. It's also important to note that if the pouches caused by diverticulosis rupture and become infected, it results in the more severe condition of diverticulitis.

Soluble versus Insoluble Fiber: Where to Get It, and What It Does

Fiber comes in two forms—insoluble and soluble. Most plant foods contain some of each kind.

- **Insoluble fiber** is mostly found in whole-grain products, such as wheat bran cereal, vegetables, and fruit. It provides "bulk" for stool formation and helps wastes move quickly through your colon.

- **Soluble fiber** is found in peas, beans, many vegetables and fruits, oat bran, whole grains, barley, cereals, seeds, rice, and some pasta, crackers, and other bakery products. It slows the digestion of carbohydrates, and can help stabilize blood sugar if you have diabetes. In addition, it helps lower "bad cholesterol." This, in turn, reduces the risk of heart disease.

Check the Nutrition Facts Label to see which foods have a higher %DV of fiber.

Label Reading Tips: Fiber

- **Read food labels.** The Nutrition Facts Label tells you the amount of dietary fiber in each serving, as well as the %DV of fiber that food contains.

When comparing the amount of fiber in food, remember:

- 5 percent DV or less is low in fiber

- 20 percent DV or more is high in fiber

The label won't indicate whether fiber is "insoluble" or "soluble," so it's best to try to get some of both.

- **Compare foods and choose the ones with higher fiber.** Look for and compare labels on whole-grain products such as bulgur, brown rice, whole wheat couscous or kasha and whole-grain breads, cereals, and pasta. In addition, compare different styles/types of canned or frozen beans and fruit.

Total Fat: Get Less Of
What It Is

Fat, or "dietary fat," is a nutrient that is a major source of energy for the body. It also helps you absorb certain important vitamins. As a food ingredient, fat provides taste, consistency, and helps you feel full.

What You Should Know

Eating too much fat can lead to a wide range of health challenges. The total amount and type of fat can contribute to and/or increase the risk of:

- Heart disease
- High cholesterol
- Increased risk of many cancers (including colon-rectum cancer)
- Obesity
- High blood pressure
- Type 2 diabetes

It is important to know that there are different types of dietary fat. Some have health benefits when eaten in small quantities, but others do not.

"Good" Fat: unsaturated fats (monounsaturated and poly-unsaturated)

- These are healthful if eaten in moderation. In fact, small amounts can even help lower cholesterol levels!
- Best Sources: Plant-based oils (sunflower, corn, soybean, cottonseed, and safflower), olive, canola and peanut oils, nuts, and soft margarines (liquid, tub or spray).

"Undesirable" Fat: saturated and trans fats. These can raise cholesterol levels in the blood, which in turn can contribute to heart disease.

- Common Sources: Meat, poultry, fish, butter, ice cream, cheese, coconut and palm kernel oils, solid shortenings, and hard margarines.
- Meat (including chicken and turkey) and fish supply protein, B vitamins, and iron. When selecting and preparing meat, poultry, fish, and milk or milk products, choose those that are lean, low-fat, or fat-free. Doing this, along with removing the skin from fish and poultry, are good strategies for limiting "undesirable" fat from your diet. In addition, dry beans, which can be used as a meat substitute, are a good source of protein and are nonfat.

Understanding Trans Fat

Trans fat is one of the newest additions to the Nutrition Facts Label, so you may be hearing more about it. Here's what you need to know:

- Most trans fat is made when manufacturers "hydrogenize" liquid oils, turning them into solid fats, like shortening or some margarines. Trans fat is commonly found in crackers, cookies, snack foods, and other foods made with or fried in these solid oils.

- Trans fat, like saturated fat and cholesterol, raises your LDL (bad) cholesterol and can increase your risk of coronary heart disease.

Trans Fat on the Label

There is no recommended total daily value for trans fat, so you won't find the %DV of trans fat on a food's Nutrition Facts Label. However, you can still use the label to see if a food contains trans fat and to compare two foods by checking to see if grams of trans fat are listed. If there is anything other than 0 grams listed, then the food contains trans fat. Because it is extremely difficult to eat a diet that is completely trans fat-free without decreasing other nutrient intakes, just aim to keep your intake of trans fat as low as possible.

Label Reading Tips: Total Fat

- When comparing foods, check the Nutrition Facts Label and choose the food with the lower %DV of total fat and saturated fat, and low or no grams of trans fat.

  - 5%DV or less of total fat is low

  - 20%DV or more of total fat is high

- When choosing foods that are labeled "fat-free" and "low-fat," be aware that fat-free doesn't mean calorie-free. Sometimes, to make a food tastier, extra sugars are added, which adds extra calories. Be sure to check the calories per serving.

Cholesterol: Get Less Of
What It Is

Cholesterol is a crystal-like substance carried through the blood-stream by lipoproteins—the "transporters" of fat. Cholesterol is required for certain important body functions, like digesting dietary fats, making hormones, and building cell walls.

Cholesterol is found in animal-based foods, like meats and dairy products.

What You Should Know

Too much cholesterol in the bloodstream can damage arteries, especially the ones that supply blood to the heart. It can build up in blood vessel linings. This is called "atherosclerosis," and it can lead to heart attacks and stroke.

However, it's important to know that not all cholesterol is bad. There are two kinds of cholesterol found in the bloodstream. How much you have of each is what determines your risk of heart disease.

High-density lipoprotein (HDL): This "good" cholesterol is the form in which cholesterol travels back to the liver, where it can be eliminated.

- HDL helps prevent cholesterol buildup in blood vessels. A higher level of this cholesterol is better. Low HDL levels increase heart disease risk. Discuss your HDL level with your healthcare provider.

Low-density lipoprotein (LDL): This "bad" cholesterol is carried into the blood. It is the main cause of harmful fatty buildup in arteries.

- The higher the LDL cholesterol level in the blood, the greater the heart disease risk. So, a lower level of this cholesterol is better.

Label Reading Tips: Cholesterol

- Cholesterol is a "nutrient to get less of." When comparing foods, look at the Nutrition Facts Label, and choose the food with the lower %DV of cholesterol. Be sure not to go above 100 percent DV for the day.
  - 5%DV or less of cholesterol is low
  - 20%DV or more of cholesterol is high
- One of the primary ways LDL ("bad") cholesterol levels can become too high in the blood is by eating too much saturated fat and cholesterol. Saturated fat raises LDL levels more than anything else in the diet.

Calcium: Get More Of
What It Is

Calcium is a mineral that has a lot of uses in the body, but it is best known for its role in building healthy bones and teeth.

What You Should Know

Lack of calcium causes osteoporosis, which is the primary cause of hip fractures. In fact, the word "osteoporosis" means "porous bones." It causes progressive bone loss as you age, and makes bones fragile—so that they can break easily. It's extremely important (especially for women) to get enough calcium throughout your life, especially after menopause. Women are at much higher risk for osteoporosis, but men can get it too.

It's true that many dairy products, which contain high levels of calcium, are relatively high in fat and calories. But keep in mind that fat-free or low-fat types of milk products are excellent calcium sources. Nutritionists recommend that you try to get most of your calcium from calcium-rich foods, rather than from calcium supplements. The Nutrition Facts Label can help you make good high-calcium choices.

Other good sources of calcium are:

- Canned salmon (with bones, which are edible)

- Calcium-fortified soy beverages

- Tofu (soybean curd that is "calcium-processed")

- Certain vegetables (for example, dark leafy greens such as collards and turnip greens)

- Legumes (black-eyed peas and white beans)

- Calcium-fortified grain products

- Calcium-fortified juice

Label Reading: Tips Calcium

- Read the label to see how much calcium is in the food you are choosing.

  - 5%DV or less is low in calcium

  - 20%DV or more is high in calcium

- Select foods that are high in calcium as often as possible.

Section 39.5

Stem Cells Build Bone

This section includes text excerpted from "New Method
Builds Bone," National Institutes of Health (NIH),
February 13, 2012. Reviewed January 2019.

Researchers have developed a way to direct the body's own stem cells to the outer bone to build new, strong bone tissue. The method, developed in mice, may lead to new treatments for osteoporosis and other bone diseases that affect millions of people.

Bones are made of a mineral and protein scaffold filled with bone cells. Bone tissues continually break down and build back up again. When the rate of bone loss outpaces the rate of bone tissue replacement, bones weaken, eventually leading to osteoporosis. This is common in people as they age.

Osteoblasts, the cells that rebuild bone, are derived from mesenchymal stem cells. These stem cells are found in bone marrow, deep inside the bone. They transform into osteoblasts and migrate to the outer bone, where they create new bone tissue.

As we age, we lose mesenchymal stem cells, so bone tissue building slows down. A team of researchers led by Dr. Wei Yao of the University of California, Davis sought to build new bone tissue by directing mesenchymal stem cells to outer bone more quickly. Their work was funded by several National Institutes of Health (NIH) components, including the National Institute of Arthritis and Musculoskeletal and Skin Diseases (NIAMS), *Eunice Kennedy Shriver* National Institute of Child Health and Human Development (NICHD) and National Institute on Aging (NIA). The results appeared in the online edition of *Nature Medicine* on February 5, 2012.

Mesenchymal stem cells express a surface protein called α4β1 integrin as they turn into osteoblasts. This protein helps them stick to bone and tissue surfaces. The scientists reasoned that a linker binding to both the α4β1 integrins and the outer bone surface would encourage the cells to stick to the outer bone.

The researchers created a hybrid compound from 2 molecules: LLP2A, a protein-like molecule that sticks to α4β1 integrins, and alendronate, an osteoporosis drug that sticks to the outer surface of bones. They called the compound LLP2A-Ale.

After 4 weeks of treatment with LLP2A-Ale, the bones of healthy mice were stronger and had more bone tissue than those of mice treated with alendronate alone or saline. In mice with weakened bone, the compound prevented further bone loss. Because mice, like humans, lose bone as they age, the scientists also treated older mice with LLP2A-Ale. The compound increased bone tissue in the older mice and prevented age-related bone loss.

The rate of bone loss can rise steeply in women after menopause. This is because levels of estrogen, a hormone important for maintaining bone health, begin to drop. To see if LLP2A-Ale could reverse bone loss when estrogen is low, the researchers infused estrogen-deficient female mice with LLP2A-Ale or parathyroid hormone, a molecule that increases bone formation. They found that LLP2A-Ale was as effective as parathyroid hormone at increasing the rate of bone formation.

"For the first time, we may have potentially found a way to direct a person's own stem cells to the bone surface where they can regenerate bone," says co-investigator Dr. Nancy Lane of UC Davis. "This technique could become a revolutionary new therapy for osteoporosis as well as for other conditions that require new bone formation."

Chapter 40

Blood Pressure Drug Improves Bone Health

People with hypertension, or high blood pressure, often have more osteoporotic fractures than those without. A study by a team including a U.S. Department of Veterans Affairs (VA) investigator found that one of the drugs frequently given to combat high blood pressure, chlorthalidone, may also improve bone strength and reduce the risk of osteoporotic fractures.

Past research had suggested that thiazide-type diuretics improve bone strength, but no studies had compared them to other blood pressure treatments. The study, a follow-up analysis of data from a large trial a few years ago, links chlorthalidone, a thiazide-like diuretic, to a lower risk of hip or pelvic fractures, compared with two other hypertension drugs, amlodipine and lisinopril.

In fact, say the researchers, it's likely that chlorthalidone actually improves bone health, in addition to another major side benefit—cardiovascular protection. Whether or not the other classes of hypertension drugs help or hurt bones is less clear. The new results could help clinicians decide which blood pressure treatment to recommend for certain patients.

The findings appeared in January 2017 in *JAMA Internal Medicine*.

This chapter includes text excerpted from "Blood Pressure Drug Found to Be Better for Bones, versus Other Treatments," U.S. Department of Veterans Affairs (VA), February 28, 2017.

Chlorthalidone Use Leads to 21 Percent Lower Fracture Risk

The study looked at three kinds of commonly prescribed hypertension medications for their effects on hip and pelvic fractures, using data from the Antihypertensive and Lipid Lowering Treatment to Prevent Heart Attack Trial (ALLHAT). The researchers focused on hip and pelvic fractures because these events almost always result in hospitalization.

Chlorthalidone is a thiazide-type diuretic, or water pill. It is sold as Hygroton. Diuretics are an older form of hypertension medication, and they are often less expensive than newer classes of drugs. They work by increasing the amount of water and salt expelled from the body as urine. Their use has been declining in favor of newer drugs.

The other two medications in the comparison were amlodipine (sold as Norvasc), a calcium channel blocker; and lisinopril (sold as Zestril), an angiotensin-converting enzyme (ACE) inhibitor.

Chlorthalidone was associated with a 21 percent lower risk of hip and pelvic fractures, compared with the other two drugs. Over five years of follow-up after ALLHAT, fracture risk continued to be lower in chlorthalidone users. The researchers say this suggests that thiazide-type diuretics have lasting effects on bone strength.

The researchers think that thiazide diuretics such as chlorthalidone may help bones because of a positive effect on the body's calcium balance. They may also directly stimulate osteoblasts, the cells that make new bone.

The results line up with other research findings. An analysis by University of Texas researchers of previous studies showed that thiazide-type diuretics were associated with a 24 percent lower risk of hip fracture, compared with other hypertension drugs.

Antihypertensive and Lipid Lowering Treatment to Prevent Heart Attack Trial

The fracture study used data from a larger study on hypertension and cardiovascular disease, known as ALLHAT. Conducted between 1994 and 2002, and sponsored by the National Institutes of Health (NIH), it was the largest clinical trial ever conducted to compare hypertension drugs. ALLHAT enrolled more than 42,000 participants, including more than 7,000 veterans at 70 VA medical centers. One of the researchers leading ALLHAT, Dr. William Cushman of the

Memphis (Tennessee) VA Medical Center, is an author on the new fracture analysis.

Among other results, ALLHAT showed that chlorthalidone was better than amlodipine, lisinopril, and doxazosin mesylate (an alpha-adrenergic blocker) at preventing cardiovascular disease. All four drugs tested had been previously shown to reduce high blood pressure. However, in ALLHAT diuretics were shown to be superior in both treating high blood pressure and preventing cardiovascular events.

Doxazosin testing was stopped early in ALLHAT, so it was not considered for the fracture study.

The main results from ALLHAT appeared in 2002 in the *Journal of the American Medical Association*.

One of the main conclusions of ALLHAT was that thiazide-type diuretics should be the drugs of choice for initial hypertension treatment in most patients, because of their low cost and cardiovascular benefits. The new findings on bone health should provide further support for their use, especially for patients at higher risk of fractures.

Chapter 41

Menopause and Bone Health

Menopause is when your periods stop permanently and you can no longer get pregnant. You have reached menopause only after it has been a full year since your last period. This means you have not had any bleeding, including spotting, for 12 months in a row. Menopause happens when you have gone 12 months in a row without a period. The average age of menopause in the United States is 52. The range for women is usually between 45 and 58. One way to tell when you might go through menopause is the age your mother went through it. After menopause your ovaries make very low levels of the hormones estrogen and progesterone. These low hormone levels can raise your risk for certain health problems.*

* *Excerpted from "Menopause," Office on Women's Health (OWH), U.S. Department of Health and Human Services (HHS), May 22, 2018.*

During the menopause transition, women may notice troublesome symptoms like hot flashes or trouble sleeping. Risk for heart disease and osteoporosis increase during this time, as well.

Here are few tips for a healthy transition:

- Staying healthy and attending to bothersome symptoms can help ease the menopause transition.

This chapter includes text excerpted from "Menopause: Tips for a Healthy Transition," National Institute on Aging (NIA), National Institutes of Health (NIH), July 3, 2017.

- It is also important to manage the increased risk of heart disease and osteoporosis that comes with menopause.
- Take care to:
  - Quit smoking and using tobacco products, if you currently do.
  - Eat a healthy diet, low in fat, high in fiber, with plenty of fruits, vegetables, and whole-grain foods.
  - Get enough calcium and vitamin D.
  - Learn what your healthy weight is, and try to stay there.
  - Do weight-bearing exercise, such as climbing stairs or dancing, at least three days each week for healthy bones. Try to be physically active in other ways for your general healthy, too.

Menopause is not a disease that has to be treated. But it is a good idea to talk to your doctor about staying healthy and things you can do if symptoms like hot flashes bother you.

Part Five

Diagnosis and Treatment of Osteoporosis

Chapter 42

How to Find a Doctor

For many people, finding a doctor who is knowledgeable about osteoporosis can be difficult. There is no physician specialty dedicated solely to osteoporosis, nor is there a certification program for health professionals who treat the disease. A variety of medical specialists treat people with osteoporosis, including internists, gynecologists, family doctors, endocrinologists, rheumatologists, physiatrists, orthopedists, and geriatricians.

There are a number of ways to find a doctor who treats osteoporosis patients. If you have a primary-care or family doctor, discuss your concerns with her or him. Your doctor may treat the disease or be able to refer you to an osteoporosis specialist.

If you are enrolled in a health maintenance organization (HMO) or a managed-care health plan, consult your assigned doctor about osteoporosis. This doctor should be able to give you an appropriate referral.

If you do not have a personal doctor or if your doctor cannot help, contact your nearest university hospital or academic health center and ask for the department that cares for patients with osteoporosis. The department will vary from institution to institution. For example, in some facilities, the department of endocrinology or metabolic bone disease treats osteoporosis patients. In other medical centers, the appropriate department may be rheumatology, orthopedics, or

This chapter includes text excerpted from "For People with Osteoporosis: How to Find a Doctor," NIH Osteoporosis and Related Bone Diseases—National Resource Center (NIH ORBD—NRC), April 2015. Reviewed January 2019.

gynecology. Some hospitals have a separate osteoporosis program or women's clinic that treats patients with osteoporosis.

Once you have identified a doctor, you may wish to ask whether the doctor has specialized training in osteoporosis, how much of the practice is dedicated to osteoporosis, and whether she or he uses bone mass measurement.

Your own primary care doctor—whether an internist, orthopedist, or gynecologist—is often the best person to treat you because she or he knows your medical history, your lifestyle, and your special needs.

Medical Specialists Who Treat Osteoporosis

After an initial assessment, it may be necessary to see an endocrinologist, a rheumatologist, or another specialist to rule out the possibility of an underlying disease that may contribute to osteoporosis:

- **Endocrinologists** treat the endocrine system, which comprises the glands and hormones that help control the body's metabolic activity. In addition to osteoporosis, endocrinologists treat diabetes and diseases of the thyroid and pituitary glands.

- **Rheumatologists** diagnose and treat diseases of the bones, joints, muscles, and tendons, including arthritis and collagen diseases.

- **Family doctors** have a broad range of training that includes internal medicine, gynecology, and pediatrics. They place special emphasis on caring for an individual or family on a long-term, continuing basis.

- **Geriatricians** are family doctors or internists who have received additional training on the aging process and the conditions and diseases that often occur among the elderly, including incontinence, falls, and dementia. Geriatricians often care for patients in nursing homes, in patients' homes, or in office or hospital settings.

- **Gynecologists** diagnose and treat conditions of the female reproductive system and associated disorders. They often serve as primary care doctors for women and follow their patients' reproductive health over time.

- **Internists** are trained in general internal medicine. They diagnose and treat many diseases. Internists provide long-term comprehensive care in the hospital and office, have expertise in many areas, and often act as consultants to other specialists.

- **Orthopedic surgeons** are doctors trained in the care of patients with musculoskeletal conditions, such as congenital skeletal malformations, bone fractures and infections, and metabolic problems.

- **Physiatrists** are doctors who specialize in physical medicine and rehabilitation. They evaluate and treat patients with impairments, disabilities, or pain arising from various medical problems, including bone fractures. Physiatrists focus on restoring the physical, psychological, social, and vocational functioning of the individual.

Chapter 43

Talking to Your Orthopedist

People with osteogenesis imperfecta (OI) usually require the services of a healthcare team that includes several specialists, along with a primary care physician. The orthopedist (a doctor who specializes in bone and joint disorders) treats fractures and recommends surgical interventions such as rodding surgery. The orthopedist plays an important role in the lives of children and adults who have OI. Some orthopedists are members of a team of specialists at an OI clinic that may also include a geneticist, an endocrinologist, a nephrologist, a neurologist, a physical therapist, an occupational therapist, and a nutritionist. In some private offices and OI clinics, a nurse or nurse practitioner is available to answer questions about cast care and orthopedic surgery.

General Principles for Good Communication

- Keep detailed medical records. Include lists of fractures, how they occurred, and how they were treated as well as information on all surgeries.

- Keep a brief summary of key points in the medical history. Include surgeries, complications, allergies, and a list of any rods, pins, or other implanted devices.

This chapter includes text excerpted from "Talking to Your Orthopaedist: A Guide for People with OI," NIH Osteoporosis and Related Bone Diseases—National Resource Center (NIH ORBD—NRC), May 2015. Reviewed January 2019.

- Find a surgeon who is knowledgeable about OI and has experience doing procedures for OI patients, or who is willing to consult with surgeons who have OI experience before doing a procedure.

- Find and meet with a new orthopedist before having a fracture or other emergency to establish a relationship and ask some general questions.

- Find a doctor who treats you with respect, listens to you, and is interested in the information about OI that you provide.

- Plan ahead for emergencies. Learn how to contact the doctor, where to go for X-rays, what to do on a weekend or holiday, and which hospital to go to. If the doctor is part of a group, find out if other members are experienced in OI as well.

- When you answer your doctor's questions, do not exaggerate, deny, or deliberately omit information.

- Be an attentive listener.

Prepare for the Appointment

- Make a list of symptoms and the events leading up to the injury.

- Be specific about the date, time, and location of the injury and the type of pain.

- Prepare a list of questions. Be ready to ask the most important question first.

- Bring paper and pencil to write down the doctor's answers.

- When possible, bring copies of previous X-rays that show the baseline status of the bone(s) in question.

- Bring a list of all drugs, vitamins, minerals, other nutritional supplements, over-the-counter (OTC) medicines, and alternative treatments you are taking. Include information about dose, reason for taking, and how long you have been on the medication.

The following list of questions is not a script. It is a list of ideas to help you have a productive conversation with your doctor. Review this list before your appointment, and select the questions that are important to you. Be sure to listen carefully during your appointment. Your doctor may answer many of these questions before you ask them.

General questions:

- What should I do if I suspect a fracture during office hours? What about on a weekend or holiday?

- What does it mean if no fracture shows up on the X-ray? Is the resolution high enough to show microfractures?

- What is the prognosis? (What can I expect might happen next?)

- Do some medications interfere with fracture healing?

- Will any of the medicines I am taking interfere with fracture healing?

- What are my treatment options?

When tests, medications, or other treatments are prescribed:

- What is the exact name of the test, drug, or treatment?

- Will my size influence the drug dose you prescribe?

- What are the costs, risks, and benefits?

- Are there any alternatives?

- What will happen to me if I don't have the treatment?

- Will this treatment affect my bone mineral density?

When surgery is recommended:

- What are the success rates for this surgery?

- What complications are possible? How often do they happen?

- How many times have you performed this operation?

- Am I a good candidate for surgery?

- How long can I wait before having this surgery?

- Should I stop taking any of my medications before surgery? How long before?

- Is the procedure done on an inpatient or outpatient basis?

- Exactly what will occur during the surgery?

- How long will the operation take?

- Is the anesthesiologist familiar with OI?

- How long will I have to stay in the hospital after the operation?

- Will the nursing staff know how to treat me? Have they ever cared for a person with OI before?

- What kind of special nursing care will I need at home?

- What will I need to take care of myself at home?

- How long will I be out of work or out of school?

- Will I need a wheelchair or other equipment while I recover?

- Will follow-up care with a physical or occupational therapist be needed?

When rodding surgery is recommended:

- What types of rods are available?

- Which one do you recommend, and why?

- What complications are possible?

- If I have been taking bisphosphonates, how long before and after surgery should I discontinue them?

When spine surgery is recommended:

- What can I do to prepare for this operation?

- What will you be doing to my spine?

- Will my spine be fused?

- If so, where will it be fused?

- Will this affect growth (if the patient is a growing child)?

- How will a fused spine affect my activities of daily living? Will I become less mobile or less able to transfer between sitting, standing, and prone positions?

- What types of rods and other instruments will be used? Will they prevent me from having an MRI (magnetic resonance imaging) in the future?

- Will this require a bone graft?

- Is there a chance my bone is too soft to use instruments? What will be done if this is the case?

- How much of the curve in my spine will the surgery be able to correct?

- Will I continue to be at risk for new compression fractures of the spine after the surgery?

- What risks are involved with this surgery? Is there a risk of paralysis?

- How long will the surgery take?

- How long will I be hospitalized after the surgery?

- How long will I need bed rest after the surgery?

- Will I need to wear a brace after surgery? For how long?

- When will I be able to return to sitting up? To walking?

- Do I need formal physical therapy? When would it start?

- Is there a risk that the rods or other instruments might break?

- How long will it take for the fusion to heal fully?

- Will I need to avoid bending, twisting, or exercising immediately after surgery? If so, for how long?

- Will I need modifications to any equipment, such as my wheelchair or bed?

When a cast, splint, or bandage is applied:

- What types of casts are available?

- Which type of cast do you recommend, and why?

- Can this get wet? Can I swim with it on?

- Will my knee, ankle, elbow, or another joint be immobilized?

- How long will the cast, splint, or Ace bandage stay on?

- What do I need to look out for while I am in the cast (i.e., changes in skin color, odors, skin sores, temperature of fingers or toes)?

- Will there be a second cast or something else to protect the bone during the healing process?

- Who can teach me how to take care of the cast and my skin?

- What will I need to take care of myself at home? Do I need to rent any equipment?

- How much weight can I put on the leg? What can I lift with my arm?

- Do I need crutches, a cane, or a wheelchair?

- How much activity can I do? When can I resume weight-bearing activity?

Other situations:

- What options are available to treat a nonunion fracture (a broken bone that has failed to heal)?

- Would transcutaneous (through the skin) electrical nerve stimulation (TENS) therapy be helpful?

- Would braces, a temporary splint, or other orthotics be helpful?

- Will the type of orthopedic rods, pins, or other implants in my body exclude me from having an MRI?

Pain management:

- What types of pain treatment are available?

- Which type do you recommend, and why?

- Will any pain medications interfere with healing?

- Can any of the pain medication you are prescribing be addictive?

Physical therapy and exercise:

- When can I resume weight-bearing activity?

- What type of physical therapy do I need to do to regain strength and function? How many times a week, how long a session, and how many sessions in total are needed?

- Do you keep in contact with the physical therapist?

- Does the therapist have experience working with a person with OI?

- If my insurance company won't cover physical therapy in a medical setting, can I go to a gym?

- When can I resume normal activities?

- What precautions should I take to prevent a second fracture?

Closing:

- How can I reach you if I have questions later today or tomorrow?
- When should I return for my next appointment?

Chapter 44

The Diagnosis of Osteoporosis

Diagnosing osteoporosis involves several steps, starting with a:

- Physical exam and a careful medical history

- General testing, such as blood tests and X-rays

- Bone mineral density testing

Physical Exam and Medical History

When recording information about your medical history, your doctor will ask questions to find out whether you have risk factors for osteoporosis and fractures. The doctor may ask about:

- Any previous fractures

- Your lifestyle (including diet, exercise habits, and whether you smoke)

This chapter contains text excerpted from the following sources: Text in this chapter begins with excerpts from "Osteoporosis," National Institute of Arthritis and Musculoskeletal and Skin Diseases (NIAMS), February 28, 2016; Text under the heading "Fracture Risk Assessment Tool (FRAX)" is excerpted from "FRAX-based Estimates of 10-year Probability of Hip and Major Osteoporotic Fracture Among Adults Aged 40 and Over: United States, 2013 and 2014," Centers for Disease Control and Prevention (CDC), March 28, 2017.

- Current or past health problems and medications that could contribute to low bone mass and increased fracture risk

- Your family history of osteoporosis and other diseases

- For women, your menstrual history

The doctor will also do a physical exam that should include checking for loss of height and changes in posture and may include checking your balance and gait (the way you walk).

General Testing

If you have back pain or have experienced a loss in height or a change in posture, the doctor may request an X-ray of your spine to look for spinal fractures or malformations caused by osteoporosis. However, X-rays cannot necessarily detect osteoporosis. The results of laboratory tests of blood and urine samples can help your doctor identify conditions that may be contributing to bone loss, such as hormonal problems or vitamin D deficiency. If the results of your physical exam, medical history, X-rays, or laboratory tests indicate that you may have osteoporosis or that you have significant risk factors for the disease, your doctor may recommend a bone density test.

Bone Mineral Density Testing

Mineral is what gives hardness to bones, and the density of mineral in the bones is an important determinant of bone strength. BMD testing can be used to:

- Definitively diagnose osteoporosis

- Detect low bone mass before osteoporosis develops

- Help predict your risk of future fractures

- Monitor the effectiveness of ongoing therapy

In general, the lower your bone density, the higher your risk for fracture. The results of a bone density test will help guide your doctor's decisions about starting therapy to prevent or treat osteoporosis.

The most widely recognized test for measuring bone mineral density is a quick, painless, noninvasive technology known as central dual-energy X-ray absorptiometry (DXA). This technique, which uses low levels of X-rays, involves passing a scanner over your body while you are lying on a cushioned table. DXA can be used to determine BMD of the entire skeleton and at various sites that are prone to fracture, such as the hip, spine, or wrist. Bone density measurement by DXA at the hip and spine is generally considered the most reliable way to diagnose osteoporosis and predict fracture risk.

Your doctor will compare your BMD test results to the average bone density of young, healthy people and to the average bone density of other people of your age, sex, and race. If you are diagnosed with osteoporosis or very low bone density, or if your bone density is below a certain level and you have other risk factors for fractures, the doctor will talk with you about options for treatment or prevention of osteoporosis.

Fracture Risk Assessment Tool (FRAX)

Fractures due to osteoporosis are a serious concern in the United States due to their economic burden as well as their negative impact on health and well-being. Osteoporosis is currently defined on the basis of bone mineral density (BMD) because BMD is a strong predictor of future fracture. However, many fractures occur in persons with BMD values that fall above the osteoporosis threshold. Thus, measuring BMD only partially identifies the population segment who are at risk of fracture.

To address this discrepancy, researchers at the World Health Organization (WHO) Collaborating Centre at Sheffield, United Kingdom, in the early 2000s developed a more global evaluation of fracture risk than that based on BMD alone. As part of the effort, a number of clinical risk factors that predict fracture independently of BMD (e.g., lifestyle and health history risk factors easily assessed in primary care settings) were identified and validated using data from a large number of international, prospective population-based cohorts. An algorithm, called FRAX, was then developed to integrate these risk factors with mortality data to estimate the 10-year absolute probability of hip and major osteoporotic (clinical spine, forearm, hip, or humerus) fracture among adults aged 40 and over. Risk factors used in the algorithm include age, sex, femur neck BMD, body mass index (BMI), prior fragility fracture, parental history of hip fracture, glucocorticoid use, rheumatoid arthritis, current smoking, excess alcohol consumption, and secondary osteoporosis. Separate FRAX algorithms have been developed for different countries using country-specific fracture and mortality data. The U.S. Food and Drug Administration has approved incorporating the FRAX algorithm into dual energy X-ray absorptiometry (DXA) systems so that FRAX estimates can be provided in addition to BMD results when DXA scans are performed. FRAX-based 10-year fracture probability estimates are currently used in many national and international osteoporosis guidelines, including several guidelines used in the United States (9–12). One of these U.S. guidelines, developed by the National Osteoporosis Foundation on the basis of a cost-effective analysis, includes criteria to define elevated fracture probabilities applicable to U.S. adults aged 50 and over.

Although FRAX-based estimates of 10-year fracture probabilities, or FRAX scores, are widely used in the United States, the distribution of these fracture probability scores among the adult U.S. population has not been previously described. This report provides detailed information about the FRAX score distribution for U.S. adults aged 40 and over using data from the National Health and Nutrition Examination Survey (NHANES) conducted in 2013 and 2014. Information on the prevalence of the risk factors used in the FRAX algorithm among adults aged 40 and over, and the prevalence of elevated FRAX scores among adults aged 50 and over, are also provided.

Chapter 45

Strong Recommendation for Bone Density Testing

What Is a Bone Density Test?

A bone mineral density (BMD) test can provide a snapshot of your bone health. The test can identify osteoporosis, determine your risk for fractures (broken bones), and measure your response to osteoporosis treatment. The most widely recognized BMD test is called a central dual-energy X-ray absorptiometry, or central dual-energy X-ray absorptiometry (DXA) test. It is painless—a bit like having an X-ray.

Peripheral bone density tests measure bone density in the lower arm, wrist, finger, or heel. These tests are often used for screening purposes and can help identify people who might benefit from additional bone density testing.

What Does the Test Do?

A BMD test measures your bone mineral density and compares it to that of an established norm or standard to give you a score. Although no bone density test is 100 percent accurate, the BMD test is an important predictor of whether a person will have a fracture in the future.

This chapter includes text excerpted from "Bone Mass Measurement: What the Numbers Mean," NIH Osteoporosis and Related Bone Diseases—National Resource Center (NIH ORBD—NRC), June 2015. Reviewed January 2019.

The T-Score

Most commonly, your BMD test results are compared to the ideal or peak bone mineral density of a healthy 30-year-old adult, and you are given a T-score. A score of 0 means your BMD is equal to the norm for a healthy young adult. Differences between your BMD and that of the healthy young adult norm are measured in units called standard deviations (SDs). The more standard deviations below 0, indicated as negative (−) numbers, the lower your BMD and the higher your risk of fracture.

As shown in the table below, a T-score between +1 and −1 is considered normal or healthy. A T-score between −1 and −2.5 indicates that you have low bone mass, although not low enough to be diagnosed with osteoporosis. A T-score of −2.5 or lower indicates that you have osteoporosis. The greater the negative number, the more severe the osteoporosis.

Table 45.1. T-Score for Bone Mineral Density

Level	Definition
Normal	Bone density is within 1 SD (+1 or −1) of the young adult mean.
Low bone mass	Bone density is between 1 and 2.5 SD below the young adult mean (−1 to −2.5 SD).
Osteoporosis	Bone density is 2.5 SD or more below the young adult mean (−2.5 SD or lower).
Severe (established) osteoporosis	Bone density is more than 2.5 SD below the young adult mean, and there have been one or more osteoporotic fractures.

World Health Organization (WHO) definitions based on bone density levels.

Low Bone Mass versus Osteoporosis

The information provided by a BMD test can help your doctor decide which prevention or treatment options are right for you.

If you have low bone mass that is not low enough to be diagnosed as osteoporosis, this is sometimes referred to as osteopenia. Low bone mass can be caused by many factors such as:

- Heredity

- The development of less-than-optimal peak bone mass in your youth

- A medical condition or medication to treat such a condition that negatively affects bone

- Abnormally accelerated bone loss

Although not everyone who has low bone mass will develop osteoporosis, everyone with low bone mass is at higher risk for the disease and the resulting fractures.

As a person with low bone mass, you can take steps to help slow down your bone loss and prevent osteoporosis in your future. Your doctor will want you to develop—or keep—healthy habits such as eating foods rich in calcium and vitamin D and doing weight-bearing exercise such as walking, jogging, or dancing. In some cases, your doctor may recommend medication to prevent osteoporosis.

Osteoporosis: If you are diagnosed with osteoporosis, these healthy habits will help, but your doctor will probably also recommend that you take medication. Several effective medications are available to slow—or even reverse—bone loss. If you do take medication to treat osteoporosis, your doctor can advise you concerning the need for future BMD tests to check your progress.

Who Should Get a Bone Density Test?

The U.S. Preventive Services Task Force (USPSTF) recommends that all women over age 65 should have a bone density test. Women who are younger than age 65 and at high risk for fractures should also have a bone density test.

Due to a lack of available evidence, the Task Force did not make recommendations regarding osteoporosis screening in men.

Various professional medical societies have established guidelines concerning when a person should get a BMD test. Many of these guidelines can be found by conducting a search in an online database established by the National Guideline Clearinghouse (NGC) at www. guideline.gov.

Chapter 46

Bone Scan and What to Expect

You are scheduled for a bone scan. It helps your doctor find out if there is a tumor, infection, or other abnormality in your bone. This scan is a safe, effective, and painless way to make pictures of your bones. For this scan, you will be given a compound containing a small amount of radioactivity. This compound is used only for diagnostic purposes. The scan is done in the Nuclear Medicine Department.

Preparation

There is no special preparation for this scan. You may eat and drink whatever you like.

Procedure

- In the morning, a small amount of the compound (radioisotope) will be given to you by vein. You may then return to your room.

This chapter contains text excerpted from the following sources: Text in this chapter begins with excerpts from "Procedures/Diagnostic Tests-Bone Scan," Clinical Center, National Institutes of Health (NIH), February 2001. Reviewed January 2019; Text under the heading "Dual Energy X-Ray Absorptiometry" is excerpted from "Radiology and Imaging Sciences," Clinical Center, National Institutes of Health (NIH), June 22, 2017.

- After the injection, try to drink extra glasses of water over the next few hours. This will help your body rid itself of the radioactivity.

- Please return to the diagnostic imaging section at the time scheduled for you by the appointment clerk: about 21/2 to 3 hours after the injection.

- Once you are in the imaging room, you will rest on a firm table with your head flat.

- During the scan, you will lie on your back.

- While you are in this position, a sensitive machine (called a "scanner") will record the radiation given off by the radioisotope. Lie very still. Many pictures will be taken as the scanner moves from your head to your toes. After the scan, more pictures will be taken of your head and hands. Stay very still while these pictures are being taken.

After the Procedure

There are no side effects, and the scan is painless. The only sensation you will feel will be the injection of the radioisotope in your vein.

If you have questions about the procedure, please ask. Your nurse and doctor are ready to assist you at all times.

Special Instructions

- Because it uses radioactivity, this scan is not performed in pregnant women. If you are pregnant or think you might be pregnant, please inform your doctor immediately so that a decision can be made about this scan.

- Also, please inform your doctor immediately if you are breastfeeding. Some scans can be performed on breastfeeding women if they are willing to stop breastfeeding for a while.

Dual Energy X-Ray Absorptiometry

DEXA stands for Dual Energy X-Ray Absorptiometry (or Densitometry). DEXA is a procedure that measures the amount of bone, muscle, and/or body fat.

The DEXA determination of bone density or body composition (muscle and fat composition) is performed with an instrument that uses low-energy X-rays. For bone density measurements, scans are typically performed of the lumbar (lower) spine, the hip, and the wrist. For body composition measurements, a scan of the entire body is performed. The DEXA instrument is very open, consisting of a table and scanning arm (in the shape of a 'C') that houses the X-ray tube on one end of the arm and the detector on the other end.

There is no specific patient preparation for these studies. However, please consider the following regarding patient eligibility for DEXA studies:

DEXA studies cannot be performed if the patient has had a nuclear medicine study within 1 week or an X-ray procedure using contrast within 72 hours. Therefore, DEXA studies should be scheduled before other X-ray or nuclear medicine procedures. If these other procedures are performed before the DEXA procedure and the time elapsed does not meet our protocol, the DEXA procedures will not be performed, and the study will be rescheduled.

A woman of child-bearing age must have pregnancy ruled out before undergoing the test.

Often, this means having a pregnancy test performed within 1 week of the DEXA procedure.

The length of time in the clinic will depend on the number of procedures that are performed. Usually, the appointment is for either 1/2 hour or 1 hour.

The patient should wear light clothing to the clinic so she/he can change into a surgical scrub uniform for the study. After changing into a scrub uniform, the patient will have weight and height measured. For such measurements and for scans, a patient will remove shoes. The individual scanning procedures are performed with the patient either lying on top of or sitting next to the scanning table.

For each scan, the technologist must perform two steps. The first step is the scan (scan acquisition); the second step is analysis of the scan (scan analysis) to determine the information contained within the scan. The DEXA scans are, therefore, more complicated than standard X-rays. The DEXA scan is performed to actually measure the amount of bone, muscle, or fat.

After the technologist has completed and satisfactorily analyzed the scans, the patient can change back into street clothes and leave the clinic.

All scans are reviewed by one of the Nuclear Medicine physicians. A report of the DEXA scan results will be entered into the hospital's computer and record system. This is usually done the same day as the scan.

Chapter 47

A Step-by-Step Approach to Osteoporosis Treatment

A comprehensive treatment program for osteoporosis includes:

- Proper nutrition

- Lifestyle changes

- Exercise

- Prevention of falls that may result in fractures

- Medications

- Alternative therapies

If you take medication to prevent or treat osteoporosis, it is still essential that you obtain the recommended amounts of calcium and vitamin D. Exercising and maintaining other aspects of a healthy lifestyle are also important.

For people with osteoporosis resulting from another condition, the best approach is to identify and treat the underlying cause. If you are taking a medication that causes bone loss, your doctor may be able to reduce the dose of that medication or switch you to another medication that is effective but not harmful to your bones. If you have a disease that

This chapter includes text excerpted from "Osteoporosis," National Institute of Arthritis and Musculoskeletal and Skin Diseases (NIAMS), February 28, 2016.

requires long-term glucocorticoid therapy, such as rheumatoid arthritis or lupus, you can also take certain medications approved for the prevention or treatment of osteoporosis associated with aging or menopause.

Nutrition

A healthy, balanced diet that includes:

- Plenty of fruits and vegetables

- Enough calories

- Adequate calcium, vitamin D, and vitamin K is essential for minimizing bone loss and maintaining overall health. Calcium and vitamin D are especially important for bone health.

Calcium

Calcium is the most important nutrient for preventing osteoporosis and for reaching peak bone mass. For healthy postmenopausal women who are not consuming enough calcium (1,200 mg per day) in their diet, calcium and vitamin D supplements help to preserve bone mass and prevent hip fracture. Calcium is also needed for the proper function of:

- The heart

- Muscles

- Nerves

- Blood clotting

We take in calcium from our diet and lose it from our body mainly through urine, feces, and sweat. The body depends on dietary calcium to build healthy new bone and avoid excessive loss of calcium from bone to meet other needs. The Institute of Medicine (IOM) of the National Academy of Sciences (NAS) recommends specific amounts of dietary calcium and vitamin D at various stages of life. Men and women up to age 50 need 1,000 milligrams of calcium per day, and the recommendation increases to 1,200 milligrams for women after age 50 and for men after age 70.

Many people in the United States consume much less than the recommended amount of calcium in their diets. Good sources of calcium include:

- Low-fat dairy products

- Dark green leafy vegetables, such as bok choy, collards, and turnip greens

- Broccoli

- Sardines and salmon with bones

- Soybeans, tofu, and other soy products

- Calcium-fortified foods such as orange juice, cereals, and breads

If you have trouble getting enough calcium in your diet, you may need to take a calcium supplement such as calcium carbonate, calcium phosphate, or calcium citrate. If you are between the ages of 19 and 50, your daily calcium intake should not exceed 2,500 milligrams because too much calcium can cause problems such as kidney stones. (After age 50, intakes should not exceed 2,000 milligrams per day.) Calcium coming from food sources provides better protection from kidney stones. Anyone who has had a kidney stone should increase their dietary calcium and decrease the amount from supplements as well as increase fluid intake.

Vitamin D

Vitamin D is required for proper absorption of calcium from the intestine. It is made in the skin after exposure to sunlight. Only a few foods naturally contain significant amounts of vitamin D, including fatty fish and fish oils. Foods fortified with vitamin D, such as milk and cereals, are a major dietary source of vitamin D. Although many people obtain enough vitamin D naturally, studies show that vitamin D production decreases in older adults, in people who are housebound, and during the winter—especially in northern latitudes.

If you are at risk for vitamin D deficiency, you can take multivitamins or calcium supplements that contain vitamin D to meet the recommended daily intake of 600 International Units (IU) for men and women up to the age of 70 and 800 IU for people over 70. Doses of more than 2,000 IU per day are not advised unless under the supervision of a doctor. Larger doses can be given initially to people who are deficient as a way to replenish stores of vitamin D.

Table 47.1. Recommended Calcium and Vitamin D Intakes

Life-Stage Group	Calcium (Mg/Day)	Vitamin D (IU/Day)
Infants 0 to 6 months	200	400
Infants 6 to 12 months	260	400
1 to 3 years old	700	600
4 to 8 years old	1,000	600
9 to 13 years old	1,300	600
14 to 18 years old	1,300	600
19 to 30 years old	1,000	600
31 to 50 years old	1,000	600
51 to 70 years old males	1,000	600
51 to 70 years old females	1,200	600
>70 years old	1,200	800
14 to 18 years old, pregnant/ lactating	1,300	600
19 to 50 years old, pregnant/ lactating	1,000	600

Definitions: mg = milligrams; IU = International Units
(Source: Food and Nutrition Board (FNB), Institute of Medicine (IOM), National Academy of Sciences (NAS), 2010.)

Lifestyle

In addition to a healthy diet, a healthy lifestyle is important for optimizing bone health. You should:

- Avoid smoking and second-hand smoke

- Drink alcohol in moderation (no more than one drink per day is a good general guideline)

- Talk to your doctor about medications you are taking. Some prescription medications can cause bone loss or increase your risk of falling and breaking a bone.

Exercise

Exercise is an important part of an osteoporosis treatment program. The evidence suggests that the most beneficial physical activities for bone health include strength training or resistance training. Physical activity can:

- Build and maintain bone throughout adulthood

- Help maintain or even modestly increase bone density in adulthood

- Reduce your risk of falling by increasing muscle mass and strength and improving coordination and balance

- Help older people improve function and delay loss of independence

Although exercise is beneficial for people with osteoporosis, it should not put any sudden or excessive strain on your bones. If you have osteoporosis, you should avoid high-impact exercise. To help ensure against fractures, a physical therapist or rehabilitation medicine specialist can:

- Recommend specific exercises to strengthen and support your back

- Teach you safe ways of moving and carrying out daily activities

- Recommend an exercise program that is tailored to your circumstances

Other trained exercise specialists, such as exercise physiologists, may also be able to help you develop a safe and effective exercise program.

Fall Prevention

Fall prevention is a critical concern for men and women with osteoporosis. Falls increase your likelihood of fracturing a bone in the hip, wrist, spine, or other part of the skeleton. Fractures can affect your quality of life (QOL) and lead to loss of independence and even premature death. A host of factors can contribute to your risk of falling.

Falls can be caused by:

- Impaired vision or balance

- Loss of muscle mass

- Chronic or short-term illnesses that impair your mental or physical functioning

- Use of four or more prescription medications

- Side effects of certain medications, such as:

- Sedatives or tranquilizer
- Sleeping pills
- Antidepressants
- Anticonvulsants
- Muscle relaxants
- Heart Medicines
- Blood pressure pills
- Diuretics
- Drinking alcoholic beverages

If you have osteoporosis, it is important to be aware of any physical changes you may be experiencing that affect your balance or gait and to discuss these changes with your doctor or other healthcare provider. It is also important to have regular checkups and tell your doctor if you have had problems with falling.

The force or impact of a fall (how hard you land) plays a major role in determining whether you will break a bone. Catching yourself so that you land on your hands or grabbing onto an object as you fall can prevent a hip fracture. You may break your wrist or arm instead, but the consequences are not as serious as if you break your hip. Studies have shown that wearing a specially designed garment that contains hip padding may reduce hip fractures resulting from falls in frail, elderly people living in nursing homes or residential-care facilities, but use of the garments by residents is often low.

Falls can also be caused by factors in your environment that create unsafe conditions. Some tips to help eliminate the environmental factors that lead to falls include:

Outdoors and Away from Home

- Use a cane or walker for added stability.
- Wear shoes that give good support and have thin nonslip soles. Avoid wearing slippers and athletic shoes with deep treads.
- Walk on grass when sidewalks are slippery; in winter, sprinkle salt or kitty litter on slippery sidewalks.
- Be careful on highly polished floors that are slick and dangerous, especially when wet, and walk on plastic or carpet runners when possible.
- Stop at curbs and check their height before stepping up or down.

Indoors

- Keep rooms free of clutter, especially on floors.

- Keep floor surfaces smooth but not slippery.

- Wear shoes that give good support and have thin nonslip soles. Avoid wearing slippers and athletic shoes with deep treads.

- Be sure carpets and area rugs have skid-proof backing or are tacked to the floor. Use double-stick tape to keep rugs from slipping.

- Be sure stairwells are well lit and that stairs have handrails.

- Install grab bars on bathroom walls near tub, shower, and toilet.

- Use a rubber bath mat or slip-proof seat in the shower or tub.

- Improve the lighting in your home. Use a nightlight or flashlight if you get up at night.

- Use stepladders that are stable and have a handrail.

- Install ceiling fixtures or lamps that can be turned on by a switch near the room's entrance.

- If you live alone (or spend large amounts of time alone), consider purchasing a cordless phone; you won't have to rush to answer the phone when it rings and you can call for help if you do fall.

- Consider having a personal emergency-response system; you can use it to call for help if you fall.

Medications

Your doctor may prescribe medications that have been shown to slow or stop bone loss or build new bone, increase bone density, and reduce fracture risk. The U.S. Food and Drug Administration (FDA) has approved several medications for prevention or treatment of osteoporosis, based on their ability to reduce fractures:

- **Bisphosphonates:** Several bisphosphonates are approved for the prevention or treatment of osteoporosis. These medications reduce the activity of cells that cause bone loss.

- **Parathyroid hormone:** A form of human parathyroid hormone (PTH) is approved for postmenopausal women and men with osteoporosis who are at high risk for having a fracture. Use of the drug for more than two years is not recommended.

- **RANK ligand (RANKL) inhibitor:** A RANK ligand (RANKL) inhibitor is approved for postmenopausal women with osteoporosis who are at high risk for fracture.

- **Estrogen agonists/antagonists:** An estrogen agonist/ antagonist (also called a selective estrogen receptor modulator or SERM) is approved for the prevention and treatment of osteoporosis in postmenopausal women. SERMs are not estrogens, but they have estrogen-like effects on some tissues and estrogen-blocking effects on other tissues.

- **Calcitonin:** Calcitonin is approved for the treatment of osteoporosis in women who are at least five years beyond menopause. Calcitonin is a hormone involved in calcium regulation and bone metabolism.

- **Estrogen and hormone therapy:** Estrogen and combined estrogen and progestin (hormone therapy) are approved for the prevention of postmenopausal osteoporosis as well as the treatment of moderate to severe hot flashes and vaginal dryness that may accompany menopause. Estrogen without an added progestin is recommended only for women who have had a hysterectomy (surgery to remove the uterus), because estrogen increases the risk of developing cancer of the uterine lining and progestin reduces that risk.

Results of the National Institutes of Health (NIH)-sponsored Women's Health Initiative, a large, long-term study of disease prevention strategies in postmenopausal women, suggest that, in most women, the harmful effects of long-term use of hormone therapy are likely to outweigh the disease-prevention benefits.

The FDA has recommended that women use hormone therapy at the lowest dose and for the shortest time, and carefully consider and discuss with their doctor other approved osteoporosis treatments.

Alternative Therapies

Isoflavones are naturally occurring compounds found in soybeans. Because they are structurally similar to estrogen, researchers have thought that they may hold promise as an alternative to estrogen therapy to protect postmenopausal women from osteoporosis. Several studies have explored the effects of soy isoflavones on bone health, but results have been mixed, ranging from a modest impact to no effect. Most of these studies had various limitations, including their short duration and small sample size, making it difficult to fully evaluate the impact of these compounds on bone health. Moreover, reports from NIH-supported clinical trials have failed to demonstrate a bone-sparing effect of soy isoflavones.

Chapter 48

Drugs for Osteoporosis

Chapter Contents

Section 48.1

Bisphosphonates

This section includes text excerpted from "Bisphosphonates," LiverTox®, National Institutes of Health (NIH), October 30, 2018.

The bisphosphonates are pyrophosphate analogues that become incorporated into bone matrix and suppress osteoclastic activity, thereby reducing bone turnover and increasing bone mass, which makes them valuable agents for the prevention and therapy of osteoporosis. Therapy with the bisphosphonates has been associated with a low rate of serum enzyme elevations during therapy and has been linked to rare instances of clinically apparent liver injury.

Background

Bisphosphonates are pyrophosphate analogues that have two phosphonate groups attached to a central carbon atom that replaces the oxygen present in pyrophosphate. The bisphosphonates bind calcium and are rapidly taken up in bone matrix where they suppress osteoclastic activity and change the balance between bone resorption and bone formation, thus increasing bone mass. The bisphosphonates have been shown to be effective in treating malignant hypercalcemia and in preventing and treating osteoporosis. Six bisphosphonates have been approved for use in the United States (pronunciation and year of approval given in parentheses) and they differ in formulation, recommended dose regimen, spectrum of activity, and clinical indications.

- **Alendronate** is available in tablets of 5 and 10 mg for daily use, 35, 40, and 70 mg (with and without vitamin D) for weekly use, and as a suspension for oral use in several generic forms and under the brand name Fosamax. Indications include prevention and treatment of osteoporosis and treatment of Paget disease of bone.

- **Etidronate** is available in tablets of 200 and 400 mg for daily use in generic forms and under the trade name Didronel. Indications include Paget disease of bone and heterotopic ossification, but it has also been used off label for therapy of osteoporosis.

- **Ibandronate** is available in tablets of 2.5 mg for daily and 150 mg for monthly use and as an intravenous formulation under the trade name Boniva. Indications include prevention and treatment of osteoporosis.

- **Pamidronate** is available as an intravenous formulation generically and under the trade name Aredia. Indications include hypercalcemia of malignancy, multiple myeloma, and Paget disease of bone.

- **Risedronate** is available in tablets of 5 mg for daily use, 30 and 35 mg for weekly use, and 75 and 150 mg for monthly use in generic forms and under the trade name Actonel. Indications include osteoporosis and Paget disease of bone.

- **Zoledronic acid** is available as several intravenous formulations generically and under the brand names Zometa and Reclast. Indications and dosage vary by preparation, but include prevention and treatment of osteoporosis, Paget disease of bone, hypercalcemia of malignancy and multiple myeloma.

The side effects of the bisphosphonates vary by route of administration, but are largely class specific. The oral formulations are generally well tolerated, but are recommended to be given on an empty stomach and with care that they enter the stomach (by drinking water and remaining upright) to avoid esophageal irritation and potential ulceration. Common side effects of oral formulations include headache, abdominal discomfort, dyspepsia, nausea, and hypocalcemia. The intravenous formulations of the bisphosphonates can be associated with local infusion reactions and in an acute phase reaction in up to 30 percent of patients. This is characterized by a flu-like syndrome primarily with the initial infusion. Symptoms arise within 10 to 20 hours after the infusion and are accompanied by increases in C reactive protein, decreases in serum zinc and, in some instances, minor elevations in serum enzymes several days later. Severe side effects of the bisphosphonates are rare, but have included esophageal ulcer, gastrointestinal bleeding, atrial fibrillation and, with long-term treatment, osteonecrosis of the jaw and atypical femoral fractures.

Hepatotoxicity

In most large prospective trials, the bisphosphonates were associated with only rare and isolated instances of serum enzyme elevations and no cases of clinically apparent liver injury. Since their general availability and wide-scale use, however, there have been occasional publications reporting clinically apparent acute liver injury due to the more commonly used bisphosphonates (alendronate, ibandronate, risedronate, zoledronate), some of which were accompanied by mild jaundice. The time to onset ranged from 2 to 6 months or more, and patients typically presented with abdominal discomfort and nausea, sometimes followed by jaundice. The pattern of serum enzyme elevations was hepatocellular and liver histology showed an acute toxic hepatitis. Immunoallergic features (fever, rash, eosinophilia) and autoantibodies were uncommon. Most cases were mild-to-moderate in severity and most published cases resolved with drug discontinuation, although full recovery was not always prompt.

In addition, the bisphosphonates given as intravenous infusions (zoledronate, ibandronate, pamidronate) have been associated with rare instances of mild hypersensitivity reactions with rash and fever which may be accompanied by transient and mild serum enzyme elevations without jaundice typically in association with an acute phase reaction occurring with the initial dose. In some cases, infusions can be tolerated using premedication with glucocorticoids or antihistamines. With repeated doses, these reactions become less severe and may disappear. No instances of acute liver failure or chronic liver disease have been convincingly linked to use of the bisphosphonates.

Likelihood scores:

Alendronate: C (probable rare cause of clinically apparent liver injury)

Etidronate: E* (unproven but suspected rare cause of clinically apparent liver injury)

Ibandronate: D (possible rare cause of clinically apparent liver injury)

Pamidronate: E* (unproven but suspected rare cause of clinically apparent liver injury)

Risedronate: D (possible rare cause of clinically apparent liver injury)

Zoledronic acid: C (probable rare cause of clinically apparent liver injury)

Mechanism of Injury

The bisphosphonates are taken up by bone matrix and rapidly cleared from the serum by renal excretion. Hepatic metabolism is minimal, and thus it is somewhat surprising that they can be associated with hepatic injury. The mechanism of injury is likely to be metabolic idiosyncrasy as immunoallergic features are not typical.

Outcome and Management

The clinically apparent acute liver injury attributed to bisphosphonates has been mild-to-moderate in severity without published instances of acute liver failure or chronic liver disease. The possibility of cross-reactivity of the hepatic injury among the various bisphosphonates has not been studied, nor is there published experience with rechallenge using the same bisphosphonates. Cross-reactivity to such injury should be assumed and switching to another agent done with caution and careful monitoring.

Section 48.2

Selective Estrogen Receptor Modulators

This section includes text excerpted from "Selective Estrogen Receptor Modulators Raloxifene, Bazedoxifene, Ospemifene," LiverTox®, National Institutes of Health (NIH), October 30, 2018.

The selective estrogen receptor modulators (SERMs) are a group of nonsteroidal compounds that have estrogen-like effects (agonism) on some tissues (such as bone, skin, heart, or vaginal epithelium), but antiestrogen effects (antagonism) on other tissues (such as breast or uterus). Depending on the tissue specificity and balance of the agonist and antagonist activities, these agents have different clinical effects, different indications and different adverse side effects.

Typical indications for SERMS include treatment or prevention of breast cancer (tamoxifen, toremifene, raloxifene), treatment or prevention of postmenopausal osteoporosis (raloxifene, bazedoxifene), and amelioration of symptoms of menopause symptoms (ospemifene). Separate documents for the SERMs that are used largely for prevention of cancer, tamoxifen, and toremifene, are available in LiverTox (livertox.nih.gov). This section summaries background information and the potential hepatotoxicity of raloxifene, bazedoxifene, and ospemifene, SERMs used for treatment of nonmalignant conditions such as osteoporosis and menopausal symptoms of hot flashes and dyspareunia.

Background

Raloxifene is a selective estrogen receptor modulator that has estrogen-like effects (agonism) on bone and the cardiovascular system but antiestrogen activity (antagonism) on breast and uterus tissue. This differential activity takes advantage of the beneficial effects of estrogens on bone in decreasing bone resorption and turnover and thus preventing osteoporosis, while avoiding the potential harmful effects of estrogen stimulation of breast and uterine tissue. In several large clinical trials, raloxifene was shown to increase bone mineral density and prevent bone fractures in postmenopausal women at high risk for osteoporosis, while decreasing serum cholesterol levels (both total and low-density lipoprotein) and without stimulating breast and uterine growth.

Raloxifene was approved for treatment and prevention of postmenopausal osteoporosis in the United States in 1997, and indications were expanded in 2007 to include reduction of risk of breast cancer in postmenopausal women with osteoporosis as well as those at high risk of breast cancer. Raloxifene is available in tablets of 60 mg generically and under the brand name Evista, and the recommended dose is 60 mg daily. Side effects are not common, but can include hot flashes, leg cramps, peripheral edema, arthralgias, and sweating. Rare, but potentially severe adverse events include deep venous thrombosis, pulmonary embolism, and ischemic strokes, side effects that it shares with estrogen.

Hepatotoxicity

In large, prelicensure clinical trials, the rate of serum enzyme elevations during raloxifene therapy was less than 1 percent and was no higher than with placebo or comparator arms. In addition, no episodes of hepatitis or clinically apparent liver injury attributable to raloxifene were reported. In the two decades since its approval and wide-scale use, there have been isolated reports of liver injury attributed to raloxifene. One report described a case of cholestatic hepatitis arising a month after starting raloxifene which resolved with stopping, but full recovery was delayed (Case 1). The injury was accompanied by mild immunoallergic features, but autoantibodies were not present. A second case of cholestatic hepatitis was reported in a patient on long-term raloxifene who had been started on fenofibrate two weeks before the onset of jaundice. The injury was attributed to the combination of the two agents and possible drug–drug interactions.

Finally, several cases of an exacerbation of nonalcoholic steato-hepatitis during raloxifene therapy have been reported, a pattern of injury that has been reported more commonly with tamoxifen. Thus, raloxifene may be a rare cause of liver injury, but the relationship to the drug has not been very well established.

Mechanism of Injury

The reason why raloxifene might cause liver injury is not known, but the isolated cholestatic cases appear to be due to an idiosyncratic hypersensitivity reaction. Raloxifene is metabolized in the liver by glucuronidation and it has minimal effects on cytochrome P450 enzymes (CYP).

Outcome and Management

Serum enzyme elevations are uncommon during raloxifene therapy and are rarely dose limiting. While clinically apparent liver injury with jaundice has been reported with raloxifene therapy, it is very rare. Evaluation should include assessment of hepatic steatosis by ultrasound or other imaging modalities. There is no known cross sensitivity to hepatic injury among the SERMs or with other agents for osteoporosis. On the other hand, restarting raloxifene after clinically apparent liver injury cannot be recommended.

Chapter 49

Hip Replacement Surgery

Hip Fractures among Older Adults[1]

One of the most serious fall injuries is a broken hip. It is hard to recover from a hip fracture and afterward many people are not able to live on their own. As the U.S. population gets older, the number of hip fractures is likely to go up.

- Each year over 300,000 older people—those 65 and older—are hospitalized for hip fractures.

- More than 95 percent of hip fractures are caused by falling, usually by falling sideways.

- Women experience three-quarters of all hip fractures.

  - Women fall more often than men.

  - Women more often have osteoporosis, a disease that weakens bones and makes them more likely to break.

- The chances of breaking your hip go up as you get older.

This chapter includes text excerpted from documents published by two public domain sources. Text under the headings marked 1 are excerpted from "Hip Fractures among Older Adults," Centers for Disease Control and Prevention (CDC), September 20, 2016; Text under the headings marked 2 are excerpted from "Hip Replacement Surgery," National Institute of Arthritis and Musculoskeletal and Skin Diseases (NIAMS), July 30, 2016.

What Is Hip Replacement Surgery?[2]

Hip replacement surgery removes damaged or diseased parts of a hip joint and replaces them with new, human-made parts.

The goals of hip replacement surgery are to:

- Relieve pain

- Help the hip joint work better

- Improve walking and other movements

Why Do People Need Hip Replacement Surgery?[2]

Common reasons for hip replacement surgery include damage to the hip joint from:

- Arthritis

- Disease that causes the bone in joints to die

- Injuries or fractures

- Bone tumors that break down the hip joint

Your doctor will likely first suggest other treatments to decrease hip pain and improve function, including:

- Walking aids, such as a cane

- An exercise program

- Physical therapy

- Medications

Sometimes the pain remains and makes daily activities hard to do. In this case, your doctor may order an X-ray to look at the damage to the joint. If the X-ray shows damage and your hip joint hurts, you may need a hip replacement.

Healthy, active people often have very good results after hip replacement surgery. But your doctor may not suggest this surgery if you have:

- A disease that causes severe muscle weakness

- Parkinson disease (PD)

- A high risk of infection

- Poor health

How Do I Prepare for Hip Replacement Surgery?[2]

To prepare for surgery, you can:

- Learn what to expect before, during, and after surgery
- Ask the doctor for booklets about the surgery
- Ask someone to drive you to and from the hospital
- Arrange for someone to help you for a week or two after coming home from the hospital
- Put things you need in one place at home. For instance, put the remote control, telephone, medicine, tissues, and wastebasket next to your chair or bed.
- Place items you use every day at arm level to avoid reaching up or bending down
- Stock up on food
- Make and freeze meals

What Happens during Hip Replacement Surgery[2]

During hip replacement, which lasts from one to two hours, your doctor will:

- Give your medicine to put your whole body to sleep so that you won't feel pain
- Makes a six- to eight-inch cut over the side of the hip. A smaller cut may be recommended in certain cases.
- Removes the diseased tissue from the hip joint, while leaving healthy parts
- Replaces the ends of the thigh bone and hip socket with new, artificial parts
- Move you to a recovery room for one to two hours until you are fully awake or the numbness goes away

What Can I Expect after Hip Replacement Surgery?[2]

Right away. Usually, people do not spend more than one to four days in the hospital after hip replacement surgery.

The following will happen while at the hospital:

- Soon after surgery, you will:
  - Breathe deeply, cough, or blow into a device to check your lungs. Deep breathing helps to keep fluid out of your lungs after surgery.
  - Work with a physical therapist, who will teach you how to sit up, bend over, and walk with your new hip. The therapist will also teach you simple exercises to help you get better.
- Within one to two days after surgery, you may be able to sit on the edge of the bed, stand, and even walk with help.

After you go home, be sure to follow the doctor's instructions. Tips for getting better quickly are:

- Work with a physical therapist
- Wear an apron to carry things around the house. This leaves your hands and arms free for balance or to use crutches.
- Use a long-handled "reacher" to turn on lights or grab things you need. Your nurse at the hospital may give you one or tell you where to buy one.

Long term. You should talk to your doctor or physical therapist about an exercise program to reduce joint pain and stiffness.

To be completely well takes about three to six months, based on:

- The type of surgery
- Your health
- How quickly exercises help

Revision surgery (replacement of an artificial joint) is becoming more common as more people are having hip replacements at a younger age. This is because new joints generally last at least 10 to 15 years. Your doctor may consider revision surgery when:

- Treatments do not relieve pain and help you move better
- X-rays show changes in the bone or artificial parts of the joint that require surgery

What Are the Risks of Hip Replacement Surgery?[2]

Risks of problems after hip replacement surgery are much lower than they used to be. More common problems that could occur include:

- The ball comes out of the socket. This is the most common problem that can happen soon after hip replacement surgery. It can happen if you are in certain positions, such as pulling your knees up to your chest.

- Swelling that cause special cells to eat away some of the bone, causing the joint to loosen. This is the most common problem that can happen later after hip replacement surgery.

Less common problems after surgery are:

- Infection

- Blood clots

- Bone growth past the normal edges of the bone

Life after Hip Replacement Surgery[2]

For most people, hip replacement surgery:

- Relieves pain

- Helps the hip joint work better

- Improves walking and other movements

Your doctor may say not to jog or play basketball or tennis. These can damage or loosen your new hip joint. Talk to your doctor about exercises that won't injure the new joint. These exercises can include:

- Walking

- Stationary bicycling

- Swimming

- Cross-country skiing

What You Can Do to Prevent Hip Fractures[1]

You can prevent hip fractures by taking steps to strengthen your bones and prevent falls:

Talk to Your Doctor

- Ask your doctor or healthcare provider to evaluate your risk for falling and talk with them about specific things you can do.

- Ask your doctor or pharmacist to review your medicines to see if any might make you dizzy or sleepy. This should include prescription medicines and over-the-counter (OTC) medicines.

- Ask your doctor or healthcare provider about taking vitamin D supplement.

Get Screened for Osteoporosis

Get screened for osteoporosis and treated if needed.

Do Strength and Balance Exercises

Do exercises that make your legs stronger and improve your balance. Tai chi is a good example of this kind of exercise.

Have Your Eyes Checked

Have your eyes checked by an eye doctor at least once a year, and be sure to update your eyeglasses if needed.

If you have bifocal or progressive lenses, you may want to get a pair of glasses with only your distance prescription for outdoor activities, such as walking. Sometimes these types of lenses can make things seem closer or farther away than they really are.

Make Your Home Safer

- Get rid of things you could trip over.

- Add grab bars inside and outside your tub or shower and next to the toilet.

- Put railings on both sides of stairs.

- Make sure your home has lots of light by adding more or brighter light bulbs.

Chapter 50

Gene Therapy for Bone Regeneration

There is no doubt that there is an increasing need worldwide for the ability of orthopedic and oral surgeons to reproducibly regenerate bone and associated tissues that are lost due to trauma, surgical resection of cancer, or pathologies that affect the skeleton. The field of tissue engineering aims to fulfill this need through a variety of approaches that utilize morphogens, growth factors, and cytokines, scaffolds and carriers, and cells. Various combinations of these different components, tailored for specific applications, have shown great promise in preclinical animal models, and there are a number of small clinical trials underway around the world. The ultimate goal is to induce endogenous repair without the need for surgical intervention. However, the right cocktail of factors has yet to be formulated that is long lasting, without potential unwanted effects (bone where it should not be), and able to regenerate large segments of bone where the number of endogenous cells (either local or recruited) are insufficient

This chapter contains text excerpted from the following sources: Text in this chapter begins with excerpts from "Reversing Bone Loss by Directing Mesenchymal Stem Cells to Bone," U.S. Department of Energy (DOE), October 21, 2013. Reviewed January 2019. Text beginning with the heading "Technology" is excerpted from "Ex Vivo and in Vivo Genetic Therapies for Bone Regeneration," U.S. Department of Veterans Affairs (VA), May 21, 2011. Reviewed January 2019.

to complete the task. Scaffolds, either alone or in combination with factors, can be used to guide regeneration by endogenous cells in certain situations, but again, may not suffice in large skeletal defects. Consequently, cell-based therapy tops the list of potential approaches by supplying sufficient numbers of cells that can not only form bone and associated tissues, but also maintain bone as it undergoes turnover throughout life. What follows is a discussion of the isolation and characterization of potential cell sources and various approaches to cell-based bone regeneration.

Technology

The U.S. Department of Veterans Affairs (VA) has developed gene therapy-based technologies designed to stimulate bone synthesis, promote stem cell renewal, and prolong therapeutic efficacy in the treatment of osteoporosis or in the rapid healing of bone fractures.

Description

The novel method developed entails importing recombinant deoxyribonucleic acid (DNA) specifically into osteoblast nuclei or osteoblast stem cells that can be stably transduced with a gene encoding a potent bone-promoting growth factor. The modified stem cells can be injected into a patient for systemic action. As an alternative to systemic treatment with modified stem cells, osteogenic growth factors can be localized to the site of a bone fracture or weakening through retrovirus or lentivirus-based gene therapy. Therapy for this particular method would be in the form of a resorbable scaffold or a solution that would be injected into the fracture site. Following gene transfer, transduced cells express the modified transgenic osteogenic factor, resulting in high-sustained levels at the fracture site and markedly increasing bone synthesis and healing.

Competitive Advantage

Ideal therapies for weak or broken bones would be minimally invasive and of sufficient duration to promote osteogenesis, damaged bone resorption, and angiogenesis (to provide newly deposited tissue with nutrients).

This therapy:

- Can be delivered locally or systemically, depending on the pathological conditions

- Can provide extended therapy for chronic osteoporosis because the stem cells used in ex vivo gene therapy regenerate

- Allows targeting to the proliferating periosteal cells that arise shortly after a fracture event resulting in high-sustained levels of the osteogenic growth factor while also promoting angiogenesis

Chapter 51

Complementary and Alternative Approaches for Osteoporosis

Tai Chi

Tai chi may be a safe alternative to conventional exercise for maintaining bone mineral density (BMD) in postmenopausal women. Bone mineral density is one of the key indicators of bone strength. Low BMD is associated with osteoporosis, a bone disease characterized by reduced bone strength that can lead to fractures, which are a significant cause of disability in older people.

Exercise is an important component of osteoporosis prevention and treatment. Tai chi is a mind-body practice that originated in China as a

This chapter contains text excerpted from the following sources: Text under the heading "Tai Chi" is excerpted from "Tai Chi May Help Maintain Bone Mineral Density in Postmenopausal Women," National Center for Complementary and Integrative Health (NCCIH), August 20, 2015. Reviewed January 2019; Text under the heading "Black Cohosh" is excerpted from "Laboratory Study Shows Black Cohosh Promotes Bone Formation in Mouse Cells," National Center for Complementary and Integrative Health (NCCIH), January 20, 2012. Reviewed January 2019; Text under the heading "Turmeric" is excerpted from "Laboratory Study Shows Turmeric May Have Bone-Protective Effects," National Center for Complementary and Integrative Health (NCCIH), October 19, 2015. Reviewed January 2019.

martial art. It consists of slow and gentle body moves, while breathing deeply and meditating (tai chi is sometimes called "moving meditation").

Peter Wayne, Ph.D., and colleagues conducted a systematic review of research looking at the effect of tai chi on BMD. They found that tai chi may be an effective, safe, and practical intervention for maintaining BMD in postmenopausal women. They note that the evidence is preliminary because the research they reviewed was of limited scope and quality, but enough evidence of effectiveness exists to warrant further research.

The benefits of tai chi appeared similar to those of conventional exercise. However, tai chi may also improve balance, reduce fall frequency, and increase musculoskeletal strength.

Black Cohosh

Results of laboratory research are the first to indicate that extracts of the herb black cohosh (Actaea racemosa) may stimulate bone formation, according to a study published in the journal *Bone*. Although results from the study suggest that black cohosh may have potential implications for the prevention or treatment of postmenopausal bone loss, there is no evidence yet that this laboratory research can be extended to treatments in people.

Researchers from the University of Hong Kong, City University of New York, and Columbia University added an extract of black cohosh to a culture of bone-forming mouse cells. The researchers observed that a high dose (1,000 ng/mL) of the extract suppressed the production of these bone-forming cells, yet a lower dose (500 ng/mL) significantly increased the formation of bone nodules. When the cells were treated with a protein whose molecules attach to estrogen receptors in place of estrogen, this effect on bone nodule formation disappeared. Thus, the researchers suggest that ingredients within black cohosh contain a component that acts through estrogen receptors.

The researchers concluded that their results provide a scientific explanation at the molecular level for claims that black cohosh may protect against postmenopausal osteoporosis. They also noted that studying extraction methods and identifying black cohosh's active components may make it possible to develop new ways to prevent and treat this condition.

Turmeric

Turmeric—an herb commonly used in curry powders, mustards, and cheeses—may protect bones against osteoporosis, according to a recent laboratory study published in the *Journal of Agricultural and Food Chemistry*. Osteoporosis is a bone disease that can lead to an increased risk of fractures. The condition is common in postmenopausal women. This study, which used an animal (rat) model of postmenopausal osteoporosis, builds on previous laboratory research examining turmeric's antiarthritic properties.

The study tested two turmeric extracts containing different amounts of curcuminoids—(components of the herb) in female rats whose ovaries had been surgically removed (ovariectomy—a procedure that causes changes associated with menopause, including bone loss). Researchers injected rats with enriched turmeric extract (94% curcuminoids by weight) or nonenriched turmeric extract (41% curcuminoids), at a dose of 60 mg/kg three times a week for 2 months. As controls, other rats received placebo injections after either ovariectomy or sham surgery. Tests showed that while nonenriched turmeric extract did not have bone-protective effects, curcuminoid-enriched turmeric extract prevented up to 50 percent of bone loss, and also preserved bone structure and connectivity. Other physiological changes associated with ovariectomy (weight gain and shrinking of the uterus) were unaffected—an indication that the bone-protective effects did not involve an estrogen-based chemical pathway.

The researchers concluded that turmeric may protect bones, but that the effect depends on the amount of curcuminoids present. If the protective effect does not involve estrogen-based pathways, turmeric may offer a safer alternative to menopausal hormone therapy or botanical phytoestrogens (compounds similar to the female hormone estrogen) for bone preservation in menopause. However, the researchers emphasized that clinical research is needed to evaluate the use of turmeric-derived curcuminoid products to guard against osteoporosis in humans.

Part Six

Living with Osteoporosis

Chapter 52

How Lifestyle Changes Can Help

Many of the things you do to prevent osteoporosis also help you to manage it. To help keep your bones strong and slow down bone loss.

Diet

A healthy diet with enough calcium and vitamin D helps make your bones strong. Many people get less than half the calcium they need. Good sources of calcium are:

- Low-fat milk, yogurt, and cheese
- Foods with added calcium such as orange juice, cereals, and bread

Vitamin D is also needed for strong bones. You may need to take vitamin D pills. The table on this page shows the amount of calcium and vitamin D you should get each day.

Exercise

Exercise helps your bones grow stronger. The best exercises for healthy bones are strength building and weight-bearing, such as:

- Walking

This chapter includes text excerpted from "Osteoporosis," National Institute of Arthritis and Musculoskeletal and Skin Diseases (NIAMS), February 28, 2016.

Table 52.1. Recommended Calcium and Vitamin D Intakes

Life-Stage Group	Calcium Mg/Day	Vitamin D (IU/Day)
Infants 0 to 6 months	200	400
Infants 6 to 12 months	260	400
1 to 3 years old	700	600
4 to 8 years old	1,000	600
9 to 13 years old	1,300	600
14 to 18 years old	1,300	600
19 to 30 years old	1,000	600
31 to 50 years old	1,000	600
51- to 70-year-old males	1,000	600
51- to 70-year-old females	1,200	600
>70 years old	1,200	800
14 to 18 years old, pregnant/lactating	1,300	600
19 to 50 years old, pregnant/lactating	1,000	600

Definitions: mg = milligrams; IU = International Units
(Source: Food and Nutrition Board (FNB), Institute of Medicine (IOM), National Academy of Sciences (NAS), 2010.)

- Hiking
- Jogging
- Climbing stairs
- Lifting weights
- Playing tennis
- Dancing

Healthy Lifestyle

Smoking is bad for bones as well as the heart and lungs. Also, people who drink a lot of alcohol are more prone to bone loss and broken bones due to poor diet and risk of falling.

Preventing Falls

Men and women with osteoporosis need to take care not to fall down. Falls can break bones. Some reasons people fall are:

- Poor vision

- Poor balance

- Certain diseases that affect how you walk

- Some types of medicine, such as sleeping pills

Some tips to help prevent falls outdoors are:

- Use a cane or walker

- Wear rubber-soled shoes so you don't slip

- Walk on grass when sidewalks are slippery

- In winter, put salt or kitty litter on icy sidewalks

Some ways to help prevent falls indoors are:

- Keep rooms free of clutter, especially on floors

- Use plastic or carpet runners on slippery floors

- Wear low-heeled shoes that provide good support

- Do not walk in socks, stockings, or slippers

- Be sure carpets and area rugs have skid-proof backs or are tacked to the floor

- Be sure stairs are well lit and have rails on both sides

- Put grab bars on bathroom walls near tub, shower, and toilet

- Use a rubber bath mat in the shower or tub

- Keep a flashlight next to your bed

- Use a sturdy step stool with a handrail and wide steps

- Add more lights in rooms

- Keep a cordless phone with you so that you don't have to rush to the phone when it rings and if you fall, you can call for help

Chapter 53

Osteoporosis and Medicare

Bone Mass Measurements

Medicare Part B (medical insurance) covers this test once every 24 months (or more often if medically necessary) if you meet one or more of these conditions:

- You're a woman whose doctor determines that you are estrogen deficient and at risk for osteoporosis, based on your medical history and other findings

- Your X-rays show possible osteoporosis, osteopenia, or vertebral fractures

- You're taking prednisone or steroid-type drugs or are planning to begin this treatment

- You've been diagnosed with primary hyperparathyroidism

- You're being monitored to see if your osteoporosis drug therapy is working

---

This chapter contains text excerpted from the following sources: Text under the heading "Bone Mass Measurements" is excerpted from "Your Medicare Coverage—Bone Mass Measurements," Centers for Medicare & Medicaid Services (CMS), November 26, 2018; Text beginning with the heading "Osteoporosis Drugs" is excerpted from "Your Medicare Coverage—Osteoporosis Drugs," Centers for Medicare & Medicaid Services (CMS), November 20, 2018.

Your Costs in Original Medicare

You pay nothing for this test if the doctor or other qualified health-care provider accepts the assignment.

What It Is

This test helps to see if you're at risk for broken bones.

Osteoporosis Drugs

Medicare Part A (Hospital Insurance) and Medicare Part B (Medical Insurance) help pay for an injectable drug for osteoporosis and visits by a home-health nurse to inject the drug if you meet these conditions:

- You're a woman

- You're eligible for Part B and meet the criteria for Medicare home-health services

- You have a bone fracture that a doctor certifies is related to postmenopausal osteoporosis

- Your doctor certifies that you're unable to learn to give yourself the drug by injection and your family members and/or caregivers are unable and unwilling to give you the drug by injection

Your Costs in Original Medicare

You pay 20 percent of the Medicare-approved amount for the cost of the drug, and the Part B deductible applies. You pay nothing for the home-health nurse visit to inject the drug.

Chapter 54

Osteoporosis Pain Management

What Is Pain?

Pain is a physical sensation produced by our body in response to tissue damage. If any sudden detectable changes such as bruising, squashing, squeezing, bone-breaking (fracture), twisting, and so on occur in the tissue, a specialized set of nerves called "nociceptors" or "danger detectors" (which are distributed throughout the body) gets activated and sends messages to the brain through the spinal cord. The brain then signals our body to say that something is damaged and our body produces a sensation as a response, which is said to be "pain."

It is an unpleasant experience, which has been categorized into three types.

- **Acute pain** occurs following surgery or trauma. It lasts for only a short period of time, improves with time, and then resolves when the actual damage heals completely. If acute pain is untreated or poorly treated, it can transition into chronic pain.

- **Chronic pain** also occurs following surgery or trauma, but lasts for a long period of time and interferes with normal life. Chronic pain persists even after the healing of an injury.

"Osteoporosis Pain Management," © 2019 Omnigraphics. Reviewed January 2019.

- **Cancer pain** occurs during an early or advanced stage of disease, and cancer survivors experience this debilitating pain as a side effect of their treatment.

What about Pain and Osteoporosis

Osteoporosis remains silent until it hurts—gentle bone loss and increased fracture risk cannot be felt as osteoporosis (OP) manifests quietly and progresses gradually. OP manifests clinically as painful fractures. Healing time for a new fracture is approximately three months, and pain that lasts for longer than three months is considered chronic pain. Chronic pain can result in disability and the affected individual may need long-term care.

Some people experience painless vertebral fractures, while others experience vertebral fractures and osteoporotic spinal fractures with intense pain and muscular spasms that last even after the healing of the fracture (i.e., they may have persistent pain in their necks, mid-backs, and lower backs even after the fracture heals).

In the absence of timely treatment of chronic pain, neuroplastic changes occur in the nervous system. This increases a person's sensitivity to pain, and people may then experience pain without any external stimuli. For example, an individual may feel pain from clothing touching the skin or even from a breeze. This is called "pain sensitization."

Chronic pain should be taken seriously as it affects all areas of our life. If you feel that you have chronic pain and need help managing it, then it is time to seek a doctor's advice and to discuss coping strategies.

What Are the Coping Strategies of Chronic Pain?

The evaluation and management of pain require a holistic approach that allows the patients to discuss their particular symptoms with a healthcare provider in order to determine the best treatment options for them. The United States now has specialized pain clinics across the country that deal with various pain-management strategies, such as:

- Medical management

- Procedural methods

- External stimuli

- Compresses

- Exercises

- Support systems
- Therapeutic methods
- Relaxation training
- Distraction techniques

Medical Management

- **Anesthetics:** Danger detectors can be turned off with the use of anesthetics (mostly for surgical and procedural use; Types include local and general anesthesias).

- **Analgesics/painkillers/pain relievers:** Based on the intensity and chronicity of pain, your healthcare provider may suggest using analgesics with or without adjuvants.

- **Adjuvants:** A set of molecules that can enhance analgesic effects and contribute to pain reduction. Some of the adjuvants include bisphosphonates, antiepileptics, corticosteroids, antidepressants, benzodiazepines, and other classes of drugs. Adjuvants that can be used as a first-line treatment on a timely basis include bisphosphonates for osteoporotic fractures and antiepileptic drugs for neuropathic pain.

  - **For mild pain:** Use NSAIDs or acetaminophen with or without the addition of adjuvants (i.e., diclofenac, etc.).

  - **For moderate pain:** Use weak opioids with or without NSAIDs or acetaminophen, along with a possible adjuvant addition (e.g., Codeine, tramadol, etc.).

  - **For severe pain:** Use opioids with NSAIDs or paracetamol, along with possible adjuvant addition (i.e., oral morphine, tapentadol, oxycodone, buprenorphine, hydromorphone, fentanyl, methadone, etc.).

- **Antiresorptive drugs:** Bisphosphonates are drugs that slow down bone loss and thereby increase bone mineral density, which reduces fracture risk. Some bisphosphonates are:

  - Alendronate—decreases pain

  - Ibandronate—decreases pain and stiffness

  - Minodronate—lowers back pain and limits bone turnover

  - Risedronate—reduces pain and disability

429

- Clodronate—high painkiller effect than paracetamol or neridronate
- Pamidronate (IV)—reduces chronic back pain
- Zoledronic acid—reduces back pain and improves activity

- **Anticonvulsant drugs:** These drugs are used for effective analgesic effect for neuropathic pain that is caused by spinal fracture or spinal-cord injury. Some examples of anticonvulsant drugs are:
  - Gabapentin
  - Pregabalin

- **Antidepressant drugs:** These drugs are used to treat neuropathic pain, muscular pain, chemotherapy-induced nerve pain, but mainly used to treat depression and anxiety. Some examples of antidepressant drugs are:
  - Tricyclic antidepressants (amitriptyline, nortriptyline, desipramine)
  - Duloxetine

- **Estrogen agonists or antagonists therapy:** Selective estrogen-receptor modulators (SERMS) reduce spinal-fracture risks in postmenopausal women (raloxifene (Evista)).

- **Hormonal therapy:** Two major hormonal therapies are recommended:
  - Parathyroid hormone (PTH)—stimulates bone formation and is mainly recommended for people with high risk of fracture (teriparatide (Forteo)).
  - Calcitonin—an endogenous peptide hormone that increases bone density, prevents spinal fracture, and helps manage postfracture pain, especially in postmenopausal women (Calcimar, Miacalcin).

- **Immunotherapy:** This new type of treatment with RANK ligand (RANKL) inhibitors reduces pain. Some example of immunotherapy drugs are:
  - Denosumab (Xgeva)
  - Romosozumab
  - Strontium ranelate

Romosozumab increases bone formation and reduces vertebral-fracture risk in postmenopausal women with osteoporosis. Strontium ranelate is approved for use in Europe to reduce back pain in postmenopausal women, but has not yet been approved for treatment of osteoporosis in the United States.

What Are the Possible Risks and Side Effects of Osteoporotic Medications?

One can reduce the following risks and side effects by avoiding over-the-counter (OTC) usage and appropriately adhering to the prescribed drug regimen.

- **Bisphosphonates** cause nausea, heartburn, stomach pain, fever, headache, muscle pain, osteonecrosis of the jaw (nonhealing jaw bone after tooth extraction), and can rarely cause fracture of the thigh bone.

- **Denosumab** lowers your calcium and can cause fever, chills, stomach pain, painful urination or burning with urination, muscular and bone pain (especially on arms, back, and legs), and skin problems such as blisters, crusting, rash, redness, itching, and dry skin.

- **Hormonal therapy** causes dizziness, headaches, nausea, and calcitonin, and sometimes may increase the risk of cancer. Some provides recommend use of Forteo as a last option.

- **Estrogen-like drugs** cause heart disease, blood clots, and contribute to some cancers (such as breast and endometrium). Also, SERMs lead to blood clots and stroke.

- **Opioids** lead to addiction, constipation, urinary retention, and imbalance. Also, long-term opioid therapy can worsen osteoporosis.

- **NSAIDs** cause stomach irritation, constipation, ulcers, gastrointestinal bleeding, cardiovascular toxicity, impaired renal function, and, in rare cases, cognitive impairment and personality changes in the elderly.

Procedural Methods

When osteoporosis is widespread, vertebral compression fractures will go hand and hand with the disease. There are two minimally invasive approaches for restoration of the height of these broken bones and posture, which can improve the quality of patients' lives. They are:

- Vertebroplasty

- Kyphoplasty

Both procedures are done generally done either on an outpatient basis or require overnight hospitalization. The procedures can be performed under twilight sedation, or general and local anesthesia. Medical professionals will insert a balloon inside the fractured bone via a needle under X-ray guidance. The balloon will then restore the shape, size, and height of the broken bone, and, once deflated, will allow the hole to be filled with quick-setting bone cement. The bone cement will harden within 15 minutes, but the surrounding muscles and tissues may take some days or weeks to heal completely. Thus, the broken bone can be realigned to its normal position. Usually, patients report rapid improvement in their pain and posture following these procedures, with variation depending on the severity of their osteoporosis. These procedures may require temporary bracing or rehabilitation therapies.

External Stimuli

In this process, electrical impulses are sent through two electrodes with very mild electrical/current supply to the site where patients experience pain. These impulses block the transmission of pain signals to the brain and thus provide pain relief, which can last for some hours. This process is called "Transcutaneous Electrical Nerve Stimulation" (TENS). The device or equipment used for this procedure is called a "TENS unit." These units should only be used under the supervision of a physical therapist or healthcare physician. Small portable TENS units are available and allow patients to hook their belts to the units for continuous relief.

These units can be purchased from a hospital or rented from the hospital or a surgical-supply company via a prescription. Patients may also receive insurance reimbursement for use of this equipment.

Compresses

Two types of compresses can be used to alleviate pain. They are heat and ice.

- **Heat** is used in the form of hot packs and hot showers and is called hot compresses. Heat relieves chronic pain and muscle stiffness.

- **Ice** is used in the form of ice packs and is called cold compresses. Ice alleviates pain by numbing the pain-sensing nerves. Ice also reduces pain and swelling in the affected area.

Depending on which method feels better, you can apply heat or cold to the affected area for around 15 to 20 minutes. It is also important to protect your skin with a towel or other materials to avoid external harm.

Support Systems

- **Braces:** Spinal support or braces will reduce inflammation and swelling by restricting movement following a fracture or injury. Back braces will relieve pain following a vertebral fracture and allow you to resume normal activities while the fracture heals. Continuous use of back braces is not recommended as this can weaken back muscles. To avoid this scenario, patients exercise in accordance with the recommendations of physiotherapists.

- **Crutches:** These are mobility aids that transfer body weight from the legs to the upper body. This equipment is often used after a leg injury to help with mobility until the injury or fracture heals and the patient adjusts progressively to more weight bearing.

Exercises

It is important to remain active because prolonged inactivity may increase weakness and loss of muscle strength and mass. Exercise mobilizes our muscles and raises our endorphin levels—the natural painkillers produced by our brain—which can improve pain. A regular exercise program helps us to:

- Regain energy
- Strengthen muscles
- Relieve tension
- Increase flexibility
- Reduce fatigue

Therapeutic Methods

- **Physical therapy:** This therapy is performed by specialists called "physical therapists" who teach appropriate strengthening and stretching exercises to enhance our muscular health.

- **Water therapy**: This therapy is performed in a pool, and improves back muscle strength and reduces pain.

- **Acupuncture:** In this therapy, special needles are inserted into the body at specific locations to stimulate nerve endings. This causes the brain to release endorphins, the natural painkillers produced by our brain. Patients attend several sessions based on the improvement of pain.

- **Acupressure:** In this therapy, direct pressure is applied to the affected areas by a specialist. With training from the specialist, one can learn to self-administer this method for pain relief.

- **Massage therapy:** In this therapy, a specialist applies very mild/gentle pressure to the affected areas with slow circular motions or a deep kneading motion to the affected areas using fingertips. This relieves pain and relaxes stiffness. Deep massages should not be done near the spine of a person with spinal osteoporosis; instead, a light circular massage will provide the best pain relief.

Relaxation Training

This training involves slow and deep breathing. Learning to relax takes practice, but keeps us focused. Relaxation training releases tension from our muscles and reduces pain.

- **Biofeedback:** With the use of special machines, the professional teaches you how to release muscle tension. If you release the tension, the machine automatically indicates success. Once you master the technique, you can practice this method without the machine.

- **Visual imagery:** This training involves repeating positive words or phrases or concentrating on pleasant events or happy scenes, which helps to reduce the pain. Recordings are available to help you learn this skill.

Distraction Techniques

- **Distraction:** You can distract your mind with some behavioral and lifestyle changes such as listening to music, reading a book, watching a movie, and so on.

- **Hypnotherapy:** Hypnosis reduces the perception of pain and is performed by a therapist who offers posthypnotic suggestions that reduce pain. The therapist can also teach you to use self-hypnosis to hypnotize yourself for pain reduction.

- **Individual, group, or family talk therapy:** Often people with chronic pain experience stress, depression, and emotional imbalance. To overcome these feelings, which influence pain, you can undergo individual, family, or group meditation therapy to help manage your pain.

No treatment can reverse established osteoporosis, medical professionals can halt its progression, and work with you to manage the pain that accompanies your condition.

References

1. "What You Should Know about Osteoporosis Meds," WebMD, October 9, 2018.

2. Watson, James C. "Treatment of Pain," MSD Manual Professional Version, August 2018.

3. Bethel, Monique. "Osteoporosis Treatment and Management," emedicine, Medscape, July 19, 2018.

4. Paolucci, Teresa; Saraceni, Vincenzo Maria; Piccinini, Giulia. "Management of Chronic Pain in Osteoporosis: Challenge and Solutions," National Center for Biotechnology Information (NCBI), April 1, 2016.

Chapter 55

Behavioral and Relaxation Techniques for Chronic Pain and Insomnia

Pain

Pain is defined by the International Association for the Study of Pain as an unpleasant sensory and emotional experience associated with actual or potential tissue damage or described in terms of such damage. It is a complex, subjective, perceptual phenomenon with a number of contributing factors that are uniquely experienced by each individual. Pain is typically classified as acute, cancer-related, and chronic nonmalignant. Acute pain is associated with a noxious event. Its severity is generally proportional to the degree of tissue injury and is expected to diminish with healing and time. Cancer-related pain presents with acute episodes plus the circumstances of chronic pain because of its duration and the psychological issues inherent with malignant disease. Chronic nonmalignant pain frequently develops following an injury but persists long after a reasonable period

This chapter includes text excerpted from "Integration of Behavioral and Relaxation Approaches into the Treatment of Chronic Pain and Insomnia," National Institutes of Health Consensus Development Program, Integration of Behavioral and Relaxation Approaches into the Treatment of Chronic Pain and Insomnia, NIH Technology Assessment Statement Online, October 16–18, 1995 [cited January 2019], 4–8. Reviewed January 2019.

of healing. Its underlying causes may not be readily discernible, and the pain is disproportionate to demonstrable tissue damage. It is frequently accompanied by alteration of sleep; mood; and sexual, vocational, and avocational function.

Insomnia

Insomnia may be defined as a disturbance or perceived disturbance of the usual sleep pattern of the individual that has troublesome consequences. These consequences may include daytime fatigue and drowsiness, irritability, anxiety, depression, and somatic complaints. Categories of disturbed sleep are:

- Inability to fall asleep
- Inability to maintain sleep
- Early awakening

Relaxation Techniques

Relaxation techniques are a group of behavioral therapeutic approaches that differ widely in their philosophical bases as well as in their methodologies and techniques. Their primary objective is the achievement of nondirected relaxation, rather than direct achievement of a specific therapeutic goal. They all share two basic components:

1. Repetitive focus on a word, sound, prayer, phrase, body sensation, or muscular activity

2. The adoption of a passive attitude toward intruding thoughts and a return to the focus

These techniques induce a common set of physiologic changes that result in decreased metabolic activity. Relaxation techniques may also be used in stress management (as self-regulatory techniques) and have been divided into deep and brief methods.

Deep Methods

Deep methods include autogenic training, meditation, and progressive muscle relaxation (PMR). Autogenic training consists of imagining a peaceful environment and comforting bodily sensations. Six basic focusing techniques are used: heaviness in the limbs, warmth in the limbs, cardiac regulation, centering on breathing, warmth in the upper abdomen, and coolness in the forehead. Meditation is a self-directed practice for relaxing the body and calming the mind. A large variety of meditation techniques are in common use; each has its own proponents. Meditation generally does not involve suggestion, autosuggestion, or trance. The goal of mindfulness meditation is development of a nonjudgmental awareness of bodily sensations and mental activities occurring in the present moment. Concentration meditation trains the person to passively attend to a bodily process, a word, and/or a stimulus. Transcendental meditation focuses on a "suitable" sound or thought (the mantra) without attempting to actually concentrate on the sound or thought. There are also many movement meditations, such as yoga and the walking meditation of Zen Buddhism. PMR focuses on reducing muscle tone in major muscle groups. Each of 15 major muscle groups is tensed and then relaxed in sequence.

Hypnotic Techniques

Hypnotic techniques induce states of selective attentional focusing or diffusion combined with enhanced imagery. They are often used to induce relaxation and also may be a part of cognitive-behavioral therapy (CBT). The techniques have pre- and post-suggestion components. The post-suggestion component involves attentional focusing through the use of imagery, distraction, or relaxation, and has features that are similar to other relaxation techniques. Subjects focus on relaxation and passively disregard intrusive thoughts. The suggestion phase is characterized by introduction of specific goals; for example, analgesia may be specifically suggested. The postsuggestion component involves continued use of the new behavior following termination of hypnosis. Individuals vary widely in their hypnotic susceptibility and suggestibility, although the reasons for these differences are incompletely understood.

Cognitive-Behavioral Therapy

Cognitive-behavioral therapy (CBT) attempts to alter patterns of negative thoughts and dysfunctional attitudes in order to foster more healthy and adaptive thoughts, emotions, and actions. These interventions share four basic components: education, skills acquisition, cognitive and behavioral rehearsal, and generalization and maintenance. Relaxation techniques are frequently included as a behavioral component in CBT programs. The specific programs used to implement the four components can vary considerably. Each of the aforementioned therapeutic modalities may be practiced individually, or they may be combined in multimodal approaches to manage chronic pain or insomnia.

Relaxation and Behavioral Techniques for Insomnia

Relaxation and behavioral techniques corresponding to those used for chronic pain may also be used for specific types of insomnia. Cognitive relaxation, various forms of biofeedback, and progressive muscle relaxation may all be used to treat insomnia. In addition, the following behavioral approaches are generally used to manage insomnia:

- **Sleep hygiene,** which involves educating patients about behaviors that may interfere with the sleep process, with the hope that education about maladaptive behaviors will lead to behavioral modification.

- **Stimulus control therapy,** which seeks to create and protect a conditioned association between the bedroom and sleep. Activities in the bedroom are usually restricted to sleep and sex.

- **Sleep restriction therapy,** in which patients provide a sleep log and are then asked to stay in bed only as long as they think they are currently sleeping. This usually leads to sleep deprivation and consolidation, which may be followed by a gradual increase in the length of time in bed.

- **Paradoxical intention,** in which the patient is instructed not to fall asleep, with the expectation that efforts to avoid sleep will in fact induce it.

Chapter 56

Osteoporosis Medicines Risks

Chapter Contents

Section 56.1

Usage of Reclast and Kidney Impairment

This section includes text excerpted from "FDA Drug Safety
Communication: New Contraindication and Updated Warning on
Kidney Impairment for Reclast (Zoledronic Acid)," U.S. Food and
Drug Administration (FDA), February 8, 2018.

The U.S. Food and Drug Administration (FDA) has approved an
update to the drug label for Reclast (zoledronic acid) to better inform
healthcare professionals and patients of the risk of kidney (renal)
failure. Kidney failure is a rare, but serious, condition associated
with the use of Reclast in patients with a history of or risk factors
for renal impairment. Cases of acute renal failure requiring dialysis
or having a fatal outcome following Reclast use have been reported
to FDA.

These labeling changes are being made to the Reclast label only,
although zoledronic acid, also sold as Zometa, is approved for treatment of cancer-related indications. Renal toxicity is already addressed
in the "Warnings and Precautions" section of the Zometa label, as well
as in the Reclast label. Dose reductions for Zometa are provided for
patients with renal impairment.

Risk factors for developing renal failure include underlying moderate-to-severe renal impairment, use of kidney-damaging (nephro-
toxic) or diuretic medications at the same time as Reclast, or severe
dehydration occurring before or after Reclast is given. The risk of
developing renal failure in patients with underlying renal impairment
also increases with age.

The revised drug label will enhance the safe use of Reclast by providing healthcare professionals updated instructions for prescribing
and patient monitoring. The revised label states that Reclast should
not be used (is contraindicated) in patients with creatinine clearance
of less than 35 mL/min or in patients with evidence of acute renal
impairment. The label also recommends that healthcare professionals screen patients prior to administering Reclast in order to identify
at-risk patients. Healthcare professionals should also monitor renal
function in patients who are receiving Reclast.

"The Reclast Medication Guide" for patients is being updated to contain information about the risk of severe kidney problems. In addition,
the manufacturer of Reclast will issue a "Dear Healthcare Provider"
letter to inform healthcare professionals about this risk.

Additional Information for Patients

- Kidney failure is a rare, but serious, side effect associated with the use of Reclast.

- Your healthcare professional will order a serum creatinine level (a blood test) before and after each dose of Reclast to assess how well your kidneys are functioning.

- If you have kidney disease, discuss the necessity of Reclast treatment with your healthcare professional. There may be other treatment choices available to you.

- Make sure your healthcare professional knows about all the medications you are taking. It is helpful to keep a list of all your current medications in your wallet or another location where it is easily retrieved.

- Report any side effects with Reclast to the FDA's MedWatch program using the information at the bottom of the page in the "Contact Us" box.

Section 56.2

Risk of Esophageal Cancer

This section includes text excerpted from "FDA Drug Safety
Communication: Ongoing Safety Review of Oral Osteoporosis Drugs
(Bisphosphonates) and Potential Increased Risk of Esophageal
Cancer," U.S. Food and Drug Administration (FDA), August 4, 2017.

The U.S. Food and Drug Administration (FDA) is continuing to review data from published studies to evaluate whether use of oral bisphosphonate drugs is associated with an increased risk of cancer of the esophagus (esophageal cancer). There have been conflicting findings from studies evaluating this risk.

At this time, the FDA believes that the benefits of oral bisphosphonate drugs in reducing the risk of serious fractures in people with osteoporosis continue to outweigh their potential risks.

The FDA's review is ongoing and the agency has not concluded that patients taking oral bisphosphonate drugs have an increased risk of esophageal cancer. It is also important to note that esophageal cancer is rare, especially in women.

The largest studies that the FDA has reviewed thus far are two epidemiologic studies using one patient database (the U.K. General Practice Research Database, or GPRD). One study found no increase in the risk of esophageal cancer. The second study found a doubling of the risk of esophageal cancer among patients who had 10 or more prescriptions of the drugs, or who had taken the drugs over 3 years. Other external researchers investigating this issue, using different patient databases, have reported no increase in risk, or reduced risk.

Patients should talk with their healthcare professionals about the benefits and risks of taking oral bisphosphonates. Patients who take oral bisphosphonates should pay particular attention to the directions for use to minimize any potential adverse events.

Additional Information for Patients

- There is conflicting information on whether oral bisphosphonate drugs can affect your chance of developing esophageal cancer.

- Directions for use of the oral bisphosphonate drug should be followed carefully. All oral bisphosphonate drugs, except Atelvia, should be taken first thing in the morning after awakening, with a full glass of plain water. Atelvia should be taken immediately following breakfast. Do not lie down or eat or drink anything for at least 30 to 60 minutes after taking any oral bisphosphonate drug.

- Talk to your healthcare professional if you develop swallowing difficulties, chest pain, new or worsening heartburn, or have trouble or pain when you swallow. These may be signs of problems of the esophagus.

- You should not take oral bisphosphonates if you have esophageal conditions that delay emptying of the esophagus, or if you cannot stand or sit upright for at least 30 to 60 minutes, or have low calcium levels in your blood.

- Talk to your healthcare professional about the benefits and risks of taking oral bisphosphonates and how long you should expect to take them.

- Discuss any questions or concerns about your oral bisphosphonate drug with your healthcare professional.

- Report any side effects you experience to the FDA MedWatch program using the information in the "Contact Us" box at the bottom of the page.

Chapter 57

Physical Activity and Exercises: Managing Osteogenesis Imperfecta

Osteogenesis imperfecta (OI) is a connective-tissue disorder characterized by fragile bones, weak muscles, and loose ligaments. Bone problems can include bowing of the long bones, scoliosis (curvature of the spine), a barrel chest, and joint problems. Varying degrees of short stature and decreased muscle mass and strength also may be present.

Not so long ago, parents were advised to "protect" their children with this disorder by carrying them on pillows and avoiding recreational activities. But this well-intentioned approach did not protect children from fractures (broken bones) and may have hindered their development and achievement of independent functioning.

Bone growth depends on muscle pull as well as loading (weight-bearing) through standing, walking, and lifting. Immobilization may result in loss of muscle and skeletal mass. It can take as long as a year to restore this bone mass following a relatively short period of

This chapter includes text excerpted from "Exercise and Activity: Key Elements in the Management of Osteogenesis imperfecta (OI)," NIH Osteoporosis and Related Bone Diseases—National Resource Center (NIH ORBD—NRC), May 2015. Reviewed January 2019.

immobilization. Over the years, it has become clear that physical activity is an important part of managing OI in both children and adults.

Research indicates that physical activity is important because it promotes:

- General health through
- Cardiovascular fitness
- Mental alertness
- Weight control
- Improved sleep quality
- Improved ability to handle infection
- Reduced risk for some cancers
- Maximum bone density
- Optimal physical function to support independence in daily activities
- Optimal psychological and social well-being by improving self-confidence and the ability to interact socially with peers

Children and adults with OI will benefit from a regular program of physical activity to promote optimal function through muscle strengthening, aerobic exercise, and recreational pursuits. Specifics of the exercise program vary depending on the person's age, level of function, the severity of OI, and needs and desires. A well-designed program can combine activities to prevent problems as well as to restore function.

Activity programs may include specific exercises recommended by rehabilitation professionals (physiatrists, physical therapists, occupational therapists, and recreation therapists) as well as sports and other recreational activities. Having fun and feeling a sense of accomplishment are legitimate goals for an exercise program. In addition, diet, weight control, and commitment to a healthy lifestyle are essential to longevity and an improved quality of life (QOL).

The optimal long-term goal for children with OI is good health and independence in all areas of function (social, educational, self-care, locomotion, and recreation), using adaptive devices as needed. Goals for adults with OI include maintaining independence, preserving bone density, and supporting cardiovascular function. To achieve these goals, it is often necessary to improve muscle strength and body alignment.

When to Begin

The first year of life includes many motor-skill transitions and is a critical window of opportunity for babies who are born with muscle weakness, alignment problems, and fragility. Physical therapy should begin as soon as the infant exhibits weakness or motor-skill delays when compared with other infants of the same age. This might be first noticed because the baby cannot hold up his or her head independently or sit without support until later than most other children.

Treatments for such problems are often aimed at proper positioning and placing children in positions that encourage their use of certain muscle groups. Proper positioning elicits specific antigravity muscular effort, which is the basis for learning to sit and later on stand. Babies with large heads will face additional challenges and limitations in developing the ability to move against gravity.

An infant or child with weakness or motor-skill delays should be working for brief periods daily or at least five days a week to improve muscle strength and motor skills. In the process, the child gains endurance and independence in self-care activities. Treatment should not be confined to "therapy hours" only. Very short exercise efforts during the day, as short as five minutes, will often result in improvement more quickly than an hour-long session once or twice a week.

Depending on the child's age, the interventions can take several forms, including positioning, specific exercises, and developmental activities (such as standing in a standing device). Ideally, family members and care providers would integrate the activities naturally into the child's day. Playtime can be purposeful, but it should still be fun for both the parent and the child.

Children with OI can excel in the water, particularly if the activity is presented as an opportunity for recreation and independent exploration, rather than a demand to exercise. Water exercise can begin during infancy, with the child lying on her or his back in two to three inches of warm water to promote independent kicking. Over time, the child can progress to independent activity in the water, first in a swim vest or other support, and then swimming without support. Walking in the water may be possible for individuals who are unable to walk outside the pool. Water activities in childhood can be the foundation for a lifelong, enjoyable fitness activity.

Adults with OI can benefit from water activity as well. It is an excellent form of aerobic conditioning and may have some benefit with respect to strengthening. Because water activities do little to promote bone health, however, adults also should try to add walking or other weight-bearing exercises to their physical activity program.

Safety

People of any age who have OI can safely exercise. Obstacles to consider when evaluating an activity include prior fracture history, the degree of bending of long bones, degree of muscle weakness, joint stiffness or laxity (looseness), joint alignment, poor exercise tolerance, and lack of stamina. Inability to accomplish daily activities without specialized equipment also can affect which activities can be done safely. For example, long-term sitting in a wheelchair may be associated with hip flexion contractures and compensatory back curvatures, which often are associated with back pain, joint stiffness, osteoporosis, and obesity. A safe physical activity program would include getting out of the chair and changing body positions at least every two hours when possible.

People who have OI should avoid some activities. These include jumping, diving, and contact sports, as well as activities that promote falls, abrupt joint compressions, or high-rotary (twisting) forces on bones.

Steps for Developing a Successful Exercise Program at Any Age

1. Determine the person's capabilities by asking: "What can the child or adult do?"

2. Determine the goal you want to pursue by asking: "What is the child or adult trying to achieve?"

3. Determine the constraints or limitations to achieving the goal by asking: "Is limited range of motion, strength, alignment, or joint instability preventing successful performance?" These limitations may have to be addressed before the goal can be accomplished, perhaps by modifying the exercise program.

4. Determine which equipment or treatments are available to help accomplish the goal. A wide range of devices can support improved function. Examples include bathroom safety equipment, walking aids, and devices for reaching objects in high or low places. A consultation with an occupational therapist may be necessary to help choose the best devices to accomplish a specific goal.

450

It's Never Too Late to Begin

Adults and older children who do not exercise are encouraged to make a new commitment to a healthy lifestyle and become more physically active. They should include enjoyable exercises that will improve strength, balance, and endurance and, if possible, promote socialization. Rehabilitation specialists or exercise specialists who are familiar with OI or osteoporosis can help design an appropriate program. Enjoyment plus improved function can be found through physical activity at every age.

Chapter 58

How to Prevent Falls and Improve Your Balance

A simple thing can change your life—like tripping on a rug or slipping on a wet floor. If you fall, you could break a bone, as thousands of older men and women do each year. For older people, a break can be the start of more serious problems, such as a trip to the hospital, injury, or even disability.

If you or an older person you know has fallen, you're not alone. More than one in three people age 65 years or older fall each year. The risk of falling—and fall-related problems—increases with age.

Many Older Adults Fear Falling

The fear of falling becomes more common as people age, even among those who haven't fallen. It may lead older people to avoid activities such as walking, shopping, or taking part in social activities.

But don't let a fear of falling keep you from being active. Overcoming this fear can help you stay active, maintain your physical health, and prevent future falls. Doing things such as getting together with

This chapter contains text excerpted from the following sources: Text in this chapter begins with excerpts from "Prevent Falls and Fractures," National Institute on Aging (NIA), National Institutes of Health (NIH), March 15, 2017; Text under the heading "Exercises to Prevent Falls and Improve Your Balance" is excerpted from "How to Prevent Falls and Improve Your Balance," *Go4Life*, National Institutes of Health (NIH), August 17, 2018.

friends, gardening, walking, or going to the local senior center helps you stay healthy. The good news is that there are simple ways to prevent most falls.

Causes and Risk Factors for Falls

Many things can cause a fall. Your eyesight, hearing, and reflexes might not be as sharp as they were when you were younger. Diabetes, heart disease, or problems with your thyroid, nerves, feet, or blood vessels can affect your balance. Some medicines can cause you to feel dizzy or sleepy, making you more likely to fall. Other causes include safety hazards in the home or community environment.

Scientists have linked several personal-risk factors to falling, including muscle weakness, problems with balance and gait, and blood pressure that drops too much when you get up from lying down or sitting (called postural hypotension). Foot problems that cause pain and unsafe footwear, such as backless shoes or high heels, can also increase your risk of falling.

Confusion can sometimes lead to falls. For example, if you wake up in an unfamiliar environment, you might feel unsure of where you are. If you feel confused, wait for your mind to clear or until someone comes to help you before trying to get up and walk around.

Some medications can increase a person's risk of falling because they cause side effects such as dizziness or confusion. The more medications you take, the more likely you are to fall.

Take the Right Steps to Prevent Falls

If you take care of your overall health, you may be able to lower your chances of falling. Most of the time falls and accidents don't "just happen." Here are a few tips to help you avoid falls and broken bones:

- **Stay physically active.** Plan an exercise program that is right for you. Regular exercise improves muscles and makes you stronger. It also helps keep your joints, tendons, and ligaments flexible. Mild weight-bearing activities, such as walking or climbing stairs, may slow bone loss from osteoporosis.

- **Have your eyes and hearing tested.** Even small changes in sight and hearing may cause you to fall. When you get new eyeglasses or contact lenses, take time to get used to them. Always wear your glasses or contacts when you need them. If you have a hearing aid, be sure it fits well and wear it.

- **Find out about the side effects of any medicine you take.** If a drug makes you sleepy or dizzy, tell your doctor or pharmacist.

- **Get enough sleep.** If you are sleepy, you are more likely to fall.

- **Limit the amount of alcohol you drink.** Even a small amount of alcohol can affect your balance and reflexes. Studies show that the rate of hip fractures in older adults increases with alcohol use.

- **Stand up slowly.** Getting up too quickly can cause your blood pressure to drop. That can make you feel wobbly. Get your blood pressure checked when lying and standing.

- **Use an assistive device if you need help feeling steady when you walk.** Appropriate use of canes and walkers can prevent falls. If your doctor tells you to use a cane or walker, make sure it is the right size for you and the wheels roll smoothly. This is important when you're walking in areas you don't know well or where the walkways are uneven. A physical or occupational therapist can help you decide which devices might be helpful and teach you how to use them safely.

- **Be very careful when walking on wet or icy surfaces.** They can be very slippery! Try to have sand or salt spread on icy areas by your front or back door.

- **Wear nonskid, rubber-soled, low-heeled shoes, or lace-up shoes with nonskid soles that fully support your feet.** It is important that the soles are not too thin or too thick. Don't walk on stairs or floors in socks or in shoes and slippers with smooth soles.

- **Always tell your doctor if you have fallen since your last checkup, even if you aren't hurt when you fall.** A fall can alert your doctor to a new medical problem or problems with your medications or eyesight that can be corrected. Your doctor may suggest physical therapy, a walking aid, or other steps to help prevent future falls.

Keep Your Bones Strong to Prevent Falls

Falls are a common reason for trips to the emergency room and for hospital stays among older adults. Many of these hospital visits are for fall-related fractures. You can help prevent fractures by keeping your bones strong.

Having healthy bones won't prevent a fall, but if you fall, it might prevent breaking a hip or other bone, which may lead to a hospital or nursing home stay, disability, or even death. Getting enough calcium and vitamin D can help keep your bones strong. So can physical activity. Try to get at least 150 minutes per week of physical activity.

Other ways to maintain bone health include quitting smoking and limiting alcohol use, which can decrease bone mass and increase the chance of fractures. Also, try to maintain a healthy weight. Being underweight increases the risk of bone loss and broken bones.

Osteoporosis is a disease that makes bones weak and more likely to break. For people with osteoporosis, even a minor fall may be dangerous. Talk to your doctor about osteoporosis.

Exercises to Prevent Falls and Improve Your Balance

Balance exercises can help you prevent falls and avoid the disability that may result from falling. You can do balance exercises almost anytime, anywhere, and as often as you like, as long as you have something sturdy nearby to hold on to for support.

Try these balance exercises:

- Stand on one foot, walk heel to toe, and walk in a straight line with one foot in front of the other.

- A number of lower-body strengthening exercises—especially those that strengthen your legs and ankles—also can help improve your balance. These include the back-leg raise, side-leg raise, knee curl, and toe-stand exercises.

In the beginning, using a chair or the wall for support will help you work on your balance safely.

Part Seven

Additional Help and Information

Chapter 59

Glossary of Important Terms

absorption: The process of taking in. For a person or an animal, absorption is the process of a substance getting into the body through the eyes, skin, stomach, intestines, or lungs.

acquired immunodeficiency syndrome (AIDS): A disease caused by the human immunodeficiency virus (HIV). People with AIDS are at an increased risk for developing certain cancers and for infections that usually occur only in individuals with a weak immune system.

acupuncture: The technique of inserting thin needles through the skin at specific points on the body to control pain and other symptoms. It is a type of complementary and alternative medicine.

acute pain: Pain that comes on quickly, can be severe, but lasts a relatively short time.

adverse effect: An unexpected medical problem that happens during treatment with a drug or other therapy. Adverse effects may be mild, moderate, or severe, and may be caused by something other than the drug or therapy being given. Also called adverse event.

This glossary contains terms excerpted from documents produced by several sources deemed reliable.

alcohol: A chemical substance found in drinks such as beer, wine, and liquor. It is also found in some medicines, mouthwashes, household products, and essential oils (scented liquid taken from certain plants). It is made by a chemical process called fermentation that uses sugars and yeast.

allergen: A substance that causes an allergic response. Examples include pollen, molds, and certain foods.

amenorrhea: The abnormal absence of menstrual periods. Early amenorrhea caused by overtraining can cause bones to become brittle and break.

amino acid: One of several molecules that join together to form proteins. There are 20 common amino acids found in proteins.

analgesics: A group of medications that reduce pain.

anemia: A condition in which the number of red blood cells is below normal.

anesthetic: A drug that causes insensitivity to pain and is used for surgeries and other medical procedures.

antibiotic: A drug used to treat infections caused by bacteria and other microorganisms.

anxiety: Feelings of fear, dread, and uneasiness that may occur as a reaction to stress. A person with anxiety may sweat, feel restless and tense, and have a rapid heartbeat.

arthritis: A general term for conditions that cause inflammation (swelling) of the joints and surrounding tissues. Some forms of arthritis may occur simultaneously with osteoporosis and Paget disease.

aspiration: The removal of fluid or tissue through a needle. Also, the accidental breathing in of food or fluid into the lungs.

assessment: The process of gathering evidence and documentation of a student's learning.

assistive device: Tools that enable individuals with disabilities to perform essential job functions, e.g., telephone headsets, adapted computer keyboards, and enhanced computer monitors.

asthma: A chronic disease in which the bronchial airways in the lungs become narrowed and swollen, making it difficult to breathe. Symptoms include wheezing, coughing, tightness in the chest, shortness of breath, and rapid breathing.

autoimmune disease: A condition in which the body recognizes its own tissues as foreign and directs an immune response against them.

backbone: The bones, muscles, tendons, and other tissues that reach from the base of the skull to the tailbone. The backbone encloses the spinal cord and the fluid surrounding the spinal cord. Also called spinal column, spine, and vertebral column.

bacteria: A large group of single-cell microorganisms. Some cause infections and disease in animals and humans.

bisphosphonates: Drugs used to treat osteoporosis and other bone diseases.

blood: A tissue with red blood cells (RBCs), white blood cells (WBCs), platelets, and other substances suspended in fluid called plasma. Blood takes oxygen and nutrients to the tissues, and carries away wastes.

bone: A living, growing tissue made mostly of collagen.

bone biopsy: A test in which a small sample of tissue for analysis is taken from bone.

bone marrow: The soft, sponge-like tissue in the center of most bones. It produces white blood cells, red blood cells, and platelets.

bone mass: A measure of the amount of minerals (mostly calcium and phosphorous) contained in a certain volume of bone. Bone mass measurements are used to diagnose osteoporosis (a condition marked by decreased bone mass), to see how well osteoporosis treatments are working, and to predict how likely the bones are to break.

bone mineral density (BMD) testing: A test that measures bone strength and fracture risk.

bone remodeling: The process of bone renewal through resorption (where old bone is removed from the skeleton) and formation (where new bone is added to the skeleton).

bone scan: A nuclear scanning test primarily used to help diagnose a number of conditions relating to bones including Paget disease.

breast cancer: A disease in which abnormal tumor cells develop in the breast. Women who have had breast cancer may be at increased risk for osteoporosis and fracture because of possible reduced levels of estrogen, chemotherapy or surgery, or early menopause.

breastbone: The long flat bone that forms the center front of the chest wall. The breastbone is attached to the collarbone and the first seven ribs. Also called sternum.

bypass: A surgical procedure in which the doctor creates a new pathway for the flow of body fluids.

calcitonin: A hormone involved in calcium regulation that is used to treat osteoporosis and Paget disease (PD).

calcium: A mineral that is an essential nutrient for bone health. It is also needed for the heart, muscles, and nerves to function properly and for blood to clot.

calorie: A measurement of the energy content of food. The body needs calories as to perform its functions, such as breathing, circulating the blood, and physical activity. When a person is sick, their body may need extra calories to fight fever or other problems.

cancer: A term for diseases in which abnormal cells divide without control and can invade nearby tissues.

carbohydrate: A sugar molecule. Carbohydrates can be small and simple (for example, glucose) or they can be large and complex (for example, polysaccharides such as starch, chitin or cellulose).

celiac disease: An inherited intestinal disorder in which the body cannot tolerate gluten, which is found in foods made with wheat, rye, and barley. Bone loss is a complication of untreated celiac disease.

chromosome: A chromosome is an organized package of deoxyribonucleic acid (DNA) found in the nucleus of the cell. Different organisms have different numbers of chromosomes. Humans have 23 pairs of chromosomes—22 pairs of numbered chromosomes, called autosomes, and one pair of sex chromosomes, X and Y.

chronic disease: A disease that has one or more of the following characteristics: is permanent; leaves residual disability; is caused by nonreversible pathological alternation; requires special training of the patient for rehabilitation; or may be expected to require a long period of supervision, observation, or care.

chronic pain: Pain that can range from mild to severe, and persists or progresses over a long period of time.

collagen: A family of fibrous proteins that are components of osteogenesis imperfecta is caused by a genetic defect that affects the body's production of collagen.

computed tomography (CT) scan: A procedure that uses a computer linked to an X-ray machine to make a series of detailed pictures of areas inside the body. The pictures are taken from different angles and are used to create 3-dimensional (3-D) views of tissues and organs.

constipation: A decrease in frequency of stools or bowel movements with hardening of the stool. Some forms of osteogenesis imperfecta are associated with increased risk for constipation caused by increased perspiration, growth impairment, pelvic malformation, and diminished physical activity.

contracture: A permanent tightening of the muscles, tendons, skin, and nearby tissues that causes the joints to shorten and become very stiff. This prevents normal movement of a joint or other body part.

diabetes: A disease in which the body does not produce or properly use insulin. Insulin is a hormone that is needed to convert sugar, starches, and other food into energy. Having diabetes may increase osteoporosis risk.

diet: What a person eats and drinks. Any type of eating plan.

dual-energy X-ray absorptiometry (DXA): A common test for measuring bone mineral density. It is painless, a bit like having an X-ray, but with much less exposure to radiation.

endocrine: Refers to tissue that makes and releases hormones that travel in the bloodstream and control the actions of other cells or organs. Some examples of endocrine tissues are the pituitary, thyroid, and adrenal glands.

endocrinologist: A doctor who treats the endocrine system, which are the glands and hormones that help control the body's metabolic activity. In addition to osteoporosis, endocrinologists treat diabetes and diseases of the thyroid and pituitary glands.

enzyme: A protein that speeds up chemical reactions in the body.

estrogen therapy: The use of the female hormone estrogen (sometimes combined with another hormone, progestin) to treat osteoporosis.

estrogen: A type of hormone made by the body that helps develop and maintain female sex characteristics and the growth of long bones.

exercise: A type of physical activity that involves planned, structured, and repetitive bodily movement done to maintain or improve one or more components of physical fitness.

463

family doctors: Doctors who have a broad range of training that includes internal medicine, gynecology, and pediatrics. They place special emphasis on caring for an individual or family on a long-term, continuing basis.

fracture: Broken bone. People with osteoporosis, osteogenesis imperfecta, and Paget disease are at greater risk for bone fracture.

geriatricians: Family doctors or internists who have received additional training on the aging process and the conditions and diseases that often occur among the elderly.

glucocorticoids: Steroid medications such as prednisone or cortisone used to reduce inflammation in many diseases. Bone loss is a very common side effect of these medications.

gynecologist: A doctor who diagnoses and treats conditions of the female reproductive system and associated disorders.

hypercalciuria: A disorder in which an excessive amount of calcium is lost through the urine.

hypogonadism: Abnormally low levels of sex hormone. Low levels of testosterone is sometimes a secondary cause of osteoporosis in men.

idiopathic: No identifiable cause. Osteoporosis may be characterized as idiopathic, particularly in children and men.

immune system: A complex system of cellular and molecular components having the primary function of distinguishing self from not-self and defense against foreign organisms or substances.

immunoglobulin: A protein that is made by B cells and plasma cells (types of white blood cells) and helps the body fight infection.

inflammatory bowel disease (IBD): Diseases, including ulcerative colitis and Crohn disease, that cause swelling in the intestine and/or digestive tract, which may result in diarrhea, abdominal pain, fever, and weight loss. People with IBD are at an increased risk for osteoporosis.

internist: A doctor trained in general internal medicine. These doctors diagnose and treat many diseases.

juvenile osteoporosis: Osteoporosis in children and adolescents.

lactose intolerance: Inability to digest lactose, the natural sugar found in milk and other dairy products. Individuals with lactose intolerance who avoid dairy products may be at increased risk for osteoporosis.

lesion: An area of abnormal tissue. A lesion may be benign (not cancer) or malignant (cancer).

lupus: A chronic inflammatory disease that occurs when the body's immune system attacks its own tissues and organs. Also called systemic lupus erythematosus (SLE). Inflammation caused by lupus can affect many different body systems including joints, skin, kidneys, blood cells, heart, and lungs. People with lupus are at increased risk for osteoporosis.

magnetic resonance imaging (MRI): A procedure in which radio waves and a powerful magnet linked to a computer are used to create detailed pictures of areas inside the body. These pictures can show the difference between normal and diseased tissue.

menopause: The cessation of menstruation in women. Bone health in women often deteriorates after menopause due to a decrease in the female hormone estrogen.

metabolism: The chemical changes that take place in a cell or an organism. These changes make energy and the materials cells and organisms need to grow, reproduce, and stay healthy. Metabolism also helps get rid of toxic substances.

mitosis: The process by which a single parent cell divides to make two new daughter cells. Each daughter cell receives a complete set of chromosomes from the parent cell. This process allows the body to grow and replace cells.

mutation: A change (damage) to the DNA, genes, or chromosomes of living organisms.

nonsteroidal anti-inflammatory drugs (NSAIDs): A class of medications available over the counter or with a prescription that ease pain and inflammation. Includes aspirin, ibuprofen, and naproxen.

organ: A part of the body that performs a specific function. For example, the heart is an organ.

orthopedist: A doctor who specializes in bone and joint disorders.

orthopedic surgeons: Doctors trained in the care of patients with musculoskeletal conditions such as congenital skeletal malformations, bone fractures and infections, and metabolic problems.

osteogenesis imperfecta (OI): Osteogenesis imperfecta is a genetic disorder characterized by bones that break easily, often from little or no apparent cause.

osteomalacia: A condition in adults in which bones become soft and deformed because they don't have enough calcium and phosphorus. It is usually caused by not having enough vitamin D in the diet, not getting enough sunlight, or a problem with the way the body uses vitamin D.

osteopenia: Low bone mass.

osteoporosis: Literally means "porous bone." This disease is characterized by too little bone formation, excessive bone loss, or a combination of both, leading to bone fragility and an increased risk of fractures of the hip, spine and wrist.

osteosarcoma: A cancer of the bone that usually affects the large bones of the arm or leg. It occurs most commonly in young people and affects more males than females. Also called osteogenic sarcoma.

outpatient: A patient who visits a healthcare facility for diagnosis or treatment without spending the night. Sometimes called a day patient.

over-the-counter (OTC): Refers to a medicine that can be bought without a prescription (doctor's order). Examples include analgesics (pain relievers), such as aspirin and acetaminophen. Also called nonprescription and OTC.

overweight: Overweight refers to an excessive amount of body weight that includes muscle, bone, fat, and water. A person who has a body mass index (BMI) of 25 to 29.9 [see body mass index] is considered overweight.

Paget disease of bone: A bone disease that causes bones to grow larger and weaker than normal.

parathyroid hormone: A form of human parathyroid hormone (PTH) is approved for the treatment of osteoporosis.

peak bone mass: The amount of bone tissue in the skeleton. Bone tissue can keep growing until around age 30. At that point, bones have reached their maximum strength and density, known as peak bone mass.

periodontitis: A chronic infection that affects the gums and the bones that support the teeth. Bacteria and the body's own immune system break down the bone and connective tissue that hold teeth in place. Teeth may eventually become loose, fall out, or have to be removed.

physiatrists: Doctors who specialize in physical medicine and rehabilitation. They evaluate and treat patients with impairments, disabilities, or pain arising from various medical problems, including bone fractures. Physiatrists focus on restoring the physical, psychological, social, and vocational functioning of the individual.

physical activity: Any bodily movement that is produced by the contraction of skeletal muscle and that substantially increases energy expenditure.

prevention: Actions that reduce exposure or other risks, keep people from getting sick, or keep disease from getting worse.

prognosis: The likely outcome or course of a disease; the chance of recovery or recurrence.

prostate cancer: A disease in which abnormal tumor cells develop in the prostate gland. Men who receive hormone deprivation therapy for prostate cancer have an increased risk of developing osteoporosis and broken bones.

protein: A molecule made up of amino acids. Proteins are needed for the body to function properly. They are the basis of body structures, such as skin and hair, and of other substances such as enzymes, cytokines, and antibodies.

radiation: Energy released in the form of particle or electromagnetic waves. Common sources of radiation include radon gas, cosmic rays from outer space, medical X-rays, and energy given off by a radioisotope (unstable form of a chemical element that releases radiation as it breaks down and becomes more stable). Radiation can damage cells.

receptor activator of nuclear factor kappa-β ligand (RANKL) inhibitors: A type of drug approved for the treatment of osteoporosis.

rheumatoid arthritis (RA): An inflammatory disease that causes pain, swelling, stiffness, and loss of function in the joints. It occurs when the immune system, which normally defends the body from invading organisms, attacks the membrane lining the joints. Studies have found an increased risk of bone loss and fracture in individuals with RA.

sclerosis: A hardening within the nervous system, especially of the brain and spinal cord, resulting from degeneration of nervous elements such as the myelin sheath.

secondary osteoporosis: Osteoporosis caused by an underlying medical disorder or by medications used to treat the disorder.

selective estrogen receptor modulator (SERM): A type of drug used to prevent or treat postmenopausal osteoporosis.

sodium: A mineral and an essential nutrient needed by the human body in relatively small amounts (provided that substantial sweating does not occur).

steroid: Any of a group of lipids (fats) that have a certain chemical structure. Steroids occur naturally in plants and animals or they may be made in the laboratory.

strengthening activities: Activities that require strenuous muscular contractions such as weight lifting, resistance training, push-ups, sit-ups, etc.

T-score: The extent to which an individual's bone density differs from the peak bone mineral density of a healthy 30-year old adult.

tolerance: A condition in which higher doses of a drug are required to produce the same effect achieved during initial use; often associated with physical dependence.

ultrasound: A procedure that uses high-energy sound waves to look at tissues and organs inside the body. The sound waves make echoes that form pictures of the tissues and organs on a computer screen (sonogram).

virus: In medicine, a very simple microorganism that infects cells and may cause disease. Because viruses can multiply only inside infected cells, they are not considered to be alive.

vitamin A: A family of fat-soluble compounds that play an important role in vision, bone growth, reproduction, cell division, and cell differentiation. Too much vitamin A (in the form of retinol) has been linked to bone loss and an increase in the risk of hip fracture.

vitamin D: A nutrient that the body needs to absorb calcium.

weight control: This refers to achieving and maintaining a healthy weight with healthy eating and physical activity.

withdrawal: Symptoms that occur after chronic use of a drug is reduced abruptly or stopped.

X-ray: A type of radiation used in the diagnosis and treatment of cancer and other diseases. In low doses, X-rays are used to diagnose diseases by making pictures of the inside of the body.

yoga: A mind and body practice with origins in ancient Indian philosophy. The various styles of yoga typically combine physical postures, breathing techniques, and meditation or relaxation.

Chapter 60

Directory of Resources

Government Organizations That Provide Information about Osteoporosis

Agency for Healthcare Research and Quality (AHRQ)
5600 Fishers Ln.
Seventh Fl.
Rockville, MD 20857
Phone: 301-427-1364
Website: www.ahrq.gov

Centers For Disease Control and Prevention (CDC)
1600 Clifton Rd.
Atlanta, GA 30329-4027
Toll-Free TTY: 888-232-6348
Website: wwwn.cdc.gov

Eunice Kennedy Shriver National Institute of Child Health and Human Development (NICHD)
P.O. Box 3006
Rockville, MD 20847
Toll-Free: 800-370-2943
Toll-Free TTY: 888-320-6942
Toll-Free Fax: 866-760-5947
Website: www.nichd.nih.gov
E-mail: NICHDInformation
ResourceCenter@mail.nih.gov

Go4Life
Toll-Free: 800-222-2225
Website: go4life.nia.nih.gov
E-mail: Go4Life@nia.nih.gov

Resources in this chapter were compiled from several sources deemed reliable; all contact information was verified and updated in January 2019.

Healthfinder
1101 Wootton Pkwy
Rockville, MD 20852
Website: healthfinder.gov
E-mail: healthfinder@hhs.gov

Livertox
8600 Rockville Pike
Bethesda, MD 20894
Website: livertox.nih.gov
E-mail: LiverTox@nih.gov

National Cancer Institute (NCI)
9609 Medical Center Dr.
Bethesda, MD 20892-9760
Toll-Free: 800-422-6237
Phone: 301-435-3848
Website: www.cancer.gov
E-mail: cancergovstaff@mail.nih.gov

National Center for Biotechnology Information (NCBI)
8600 Rockville Pike
Bethesda, MD 20894
Website: www.ncbi.nlm.nih.gov
E-mail: info@ncbi.nlm.nih.gov

National Heart, Lung, and Blood Institute (NHLBI)
Bldg. 31, 31 Center Dr.
P.O. Box 30105
Bethesda, MD 20892
Phone: 301-251-1222
Fax: 301-251-1223
Website: www.nhlbi.nih.gov

National Institute of Arthritis and Musculoskeletal and Skin Diseases (NIAMS)
1 AMS Cir.
Bethesda, MD 20892-3675
Toll-Free: 877-226-4267
Phone: 301-495-4484
TTY: 301-565-2966
Fax: 301-718-6366
Website: www.niams.nih.gov
E-mail: NIAMSinfo@mail.nih.gov

National Institute of Diabetes and Digestive and Kidney Diseases (NIDDK)
31 Center Dr., MSC 2560
Bldg. 31, Rm. 9A06
Bethesda, MD 20892-2560
Toll-Free: 800-860-8747
Toll-Free TTY: 866-569-1162
Website: www.niddk.nih.gov
E-mail: healthinfo@niddk.nih.gov

National Institute of Mental Health (NIMH)
6001 Executive Blvd.
Rm. 6200, MSC 9663
Bethesda, MD 20892-9663
Toll-Free: 866-615-6464
TTY: 301-443-8431
Toll-Free TTY: 866-415-8051
Fax: 301-443-4279
Website: www.nimh.nih.gov
E-mail: nimhinfo@nih.gov

National Institute on Aging Information Center (NIA)
Information Center
Bldg. 31, Rm. 5C27
31 Center Dr., MSC 2292
Bethesda, MD 20892
Toll-Free: 800-222-2225
Toll-Free TTY: 800-222-4225
Website: www.nia.nih.gov
E-mail: niaic@nia.nih.gov

National Institute on Deafness and Other Communication Disorder (NIDCD) Clearinghouse
31 Center Dr. MSC 2320
Bethesda, MD 20892-2320
Toll-Free: 800-241-1044
Phone: 301-827-8183
Toll-Free TTY: 800-241-1055
Website: www.nidcd.nih.gov
E-mail: nidcdinfo@nidcd.nih.gov

National Institutes of Health (NIH)
9000 Rockville Pike
Bethesda, MD 20892
Phone: 301-496-4000
TTY: 301-402-9612
Website: www.nih.gov

NIH Osteoporosis and Related Bone Diseases— National Resource Center (NIH OBRD—NRC)
Toll-Free: 800-624-BONE
(800-624-2663)
Phone: 202-223-0344
TTY: 202-466-4315
Fax: 202-293-2356
Website: www.bones.nih.gov
E-mail: NIHBoneInfo@mail.nih.gov

Office of Research and Development (ORD)
U.S. Environmental Protection
Agency (EPA)
Toll-Free: 844-698-2311
Toll-Free TTY: 844-698-2711
Website: www.va.gov

Office on Women's Health (OWH)
U.S. Department of Health and
Human Services (HHS)
200 Independence Ave. S.W.
Rm. 712E
Washington, DC 20201
Toll-Free: 800-994-9662
Phone: 202-690-7650
Toll-Free TDD: 888-220-5446
Fax: 202-205-2631
Website: www.womenshealth.
gov
E-mail: womenshealth@hhs.gov

President's Council on Fitness, Sports & Nutrition (PCSFN)
1101 Wootton Pkwy
Ste. 560
Rockville, MD 20852
Phone: 240-276-9567
Website: www.fitness.gov
E-mail: fitness@hhs.gov

U.S. Department of Agriculture (USDA)
1400 Independence Ave. S.W.
Washington, DC 20250
Phone: 202-720-2791
Website: www.usda.gov

U.S. Food and Drug Administration (FDA)
10903 New Hampshire Ave.
Silver Spring, MD 20993
Toll-Free: 888-INFO-FDA
(888-463-6332)
Website: www.fda.gov

U.S. National Library of Medicine (NLM)
8600 Rockville Pike
Bethesda, MD 20894
Toll-Free: 888-346-3656
Phone: 301-594-5983
Website: www.nlm.nih.gov

Weight-control Information Network (WIN)
Website: www.win.niddk.nih.gov
E-mail: healthinfo@niddk.nih.gov

Private Organizations That Provide Information about Osteoporosis

American Academy of Orthopaedic Surgeons (AAOS)
9400 W. Higgins Rd.
Rosemont, IL 60018
Phone: 847-823-7186
Fax: 847-823-8125
Website: www.aaos.org

American Academy of Otolaryngology—Head and Neck Surgery (AAO—HNS)
1650 Diagonal Rd.
Alexandria, VA 22314-2857
Phone: 703-836-4444
Website: www.entnet.org

American Association of Retired Persons (AARP) Women's Initiative
601 E. St. N.W.
Washington, DC 20049
Toll-Free: 888-OUR-AARP
(888-687-2277)
Phone: 202-434-3525
Toll-Free TTY: 877-434-7598
Website: www.aarp.org

The American College of Obstetricians and Gynecologists (ACOG)
409 12th St. S.W.
P.O. Box 70620
Washington, DC 20024-9998
Toll-Free: 800-673-8444
Phone: 202-638-5577
Website: www.acog.org
E-mail: info@ny.acog.org

American College of Sports Medicine (ACSM)
401 W. Michigan St.
Indianapolis, IN 46202-3233
Phone: 317-637-9200
Fax: 317-634-7817
Website: www.acsm.org

The American Society for Bone and Mineral Research (ASBMR)
2025 M St. N.W.
Ste. 800
Washington, DC 20036-3309
Phone: 202-367-1161
Fax: 202-367-2161
Website: www.asbmr.org
E-mail: asbmr@asbmr.org

American Speech-Language-Hearing Association (ASHA)
2200 Research Blvd.
Rockville, MD 20850-3289
Toll-Free: 888-321-ASHA
(888-321-2742)
Phone: 301-296-5700
TTY: 301-296-5650
Fax: 301-296-8580
Website: www.asha.org

Children's Brittle Bone Foundation (CBBF)
P.O. Box 619
Zion, IL 60099
Phone: 773-236-2223
Website: www.cbbf.org

Dairy Council of California
1418 N. Market Blvd.
Ste. 500
Sacramento, CA 95834
Toll-Free: 877-324-7901
Phone: 916-263-3560
Website: www.dairycouncilofca.org
E-mail: Staff@DairyCouncilofCA.org

ERIC Clearinghouse on Disabilities and Gifted Education Council for Exceptional Children
1920 Association Dr.
Reston, VA 20191-1589
Toll-Free: 800-328-0272
Website: www.icdri.org/Education/eric.htm
E-mail: ericec@cec.sped.org

Hip Society
9400 W. Higgins Rd.
Ste. 500
Rosemont, IL 60018
Phone: 847-698-1638
Fax: 847-268-9745
Website: www.hipsoc.org
E-mail: hip@aaos.org

International Bone and Mineral Society (IBMS)
330 N. Wabash
Ste. 1900
Chicago, IL 60611
Phone: 312-321-5113
Fax: 312-673-6934
Website: www.ibmsonline.org

The International Society for Clinical Densitometry (ISCD)
955 S. Main St.
Bldg. C
Middletown, CT 06457
Phone: 860-259-1000
Fax: 860-259-1030
Website: www.iscd.org
E-mail: iscd@iscd.org

MAGIC Foundation
4200 Cantera Dr.
Ste. 106
Warrenville, IL 60555
Toll-Free: 800-362-4423
Phone: 630-836-8200
Fax: 630-836-8181
Website: www.magicfoundation.
org
E-mail: contactus@
magicfoundation.org

National Association of Anorexia Nervosa and Associated Disorders (ANAD)
220 N. Green St.
Chicago, IL 60607
Phone: 630-577-1333
Website: www.anad.org
E-mail: hello@anad.org

The National Collegiate Athletic Association (NCAA)
700 W. Washington St.
P.O. Box 6222
Indiana, IN 46206-6222
Phone: 317-917-6222
Fax: 317-917-6888
Website: www.ncaa.org

National Eating Disorders Organization (NEDA)
1500 Bdwy.
Ste. 1101
New York, NY 10036
Toll-Free: 800-931-2237
Phone: 212-575-6200
Fax: 212-575-1650
Website: www.
nationaleatingdisorders.org
E-mail: info@
NationalEatingDisorders.org

National Gaucher Foundation (NGF)
5410 Edson Ln.
Ste. 220
Rockville, MD 20852
Toll-Free: 800-504-3189
Website: www.gaucherdisease.
org

National Organization for Rare Disorders (NORD)
1779 Massachusetts Ave.
Ste. 500
Washington, DC 20036
Toll-Free: 800-999-6673
Phone: 202-588-5700
Fax: 202-588-5701
Website: www.rarediseases.org
E-mail: orphan@rarediseases.org

National Osteoporosis Foundation (NOF)
251 18th St. S.
Ste. 630
Arlington, VA 22202
Toll-Free: 800-231-4222
Website: www.nof.org
E-mail: info@nof.org

National Tay-Sachs and Allied Diseases Association (NTSAD)
2001 Beacon St.
Ste. 204
Boston, MA 02135
Toll-Free: 800-90-NTSAD
(800-906-8723)
Phone: 617-277-4463
Website: www.ntsad.org
E-mail: info@ntsad.org

National Women's Health Network (NWHN)
1413 K St. N.W.
Fourth Fl.
Washington, DC 20005
Phone: 202-682-2640
Fax: 202-682-2648
Website: www.nwhn.org
E-mail: nwhn@nwhn.org

North American Menopause Society (NAMS)
30100 Chagrin Blvd.
Ste. 210
Pepper Pike, OH 44124
Phone: 440-442-7550
Fax: 440-442-2660
Website: www.menopause.org
E-mail: info@menopause.org

Older Women's League (OWL)
1625 K St. N.W.
Ste. 1275
Washington, DC 20006
Toll-Free: 877-OLDRWMN
(877-653-7966)
Phone: 202-783-6686
Fax: 202-833-3472
Website: www.owlillinois.org

Osteogenesis Imperfecta (OI) Foundation
804 W. Diamond Ave.
Ste. 210
Gaithersburg, MD 20878
Toll-Free: 844-889-7579
Phone: 301-947-0083
Fax: 301-947-0456
Website: www.oif.org
E-mail: bonelink@oif.org

Index

Index